Fungal Dimorphism
With Emphasis on Fungi Pathogenic for Humans

Fungal Dimorphism

With Emphasis on Fungi Pathogenic for Humans

Edited by

Paul J. Szaniszlo
University of Texas at Austin
Austin, Texas

Assistant Editor
James L. Harris
Texas Department of Health
and University of Texas at Austin
Austin, Texas

Plenum Press • New York and London

Library of Congress Cataloging in Publication Data

Main entry under title:

Fungal dimorphism.

Bibliography: p.
Includes index.
1. Fungi, Pathogenic—Morphology. 2. Dimorphism (Plants) I. Szaniszlo, Paul J. II. Harris, James L.
QR245.F85 1985 616′.015 85-12412
ISBN 0-306-42020-1

A Division of Plenum Publishing Corporation
233 Spring Street, New York, N.Y. 10013

Printed in the United States of America

Affectionately dedicated

to my mother and father;

their example has always been
my guiding principle.

Contributors

Ronald L. Cihlar Microbiology Department, Schools of Medicine and Dentistry, Georgetown University, Washington, D.C. 20007

Garry T. Cole Department of Botany, The University of Texas at Austin, Austin, Texas 78712

Billy H. Cooper Department of Pathology, Baylor University Medical Center, Dallas, Texas 75246

Judith E. Domer Tulane University School of Medicine, New Orleans, Louisiana 70112

Robert G. Garrison The Research Service, Veterans Administration Medical Center, Kansas City, Missouri 64128

Philip A. Geis Sharon Woods Technical Center, Procter and Gamble Company, Cincinnati, Ohio 45241

James L. Harris Mycobacteriology/Mycology Section, Bureau of Laboratories, Texas Department of Health, Austin, Texas 78756; Department of Microbiology, The University of Texas at Austin, Austin, Texas 78712

Milan Hejtmánek Department of Biology, Medical Faculty, Palacky University, 775 00 Olomouc, Czechoslovakia

Clark B. Inderlied Clinical Microbiology, Children's Hospital of Los Angeles, University of Southern California, School of Medicine, Los Angeles, California 90027

Charles W. Jacobs Division of Biological Sciences, University of Michigan, Ann Arbor, Michigan 48109

G. S. Kobayashi Divisions of Infectious Diseases, Dermatology, and Laboratory Medicine, Washington University School of Medicine, St. Louis, Missouri 63110

B. V. Kumar Division of Infectious Diseases, Washington University School of Medicine, St. Louis, Missouri 63110

B. Maresca International Institute of Genetics and Biophysics, CNR, 10 Naples, Italy

G. Medoff Division of Infectious Diseases, Washington University School of Medicine, St. Louis, Missouri 63110

Julius Peters Department of Pediatrics, UCLA School of Medicine, Harbor-UCLA Medical Center, Torrance, California 92717

José Ruiz-Herrera Department of Genetics and Molecular Biology, Center for Investigation and Advanced Studies, I.P.N., and Institute for Investigation in Experimental Biology, Faculty of Chemistry, University of Guanajuato, Guanajuato, Gto. 36000, Mexico

M. Sacco International Institute of Genetics and Biophysics, CNR, 10 Naples, Italy

Felipe San-Blas Department of Microbiology and Cellular Biology, Venezuelan Institute of Scientific Investigations (I.V.I.C.), Caracas 1010A, Venezuela

Gioconda San-Blas Department of Microbiology and Cellular Biology, Venezuelan Institute of Scientific Investigations (I.V.I.C.), Caracas 1010A, Venezuela

David R. Soll Department of Biology, University of Iowa, Iowa City, Iowa 52242

S. H. Sun Mycology Research Laboratory, Veterans Administration Hospital, San Antonio, Texas 78284

Paul J. Szaniszlo Department of Microbiology, The University of Texas at Austin, Austin, Texas 78712

Luiz R. Travassos Department of Mycology, Paulista School of Medicine, São Paulo, SP 04023, Brazil

Preface

The tendency of fungi pathogenic for humans to have shapes in tissue distinct from their usual saprophytic morphologies has fascinated the pathologist and medical mycologist for almost a century. A primary reason for this fascination is the possibility that fungal duality of form, or dimorphism, may be an important virulence factor that allows the zoopathogenic fungus to survive host defenses. A second reason relates to the desire to gain basic insights into the regulation of cellular development and morphogenesis among the etiological agents of human mycoses.

Many excellent treatises have appeared within the recent past dealing with fungal dimorphism. However, it is becoming increasingly clear that it may be beyond the capability of one or a few authors to review this subject adequately. Instead, the ever-increasing volume of literature associated with fungal dimorphism and the diversity of fungi now recognized to exhibit a type of dimorphism suggest that a volume comprised of contributions by numerous researchers may be more appropriate. This perception provided me with the motivation to compile a multiauthor volume.

The aim of this book is to present in a single volume a review as current as possible of dimorphism among zoopathogenic fungi. The book is organized in a way that attempts to enhance readability by grouping the fungi according to their predominant tissue morphologies. It is hoped that this approach highlights common trends of fungal development more than might be indicated by groupings made according to physiological or taxonomical criteria, or not made at all. My splendid group of contributing authors graciously accommodated these groupings by generally focusing their attention on aspects of morphogenesis *in vivo* or *in vitro* that are characteristics of pathogenic states. For their help and their indulgence I am very grateful.

I am also grateful to a number of other individuals who provided invaluable assistance during the preparation of this book. Paramount among these is Dr. James L. Harris, who not only contributed a chapter, but also served as my assistant editor. His attention to the requirements of the publisher greatly facilitated my efforts and helped to ensure chapter uniformity. I am also very indebted to Dr. Garry T. Cole, who diligently rescued the chapter on *Coccidioides immitis* after the untimely death of Dr. Milton Huppert. His quick efforts were heroic and can only be considered a true act of friendship. Finally, I would especially like to thank Susan Crossland, Cathy Potter and Mindy Peterson for helping with the considerable retyping done at the University of Texas, Chester R. Cooper for the innumerable favors he did for me during the book's final preparation, and my family for tolerating my considerable irritability and lack of patience while engaged in this endeavor.

Paul J. Szaniszlo

Austin, Texas

Contents

PART I. INTRODUCTION AND GENERAL MORPHOLOGY

PART II. FUNGI WITH YEAST TISSUE MORPHOLOGIES

PART III. FUNGI WITH YEAST AND HYPHAL TISSUE MORPHOLOGIES

Chapter 12

Arthroconidium–Spherule–Endospore Transformation in *Coccidioides immitis*

Garry T. Cole and S. H. Sun

PART V. DIMORPHIC MUCORS

Chapter 13

Mucor racemosus

Clark B. Inderlied, Julius Peters, and Ronald L. Cihlar

Part I

Introduction and General Morphology

Chapter 1

An Introduction to Dimorphism among Zoopathogenic Fungi

Paul J. Szaniszlo

1. DIMORPHISM: APPLICATION OF THE TERM

Many fungi have a remarkable ability to alter normal vegetative developmental sequences in response to environmental change. This ability is common among the fungi responsible for the majority of different human mycoses. With the invasion of tissue and the establishment of infection, certain fungi that are pathogenic for humans differentiate into morphologically distinct growth forms. These forms are usually budding yeasts, related blastically derived forms such as pseudohyphae, or isotropically enlarged entities known as adiaspores, sclerotic bodies, or spherules. The relatively simple *in vivo* phenotypes appear to have qualities that enhance their survival and facilitate their dissemination in host tissue. In contrast, most of the same fungi growing saprophytically in nature or under standard *in vitro* culture conditions tend to produce extensive hyphae with well-differentiated sporulation structures.

The term *dimorphism* has been employed for many years in medical mycology to describe the phenotypic duality of form in which a fungus exhibits distinct saprophytic and parasitic phases (Ainsworth, 1955; Howard, 1962; Mariat, 1964). Often the term is used in a manner that implies that the saprophytic phase is hyphal, whereas the tissue phase is a yeast (Scherr and Weaver, 1953; Cochrane, 1958; Emmons *et al.*, 1977;

Paul J. Szaniszlo • Department of Microbiology, The University of Texas at Austin, Austin, Texas 78712.

Cole and Samson, 1983; Garraway and Evans, 1984). However, the use of the term is varied. For example, some medical mycologists also include among the medically important dimorphic fungi species with tissue phases that are either yeasts or spherules (McGinnis, 1980; Campbell and Stewart, 1980; Rippon, 1982), whereas others include any human pathogenic fungus with a tissue phase distinct from its predominant saprophytic morphology (Howard, 1962; Mariat, 1964). The latter, less restrictive application is similar to the use of the word dimorphism by general mycologists and fungal developmental biologists when they describe environmentally controlled interconversions of the different vegetative growth forms of a fungus, regardless of its medical importance (Romano, 1966; Stewart and Rogers, 1978; Szaniszlo *et al.*, 1983).

It is well known that environmental perturbations induce certain saprophytic and plant pathogenic fungi to undergo distinct phase transitions (Garrison and Boyd, 1973; Barathova *et al.*, 1977; Marshall *et al.*, 1979; Kulkarni and Nickerson, 1981; Park, 1982, 1984; McNeel *et al.*, 1983) (see also Chapters 13 and 14). The molecular regulation that causes these nonzoopathogenic fungi to modify their metabolism and cell-wall construction in a manner that leads to altered vegetative morphology may sometimes be the same as that responsible for phase transitions of zoopathogens *in vivo*. Thus, an argument can be made that it is not necessary, or even appropriate, to restrict the application of the word dimorphism in some contexts to specific types of vegetative transitions (i.e., yeast–hyphal dimorphism) or in others to certain medically important fungi. Surely, if the concept of dimorphism can accommodate a spherule, then it should also easily accommodate other *in vivo* forms that develop predominantly by isotropic growth mechanisms. Furthermore, a restrictive use of the term dimorphism in medical mycology ignores the facts that medically important fungi, when growing in human tissue, usually represent misplaced saprophytes and are primarily free-living organisms (Rippon, 1980). Thus, the genetic potential for phase transition among the zoopathogens was likely acquired by exposure to natural environmental conditions, similar to those that selected for dimorphism among the nonpathogens, and not by repeated contact with *in vivo* tissue conditions. The general saprophytic nature of the zoopathogens also suggests that the ability to carry out vegetative-phase transitions is not a unique characteristic of medically important fungi, but only one of particular relevance because of its prevalence. For these speculative reasons, I have chosen to consider dimorphism broadly in this volume to involve the ability of a fungus to grow in at least two vegetative forms and to carry out any type of distinct vegetative-phase transition.

2. DIMORPHIC PATHOGENIC FUNGI

Whether or not the broader usage of the term dimorphism is appropriate, it allows for the review of vegetative morphogenesis in a greater variety of human pathogenic fungi. An ordered listing of the fungi included in the following chapters, together with a brief description of their saprophytic and parasitic morphology, is presented in Table I (modified from Szaniszlo *et al.*, 1983). The fungi are subdivided into three groups according to their morphology *in vivo.* The first group consists of four fungi that exhibit predominantly yeast development *in vivo* and have extensive sporulating hyphal phases under saprophytic conditions. Most, if not all, medical mycologists consider these fungi to be dimorphic. Two of the species, *Ajellomyces (Blastomyces) dermatitidis* and *Emmonsiella capsulata (Histoplasma capsulatum),* are cleistothecial ascomycetes, whereas the other two, *Paracoccidioides brasiliensis* and *Sporothrix schenckii,* are form-species of the Fungi Imperfecti that appear to have ascomycetous affinities (Rippon, 1982).

The second group consists of *Candida albicans, Exophiala werneckii,* and *Wangiella dermatitidis.* Each of these three form-species has a predominantly yeastlike saprophytic phase, can be induced *in vitro* to carry out distinct yeast–hyphal transitions, and tends to exhibit both yeasts and hyphae *in vivo.* With these particular species, the host environment is not always completely restrictive for the saprophytic phase or totally permissive for the parasitic phase. As a general rule, transitions *in vivo* by these dimorphic fungi involve morphogenesis from yeasts to hyphae, whereas transitions *in vivo* exhibited by fungi in the first group are from hyphae or conidia to yeasts.

The form-species in the third group, like those fungi in the first group, all have well-developed saprophytic hyphal phases, but do not develop yeast phases *in vivo* or *in vitro.* The *in vivo* morphologies are instead mostly isotropically enlarged forms. The development of these forms begins by mechanisms reminiscent of the initial swelling stage that accompanies normal spore germination or of the abnormal swelling of spores that can be induced by elevated temperatures among various saprophytic fungi prior to microcycle conidiation (Anderson, 1978). In the form-species of *Chrysosporium,* isotropic growth and nuclear divisions are extensive *in vivo,* but not coupled with further differentiation. This type of development by *Chrysosporium* form-species results in the production of an adiaspore (see Chapter 10). Conversely, in *Phialophora verrucosa* and other agents of chromoblastomycosis and in *Coccidioides immitis,* the isotropic growth and nuclear divisions accompany, or are

Table I
Growth Phases of Dimorphic Zoopathogenic Fungi[a]

In vivo group	Fungus	Saprophytic phase	Parasitic phase
Yeasts	*Ajellomyces (Blastomyces) dermatitidis*	Septate hyphae; white or beige, fluffy or glabrous colonies; microconidia; cleistothecia and ascospores in sexual state	Budding yeasts, size 8–20 μm; neck between mother cell and daughter bud very broad
	Emmonsiella capsulata (Histoplasma capsulatum)	Septate hyphae; white or tan, fluffy or flat colonies; microconidia and tuberculate macroconidia; cleistothecia and ascospores in sexual state	Budding yeasts, size 2–4 μm; neck between mother cell and daughter bud very narrow
	Paracoccidioides brasiliensis	Septate hyphae; white to beige, glabrous, leathery, flat, raised, or velvety colonies; no characteristic conidia; sexual state unknown	Budding yeasts, size variable, 2–30 μm or more; buds one to many per mother cell with neck between mother cell and daughter bud very narrow
	Sporothrix schenckii	Septate hyphae; white, black, or gray, glabrous or fuzzy, wrinkled colonies; conidiogenesis similar to that of some *Ceratocystis* species; sexual state unknown	Budding yeasts, size variable, 2–10 μm or more; sometimes cigar-shaped and up to 30 μm long; buds one to many per mother cell
Interconverting yeasts and hyphae	*Candida albicans*	Budding yeasts predominate, size 4–6 μm; smooth and creamy, white colonies; true hyphae, pseudohyphae, and chlamydospores not infrequent under certain environmental conditions; sexual state unknown	Mixtures of true hyphae, pseudohyphae, and yeasts

	Exophiala werneckii	Budding yeasts predominate in young cultures, size 6–12 μm; septate hyphae arise in older cultures, many intermediate forms; white, gray, or green-black, glabrous or fuzzy colonies; sexual state unknown	Mixtures of hyphae and yeasts
	Wangiella dermatitidis	Budding yeasts predominate in young cultures, size 6–8 μm; septate moniliform and true hyphae arise in older cultures; phialoconidia and annelloconidia; sexual state unknown	Mixtures of hyphae and yeasts; thick-walled, swollen cells and occasional multicellular (sclerotic) forms
Isotropic forms	*Phialophora verrucosa* and other chromoblastomycotic fungi	Septate hyphae; green-brown to green-black, fluffy colonies; phialoconidia, annelloconidia, etc.; sexual state unknown	Sclerotic bodies, which represent swollen, thick-walled cells and thick-walled, septated, multicellular forms
	Chrysosporium parvum var. parvum; C. parvum var. crescens	Septate hyphae; clear to white, glabrous to tufted colonies; smooth or spiny aleurioconidia; sexual state unknown	Adiaspores, which represent very swollen aleurioconidia; size varies from 10 to 400 μm in diameter; growth in tissue only by enlargement
	Coccidioides immitis	Septate hyphae that yield arthroconidia on fragmentation; white, tan, or brown, glabrous or fluffy, smooth or wrinkled colonies; arthroconidia typically barrel-shaped with disjuncters; sexual state unknown	Spherules, which represent very swollen arthroconidia that produce numerous endospores; size of spherules at maturity 30–60 μm in diameter; endospores formed by septation of cytoplasm

[a]Modified from Szaniszlo *et al.* (1983).

followed by, one or more cell divisions by septum formation (see Chapters 11 and 12). Among the agents of chromoblastomycosis, no subsequent development occurs after septation, and cell separation is infrequent. The resulting *in vivo* terminal morphology is the muriform, multicellular phenotype identified as a "sclerotic body" (McGinnis, 1983). However, in *C. immitis,* septation is followed by further differentiation of cytoplasm into endospores. The highly differentiated structure that results is known as a spherule. In time, the outer spherule wall is disrupted, bringing about endospore release.

3. GENERAL INTRODUCTORY THOUGHTS

The reviews included in this volume make it convincingly evident that few common themes have been discovered concerning the regulatory basis of dimorphism among medically important fungi. This may either reflect the taxonomic divergence of the fungi involved or indicate that few common themes exist. Alternatively, our inability to discern common themes may only suggest that the "critical mass" of multidisciplinary scientists required to supply the requisite data base for such insight is not available. In fact, only when one considers how few contemporary cell biologists and "modern" developmental mycologists actually study in depth the dimorphism of any particular zoopathogenic fungus, can the progress described in the chapters that follow be truly appreciated.

To discover the common regulatory aspects of dimorphism, if they exist, it is necessary to apply integrated experimental approaches, such as those being used to elucidate the determinants of morphogenesis in *Saccharomyces cerevisiae* and to a lesser degree in *Neurospora crassa.* Many of the insights into the growth and development gained with these monomorphic fungi are directly applicable to the dimorphic fungi and therefore make *S. cerevisiae* and *N. crassa* invaluable models. The pioneering investigations of Hartwell and his associates (Hartwell, 1974; Hartwell *et al.,* 1974; Pringle and Hartwell, 1981) and subsequent related investigations (Nurse, 1981; Thorner, 1981; Sheckman and Novick, 1982) with the budding yeast *S. cerevisiae* and related fungi have provided excellent road maps for cell-cycle-oriented studies of yeast development in dimorphic fungi. Similar studies of the growth and of the nuclear division cycle in *N. crassa* (Brody, 1973; Scott, 1976; Alberghina and Sturani, 1981) have suggested how developmental themes among the hyphal phases of dimorphic fungi might also be discovered. The rapid advances in the understanding of development in *S. cerevisiae* and *N. crassa* were greatly accelerated and facilitated by the extensive genetic literature associated with each fungus (Mortimer and Schild, 1980; Perkins *et al.*, 1982). The beginning efforts being expended to establish genetic systems among zoopathogenic fungi (see Chapters 7 and 9) most likely will similarly augment dimorphism research. Other routes to the discovery of common themes in the regulation of dimorphism among the medically important fungi have been suggested by the very enlightening chemical studies of Cabib and his co-workers (Cabib, 1975, 1981; Cabib and Shematek, 1981; Cabib *et al.*, 1982) and Bartnicki-Garcia and his associates (Bartnicki-Garcia, 1973; Bartnicki-Garcia *et al.*, 1979). Their exhaustive investigations into the nature and control of cell-wall biosynthesis are particularly relevant to the study of dimorphism, because it is the cell wall that ultimately imparts morphology to a fungus.

A theme that does become apparent after study of the morphological aspects of dimorphism and of phase transitions (Cole and Samson, 1983; Garrison, 1983; Szaniszlo *et al.*, 1983) (see also Chapter 2) is that zoopathogenic fungi, as a group, are manipulating three basic cell-wall deposition patterns. When hyphae are produced by apical growth, wall deposition is continuous and polarized and involves very little isotropism. In contrast, yeasts are produced by blastic growth, which involves discontinuous but polarized wall deposition, coupled with a moderate amount of isotropic enlargement. Complete deregulation of polarized cell-wall deposition, without the inhibition of growth itself, induces the formation of a variety of isotropically enlarged forms that may develop from yeasts, hyphae, or conidia. In general, the dimorphic zoopathogenic fungi extensively manipulate only two of the three deposition patterns. However, it is a common feature of *P. brasiliensis* yeasts to isotropically enlarge many diameters and become multinucleate prior to bud initiation (see Chapter 5), much in the manner of budding yeasts of the dimorphic mucors (see Chapters 13 and 14). Similarly, under some conditions, cells of hyphae and pseudohyphae of *C. albicans* significantly enlarge to produce spherical, thick-walled, nondeciduous, intercalary or terminal chlamydospores (Jansons and Nickerson, 1970a,b). Finally, at least one zoopathogenic fungus, *W. dermatitidis,* is distinctly polymorphic and is easily induced *in vitro* to produce terminal vegetative phenotypes that are yeasts, hyphae, or isotropically enlarged multicellular forms (see Chapter 9); the latter appear to be both structurally and functionally equivalent to the sclerotic bodies of the agents of chromoblastomycosis (see Chapter 11). A few reports have recently documented that *W. dermatitidis* infrequently produces isotropically enlarged, thick-walled cells and multicellular forms *in vivo,* as well as yeasts and hyphae (McGinnis, 1983; Nishimura and Miyaji, 1983; Matsumoto *et al.*, 1984).

It may be important to note that most fungi have the ability to manipulate the expression of all three of the cell-wall deposition patterns. For example, in some vegetatively monomorphic hyphal fungi, blastic and isotropic growth are expressed during specific life-cycle periods, most notably when conidia develop and germinate, respectively. This suggests that expression of the different deposition patterns is not restricted to dimorphic fungi, but is instead a unique property of the vegetative phases of these organisms, and even then only when development leads to distinct vegetative phenotypes; this implies that only one basic pattern is being extensively expressed at any one time. The simultaneous expression of more than one pattern in a vegetative cell gives rise to a variety of morphologies ranging from relatively nondescript transition cells to well-characterized entities such as pseudohyphae and moniliform hyphae (Szaniszlo *et al.*, 1983). With the dimorphic fungi, it is the plasticity and extreme expression of the wall-deposition patterns during vegetative growth that is so striking.

It may also be important to suggest that although changes in the wall-deposition patterns are readily reversible in a few pathogenic dimorphic fungi, in most this does not appear to be the case. Instead, transition frequently seems to depend on the acquisition or loss of inherent properties prior to phase change. Such a suggestion is particularly relevant to many yeast-to-hyphal transitions, which tend to resemble spore-germination events (Dabrowa and Howard, 1983) (see also Chapter 2). This type of dimorphism is sometimes dependent on the yeast having a stationary-phase metabolism, or at least being transiently arrested in G_1 phase of the cell cycle, prior to hyphal outgrowth (Szaniszlo *et al.*, 1983). In this regard, it is clear that many factors used by investigators to induce dimorphic transistions *in vitro,* such as shifts of cells to elevated or lowered temperatures, acidity, and various conditions of nutrient deprivation, often result in transient or prolonged G_1 arrest. Such arrests may so significantly alter fungal metabolism that new phenotypes result (see Chapter 7). In contrast, isotropic growth is more related to the continuation of balanced growth, in the absence of polarized wall deposition (see Chapters 9, 10, and 12). In systems expressing transition to isotropic forms, polarized apical and budding growth are inhibited without the inhibition of other growth activities. Alternatively, hyphal-to-yeast transitions may either represent a normal aspect of vegetative growth or require complex changes in metabolism. In fungi such as *C. albicans, E. werneckii, S. schenckii,* and *W. dermatitidis,* lateral hyphal bud cells (blastospores) are freely disarticulated from vegetative hyphae under most growth conditions and establish a yeast phase by budding (see Chapters 6, 7, 8, and 9). However, in fungi such as *B. dermatitidis, H. capsulatum,* and *P. brasiliensis,* environmental perturbations are required to induce complex metabolic changes in hyphae before they can produce yeast cells (see Chapters 3, 4, and 5). The differences associated with dimorphic transitions by medically important fungi suggest that the regulatory mechanisms involved are more complicated than simple reversals of single metabolic sequences.

A comprehensive reading of the chapters that follow should clarify the brief remarks presented in this introduction. My intention was not to describe all aspects of dimorphism, but instead to set the stage for the state-of-the-art reviews concerning the dimorphism of the medically important fungi chosen for inclusion in this particular volume. As will be very apparent, not all the zoopathogenic fungi reviewed have been equally well studied. This is unfortunate, but should document that much exciting work is still left to be done. The extent and breadth of the kinds of studies that are yet possible and might prove fruitful should become very apparent after a reading of Chapters 13 and 14, which present reviews of dimorphism as exhibited among species of dimorphic mucors. These particular reviews of nonpathogenic species were included in this volume because the dimorphic mucors represent the most intensely studied dimorphic fungi. The distinct periods of apical, budding, and isotropic vegetative development exhibited by the dimorphic mucors suggest that they too can serve, with *S. cerevisiae* and *N. crassa,* as models for discovering the regulatory aspects of dimorphism. My hope is that investigators of the zoopathogenic fungi will gain important insights from the mucors into how adept dimorphic fungi are at manipulating their vegetative morphology in response to environmental change.

REFERENCES

Ainsworth, G. C., 1955, Pathogenicity of fungi in man and animals, in: *Mechanisms of Microbial Pathogenicity* (J. W. Howie and A. J. O'Hea, eds.), Cambridge University Press, Cambridge, pp. 242–262.

Alberghina, L., and Sturani, E., 1981, Control of growth and of the nuclear division cycle in *Neurospora crassa, Microbiol. Rev.* **45**:99–122.

Anderson, J. G., 1978, Temperature-induced fungal development, in: *The Filamentous Fungi,* Vol. 3 (J. E. Smith and D. R. Berry, eds.), John Wiley, New York, pp. 358–375.

Barathova, H., Betina, V., and Ulicky, L., 1977, Regulation of differentiation of the dimorphic fungus *Paecilomyces viridis* by nitrogen sources, antibiotics and metabolic inhibitors, *Folia Microbiol.* **22**:222–231.

Bartnicki-Garcia, S., 1973, Fundamental aspects of hyphal morphogenesis, in: *Microbial Differentiation,* Vol. 23 (J. M. Ashworth and J. E. Smith, eds.), Cambridge University Press, Cambridge, pp. 245–267.

Bartnicki-Garcia, S., Ruiz-Herrera, J., and Bracker, C. E., 1979, Chitosomes and chitin synthesis, in: *Fungal Walls and Hyphal Growth* (J. H. Burnett and A. P. J. Trinci, eds.), Cambridge University Press, Cambridge, pp. 149–168.

Brady, S., 1973, Metabolism, cell walls and morphogenesis, in: *Developmental Regulation: Aspects of Cell Differentiation* (S. J. Coward, ed.), Academic Press, New York, pp. 107–154.

Cabib, E., 1975, Molecular aspects of yeast morphogenesis, *Annu. Rev. Microbiol.* **29:**191–214.

Cabib, E., 1981, Chitin: Structure, metabolism, and regulation of biosynthesis, in: *Encyclopedia of Plant Physiology,* New Series, Vol. 13B (W. Tanner and F. A. Loewus, eds.), Springer-Verlag, Berlin, pp. 395–415.

Cabib, E., and Shematek, E. M., 1981, Structural polysaccharides of plants and fungi: Comparative and morphogenetic aspects, in: *Biology of Carbohydrates,* Vol. 1 (V. Ginsburg, ed.), John Wiley, New York, pp. 51–90.

Cabib, E., Roberts, R., and Bowers, B., 1982, Synthesis of the yeast cell wall and its regulation, *Annu. Rev. Biochem.* **51:**763–793.

Campbell, M. C., and Stewart, J. L., 1980, *The Medical Mycology Handbook,* John Wiley, New York.

Cochrane, V. W., 1958, *Physiology of Fungi,* John Wiley, New York.

Cole, G. T., and Samson, R. A., 1983, Conidium and sporangiospore formation in pathogenic microfungi, in: *Fungi Pathogenic for Humans and Animals,* Part A, *Biology* (D. H. Howard, ed.), Marcel Dekker, New York, pp. 437–524.

Dabrowa, N., and Howard, D. H., 1983, Blastoconidium germination, in: *Fungi Pathogenic for Humans and Animals,* Part A, *Biology* (D. H. Howard, ed.), Marcel Dekker, New York, pp. 525–545.

Emmons, C. W., Binford, C. H., Utz, J. P., and Kwon-Chung, K. J., 1977, *Medical Mycology,* 3rd ed., Lea and Febiger, Philadelphia.

Garraway, M. O., and Evans, R. C., 1984, *Fungal Nutrition and Physiology,* John Wiley, New York.

Garrison, R. G., 1983, Ultrastructural cytology of pathogenic fungi, in: *Fungi Pathogenic for Humans and Animals,* Part A, *Biology* (D. H. Howard, ed.), Marcel Dekker, New York, pp. 229–321.

Garrison, R. G., and Boyd, K. S., 1973, Dimorphism of *Penicillium marniffei* as observed by electron microscopy, *Can. J. Microbiol.* **19:**1305–1309.

Hartwell, L. H., 1974, *Saccharomyces cerevisiae* cell cycle, *Bacteriol. Rev.* **38:**164–198.

Hartwell, L. H., Culotti, H. J., Pringle, J. R., and Reid, B. J., 1974, Genetic control of the cell division cycle in yeast, *Science* **183:**46–51.

Howard, D. H., 1962, The morphogenesis of the parasitic form of the dimorphic fungi, *Mycopathol. Mycol. Appl.* **18:**127–139.

Jansons, V. K., and Nickerson, W. J., 1970a, Induction, morphogenesis, and germination of the chlamydospores of *Candida albicans, J. Bacteriol.* **104:**910–921.

Jansons, V. K., and Nickerson, W. J., 1970b, Chemical composition of chlamydospores of *Candida albicans, J. Bacteriol.* **104:**922–932.

Kulkarni, R. K., and Nickerson, K. W., 1981, Nutritional control of dimorphism in *Ceratocystis ulmi, Exp. Mycol.* **5:**148–154.

Mariat, F., 1964, Saprophytic and parasitic morphology of pathogenic fungi, in: *Microbial Behavior, In Vivo and In Vitro* (H. Smith, ed.), Cambridge University Press, Cambridge, pp. 85–111.

Marshall, M., Russo, G., Van Etten, J., and Nickerson, K., 1979, Polyamines in dimorphic fungi, *Curr. Microbiol.* **22:**187–190.

Matsumoto, T., Padhye, A. A., Ajello, L., Standard, P. G., and McGinnis, M. R., 1984, Critical review of human isolates of *Wangiella dermatitidis, Mycologia* **76:**232–249.

McGinnis, M. R., 1980, *Laboratory Handbook of Medical Mycology,* Academic Press, New York.
McGinnis, M. R., 1983, Chromoblastomycosis and phaeohyphomycosis: New concepts, diagnosis, and mycology, *J. Am. Acad. Dermatol.* **8:**1–16.
McNeel, D. J., Kulkarni, R. K., and Nickerson, K. W., 1983, Pleomorphism in *Ceratocystis ulmi:* Chlamydospore formation, *Can. J. Bot.* **61:**1349–1352.
Mortimer, R. K., and Schild, D., 1980, Genetic map of *Saccharomyces cerevisiae, Microbiol. Rev.* **44:**519–571.
Nishimura, K., and Miyaji, M., 1983, Defense mechanisms of mice against *Exophiala dermatitidis* infection, *Mycopathologia* **81:**9–21.
Nurse, P., 1981, Genetic analysis of the cell cycle, in: *Genetics as a Tool in Microbiology* (S. W. Glover and D. A. Hopwood, eds.), Cambridge University Press, London, pp. 291–314.
Park, D., 1982, Inorganic nitrogen nutrition and yeast–mycelial dimorphism in *Aureobasidium pullulans, Trans. Br. Mycol. Soc.* **81:**168–172.
Park, D., 1984, Low pH and the development of large cells in *Aureobasidium pullulans, Trans. Br. Mycol. Soc.* **82:**717–720.
Perkins, D. D., Radford, A., Newmeyer, D., and Bjorkman, M., 1982, Chromosomal loci of *Neurospora crassa, Microbiol. Rev.* **46:**426–570.
Pringle, J. R., and Hartwell, L. H., 1981, The *Saccharomyces cerevisiae* cell cycle, in: *Molecular Biology of the Yeast Saccharomyces: Life Cycle and Inheritance* (J. N. Strathern, E. W. Jones, and J. R. Broach, eds.), Cold Spring Harbor Laboratory, New York, pp. 97–142.
Rippon, J. W., 1980, Dimorphism in pathogenic fungi, *Crit. Rev. Microbiol.* **8:**49–97.
Rippon, J. W., 1982, *Medical Mycology: The Pathogenic Fungi and Pathogenic Actinomycetes,* 2nd ed., W. B. Saunders, Philadelphia.
Romano, A. H., 1966, Dimorphism, in: *The Fungi: An Advanced Treatise,* Vol. 2 (G. C. Ainsworth and A. S. Sussman, eds.), Academic Press, New York, pp. 181–209.
Scherr, G. H., and Weaver, R. H., 1953, The dimorphism phenomena in yeasts, *Bacteriol. Rev.* **17:**51–92.
Scott, W. A., 1976, Biochemical genetics of morphogenesis in *Neurospora, Annu. Rev. Microbiol.* **30:**85–104.
Sheckman, R., and Novick, P., 1982, The secretory process and yeast cell-surface assembly, in: *Molecular Biology of the Yeast Saccharomyces: Metabolism and Gene Expression,* (J. N. Strathern, E. W. Jones, and J. R. Broach, eds.), Cold Spring Harbor Laboratory, New York, pp. 361–398.
Stewart, P. R., and Rogers, P. J., 1978, Fungal dimorphism: A particular expression of cell wall morphogenesis, in: *The Filamentous Fungi,* Vol. 3 (J. E. Smith and D. R. Berry, eds.), John Wiley, New York, pp. 164–196.
Szaniszlo, P. J., Jacobs, C. W., and Geis, P. A., 1983, Dimorphism: Morphological and biochemical aspects, in: *Fungi Pathogenic for Humans and Animals,* Part A, *Biology* (D. H. Howard, ed.), Marcel Dekker, New York, pp. 323–436.
Thorner, J., 1981, Pheromonal regulation of development in *Saccharomyces cerevisiae,* in: *Molecular Biology of the Yeast Saccharomyces: Life Cycle and Inheritance* (J. N. Strathern, E. W. Jones, and J. R. Broach, eds.), Cold Spring Harbor Laboratory, New York, pp. 143–180.

Chapter 2

Cytological and Ultrastructural Aspects of Dimorphism

Robert G. Garrison

1. INTRODUCTION

Until the late 1960s, when the electron microscope became widely available to the mycologist, methods of light microscopy were used for the study of the dimorphic fungi. Such studies employed fixed cellular suspensions or slide cultures to observe the transition from one growth form to the other. However, these studies were confined to gross observations of the transition process due to the resolution limitations of the light instrument. Nevertheless, one must be impressed with the careful attention given to the subject by the various investigators, since many of their findings have been subsequently confirmed by more recent studies using the electron microscope.

Various aspects of the sequential fine-structural changes that occur during mold–yeast–mold dimorphism have been described for certain of the pathogenic dimorphic fungi. On the basis of morphological changes alone, it is not entirely possible to speculate on the nature of the biochemical events or the regulatory mechanisms that characterize fungal dimorphism. Yet it is obvious that the electron microscope has provided a body of information about fungal dimorphism that could not be obtained by any other analytical means.

This chapter is concerned with aspects of the ultrastructural cytology

Robert G. Garrison • The Research Service, Veterans Administration Medical Center, Kansas City, Missouri 64128.

of the dimorphic fungal cell and of the ultrastructural events that occur during the transition from one growth phase to the other. A detailed treatment of the various techniques of electron microscopy employed for the study of the fungal organism is beyond the scope of this chapter. Many of the basic techniques for the electron microscopy of fungal tissue have been reviewed by Greenhalgh and Evans (1971) and by Kopp (1975). A comprehensive account of the ultrastructural cytology of the pathogenic fungi in general may be found in a review by the present author (Garrison, 1983).

This review emphasizes aspects of the ultrastructural cytology of dimorphism as exhibited by *Blastomyces dermatitidis, Histoplasma capsulatum,* and *Sporothirix schenckii* inasmuch as considerable information is now available that details the sequential ultrastructural events associated with the dimorphic nature of these species. Further, such emphasis is a reflection of our own interest in the subject. Consequently, all the electron micrographs assembled herein were obtained on specimens grown and processed in the author's laboratory and for which responsibility for image quality and interpretation is taken. A number of these micrographs have not been published previously. Our illustrative materials aim at providing a morphological background for subsequent chapters.

2. ASPECTS OF ULTRASTRUCTURAL CYTOLOGY

A great variety of fungi have now been examined by electron microscopy. These organisms are represented by all the major taxonomic divisions, and as might be expected, such fine-structural studies reveal the fungi to be a diverse group. All the pathogenic dimorphic fungi are typically eukaryotic cells. This term implies the utilization of a highly organized system of cell entities, thus permitting each cytological component to have distinct functions. However, there are no unique cytological features that specifically characterize or otherwise distinguish the pathogenic dimorphic fungi from other fungal pathogens (Garrison, 1983) or from nonpathogenic species (Bracker, 1967). Many organelles and inclusions found in fungal cells are also present in cells of higher eukaryotic organisms. Other cytological components of the fungi seem to be unique to the group in general.

2.1. Yeast Cell

A schematic composite of a thin section of a yeast cell is shown in Figure 1. The cell wall proper is generally thin in medial cross section,

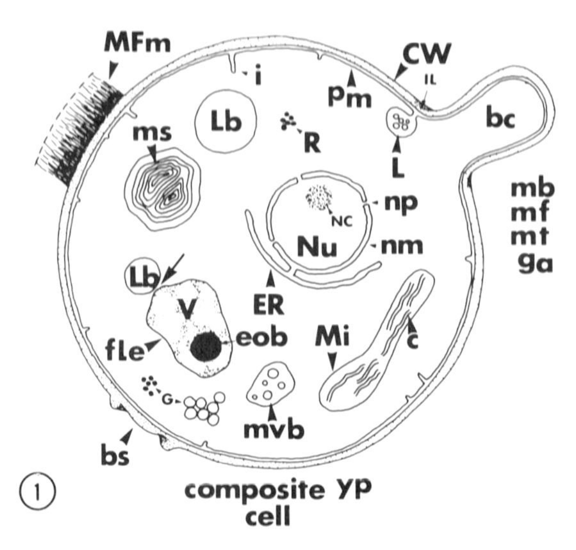

Figure 1. Composite representation of a yeast cell showing microfibrillar material (MFm) at the cell wall (CW) surface, a bud scar (bs), a bud cell (bc) and the origin of its wall from an inner layer (IL) of the parent wall, lomasome (L), plasma membrane (pm) and its invaginations (i), nucleus (Nu), nucleolus (NC), nuclear membrane (nm), nuclear pore (np), endoplasmic reticulum (ER), ribosomes (R), lipid body (Lb), membrane system (ms), multivesicular body (mvb), mitochondrion (Mi) and its cristae (c), glycogenlike material (G), vacuole (V), and fungal lysosomal-like equivalent (fLe) containing an electron-opaque body (eob). A highly structured Golgi apparatus (ga) does not occur. Microbodies (mb), microfilaments (mf), and microtubules (mt) likely occur, but have yet to be described in detail.

and its constitutive wall layers are usually not well contrasted by the conventional methods of chemical fixation and staining. In two notable examples (*Candida albicans* and *S. schenckii*), the outermost wall surface is covered with a layer of microfibrils (Lane *et al.,* 1969; Persi and Burnham, 1981; Garrison *et al.,* 1982). In at least some strains of these fungi, an electron-transparent capsule is present in more or less direct communication with the microfibrillar layer (Tronchin *et al.,* 1981; Garrison and Mirikitani, 1983). The wall microfibrils may also be associated with certain enzymatic activities such as acid phosphatase (Tronchin *et al.,* 1980; Garrison and Arnold, 1983). These wall microfibrils seem rich in mannan-containing polymers as evidenced by their binding affinity for concanavalin A (Travassos *et al.,* 1977; Cassone *et al.,* 1978; Travassos and Lloyd, 1980) and their staining reactivity toward electron cytochemical methods that detect structural polysaccharides having periodic acid-sensitive vicinal hydroxyl or α-amino groups. We have found the periodic acid–thiocarbohydrazide–silver proteinate (PATAg) method of Thiéry (1967) to be a satisfactory procedure for the detection of these substances at the fine structural level (see Figures 4, 6, 25, and 26). Although the precise nature and function(s) of wall microfibrils are not now known, it is possible that in some fungi they may be involved in some manner with mechanisms of cellular adhesion.

Most yeast cells of the dimorphic fungi reproduce by multipolar budding in which the bud cell wall arises as an extension of an innermost layer of the parental cell wall. Bud scars may be observed on occasion, but they are rarely seen in most thin sections of yeast-phase cells. The plasma membrane is usually stained by the routine methods of preparation, but its fine structure is best characterized by methods of freeze–fracture or freeze–etching (Garrison, 1981). Lomasomes (plasmalemmasomes) are characteristically membranous to vesicular structures located between the plasma membrane and the cell wall of the yeast and/or hyphal cells of a great many fungi. The exact function of these structures is as yet not clear, but they have been implicated in cell-wall synthetic activities (Wilsenach and Kessel, 1965). The periplasmic space is not readily visualized by conventional thin section.

Electron microscopy reveals a variety of organelles and inclusions in the cytoplasm of the yeast cell. In typical thin sections, the nuclear apparatus consists of the nuclear membrane, nuclear pores, nucleoplasm, and usually an eccentrically located nucleolus. Yeast cells of *B. dermatitidis* and *Paracoccidioides brasiliensis* are typically multinucleate. At present, there are no detailed studies that describe the behavior of the nucleus and its content during phase transition. Profiles of smooth endoplasmic reticulum are scattered throughout the cytoplasm, and some of these may communicate directly with the nuclear membrane in a manner that suggests that these cytomembranes actually consist of one continuous system. Ribosomes are located in a random manner throughout the cytoplasmic ground substance. They are demonstrated after fixation in glutaraldehyde–osmium tetroxide, but they are destroyed during fixation with permanganate.

Several mitochondria may be observed in a given plane of section. They are usually elongate, with the cristae parallel to the long axis. Fungal mitochondria do not differ significantly in substructure from those observed in higher eukaryotic cells. Vacuoles occur in the cytoplasm and are especially common in older cells. They may contain unorganized amorphous materials. Vacuoles of the pathogenic dimorphic fungi seem to possess lysosomal-like functions, since certain lysosomal marker enzymes have been demonstrated cytochemically to be localized within (Garrison and Tally, 1981).

Reserve polysaccharide occurring as glycogen granules or as electron-translucent aggregates of glycogenlike polymers are common in older cells. These materials react strongly to the PATAg stain and are sensitive, at least in part, to treatment with α-amylase (Garrison and Mirikitani, 1981). Other reserve materials in the form of lipid bodies are generally present.

Intracytoplasmic membrane systems may be present, but their status as true functional organelles remains to be clearly established; some workers regard them as preparational artifacts (Garrison, 1983). A class of small membranous structures referred to as multivesicular bodies have been identified in yeast cells of *B. dermatitidis* (G. A. Edwards and M. R. Edwards, 1960). Somewhat analogous structures may be seen in thin sections of *Wangiella dermatitidis* (Grove *et al.*, 1973). It is thought that these entities might represent primitive fungal equivalents of the Golgi apparatus of higher eukaryotic cells. This highly organized organelle is not found among the pathogenic fungi.

Microbodies such as glyoxysomes and peroxisomes have not been reported to occur or have not been otherwise identified in the yeast cell of the pathogenic dimorphic fungi. Little definitive information is available on the occurrence of microtubules and microfilaments among the pathogenic dimorphic fungi, although Oujezdsky *et al.* (1973) mention

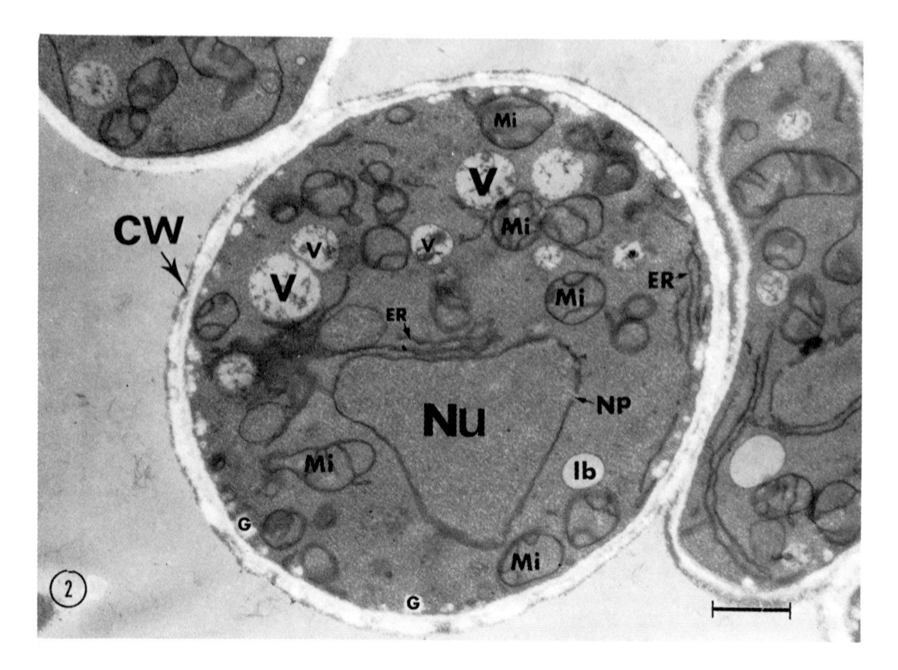

Figure 2. Thin section of *H. capsulatum* yeast showing cell wall (CW), nucleus (Nu) and nuclear pore (NP), mitochondria (Mi), lipid body (lb), vacuoles (V), glycogenlike material (G), and endoplasmic reticulum (ER). Glutaraldehyde–barium permanganate. Scale bar: 0.5 μm.

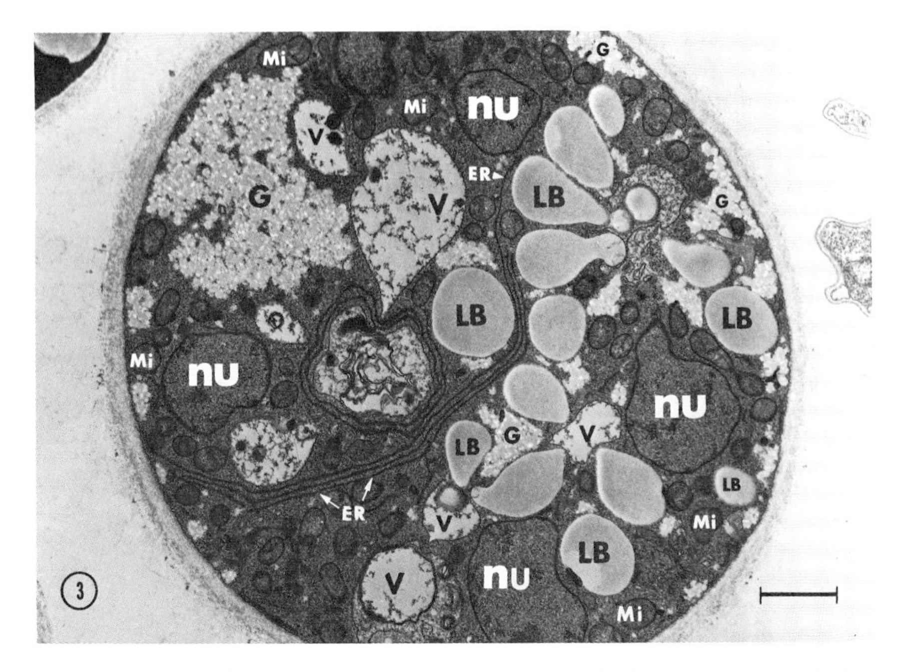

Figure 3. Thin section of *P. brasiliensis* yeast showing multiple nuclei (nu), lipid bodies (LB), glycogenlike material (G), vacuoles (V), numerous mitochondria (Mi), and profiles of endoplasmic reticulum (ER). Glutaraldehyde–osmium tetroxide. Scale bar: 1.0 μm.

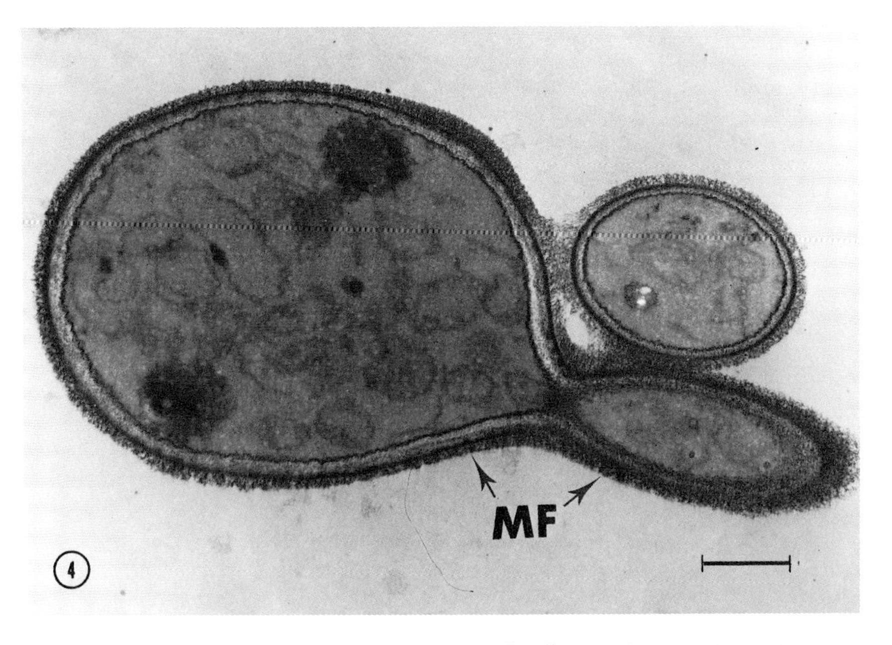

Figure 4. Thin section of a budding yeast of *S. schenckii* showing an enhanced electron opacity and disposition of microfibrils (MF) over the outer cell-wall surface. PATAg stain. Scale bar: 0.5 μm. (Adapted from Garrison *et al.*, 1982.)

the possible demonstration of microtubules in thin sections of *W. dermatitidis* yeasts. Recently, Soll and Mitchell more convincingly demonstrated microtubules in *C. albicans* (see Chapter 7). Detailed studies on the occurrence and disposition of these structures in other pathogenic fungi would be of considerable interest.

The cytology of some yeast cells of the pathogenic dimorphic fungi is rather simple (e.g., *H. capsulatum*), whereas in other species (e.g., *B. dermatitidis* and *P. brasiliensis*), the cytological organization within the cytoplasm is considerably more complex. Figures 2–4 illustrate representative electron images of thin sections of the yeast cells of *H. capsulatum, P. brasiliensis,* and *S. schenckii,* respectively.

2.2. Hypha

The content and distribution of organelles and inclusions within the hyphal cytoplasm are generally quite similar to those seen in thin sections of its homologous yeast cell. A schematic composite of a thin section of a vegetative hypha is illustrated in Figure 5.

As is the general case with yeast cells, the substructural components of the hyphal wall are poorly differentiated by the usual methods of chemical fixation and heavy-metal staining. In certain cases, cell-wall layering in both yeast and hyphal cells may be enhanced by use of the PATAg cytochemical reaction (see Figure 26). The structure of the septal area of a filamentous fungus has broad taxonomic implications (Garrison, 1983). The vegetative hyphae of all the pathogenic dimorphic fungi have asco-

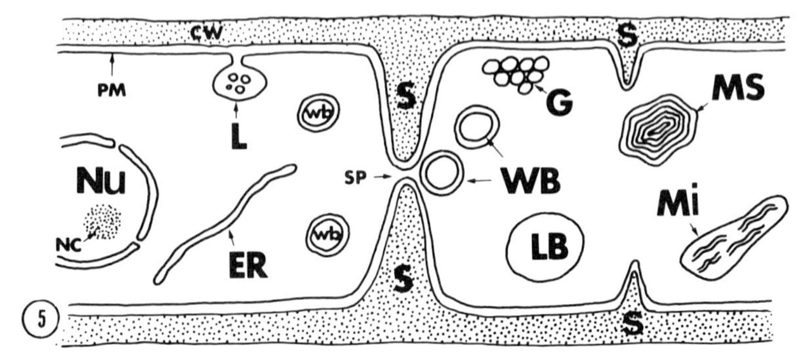

Figure 5. Composite representation of an ascomycetous hypha showing wedge-shaped septal plates (S), septal pore (SP) and associated Woronin bodies (WB/wb), cell wall (CW), plasma membrane (PM), lomasome (L), glycogenlike aggregates (G), lipid body (LB), endoplasmic reticulum (ER), mitochondrion (Mi), membrane system (MS), and nucleus (Nu) and nucleolus (NC).

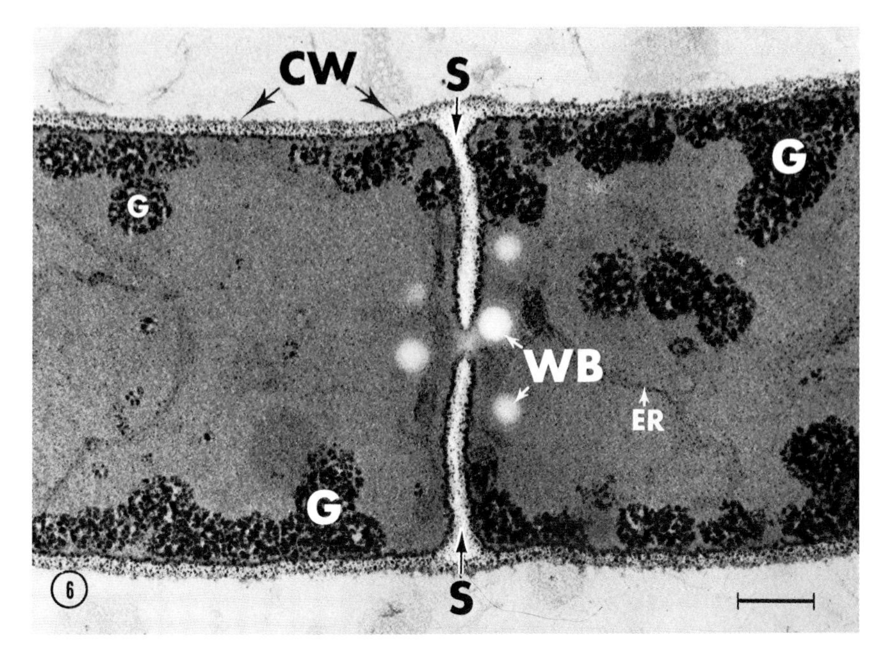

Figure 6. Septal area of *H. capsulatum* showing electron cytochemical localization of periodic acid-sensitive components. Note staining reactivities of the cell wall (CW), glycogenlike aggregates (G), endoplasmic reticulum (ER), septal plates (S), and the negative staining reactivity of the Woronin bodies (WB). PATAg stain. Scale bar: 0.25 μm. (Adapted from Garrison and Mirikitani, 1981.)

mycetous-type septa. These septa are relatively simple. The septal plates are wedge-shaped and may be more electron-translucent than the cell wall proper. It is possible that in some fungi the septal plates may be comprised in part by structural polysaccharide(s) of a somewhat different biochemical nature from those found in the main wall layers (Garrison and Mirikitani, 1981). This concept is evidenced by variations in PATAg-staining reactivities between the septal plates and main wall as shown in Figure 6. The septum of hyphal *C. albicans* is unusual in that it has a 25-nm central micropore that will not permit organellar migration and thus delimits these structures within the hyphal compartments without preventing cytoplasmic continuity (Gow *et al.*, 1980).

The septum and septal pore of the ascomycetous septal area are generally associated with a class of organelles termed Woronin bodies. These round to ovate structures are bound by a unit membrane, and they appear to act as plugs the presence or absence of which will thus regulate cytoplasmic flow between adjacent hyphal cells. There is no convincing evidence to indicate specific physiological function for the Woronin body.

2.3. Conidium

Conidia produced by certain of the pathogenic dimorphic fungi have external morphological features that may serve in the laboratory identification of the species. Some of these conidia may also participate in dimorphism (see Section 3.3). Ultrastructural analyses of the tuberculate conidia of *H. capsulatum* (M. R. Edwards *et al.*, 1960; Garrison and Lane, 1973), the hyaline and pigmented conidia of *S. schenckii* (Mariat *et al.*, 1978; Garrison *et al.*, 1982), and the conidia of *B. dermatitidis* (Garrison and Lane, 1974; Vermeil *et al.*, 1982) are available. A schematic composite of a thin section that illustrates typical conidial cytology is presented in Figure 7.

Hyphal cultures of *S. schenckii* may produce two types of conidia that differ in size, shape, and coloration. The usual *Sporothrix* conidial type is characterized by easily detached, round to oval hyaline cells that are produced sympodially at apices of conidiophores in rosettelike arrangements or inserted directly onto the filaments. At other times, pigmented, triangular, flattened macrospores may occur. Secondary conidia may arise more or less directly from the parent sympodulospores (Nicot and Mariat, 1973). The pigmented macrospores possess numerous elec-

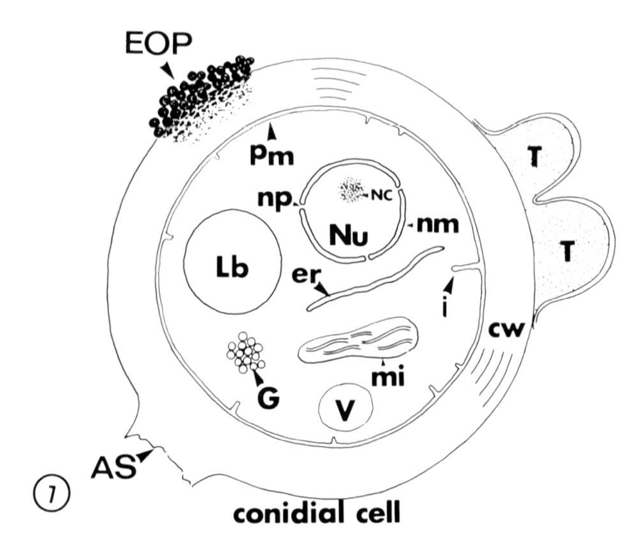

Figure 7. Composite representation of a conidium showing electron-opaque particles (EOP) and tubercles (T) at the outer cell wall (cw), abcission scar (AS), plasma membrane (pm) and its invaginations (i), lipid body (Lb), glycogenlike material (G), vacuole (V), mitochondrion (mi), endoplasmic reticulum (er), nucleus (Nu) and nucleolus (NC), nuclear membrane (nm), and nuclear pores (np).

tron-opaque aggregates at the outer wall surface (Figure 8). We believe these aggregates to be responsible for the dark coloration of the cell. The wall of the hyaline conidium appears smooth on light microscopy, but examination of thin sections reveals the presence of a thin, sparse microfibrillar layer at the wall surface (Garrison *et al.,* 1982).

Generally, the spore wall is thick and apparently finely laminated. The conidial wall of *H. capsulatum* is usually adorned with tubercules of various length (Figure 9). The wall is described as varying from a structureless material of low electron opacity, through a gradually increasing number of fibrils, to a densely packed, radially oriented, peripheral layer of increased electron opacity (G. A. Edwards and M. R. Edwards, 1960). The tubercles are of uniform and often increased electron opacity, are finely fibrillar in substructure, and arise as direct extensions of the outer zone of the wall proper. The wall and its tubercles are of low PATAg-staining reactivity (Garrison and Mirikitani, 1981). Abscission scars may be evident, as is often the case with conidia of *B. dermatitidis* (Figure 10).

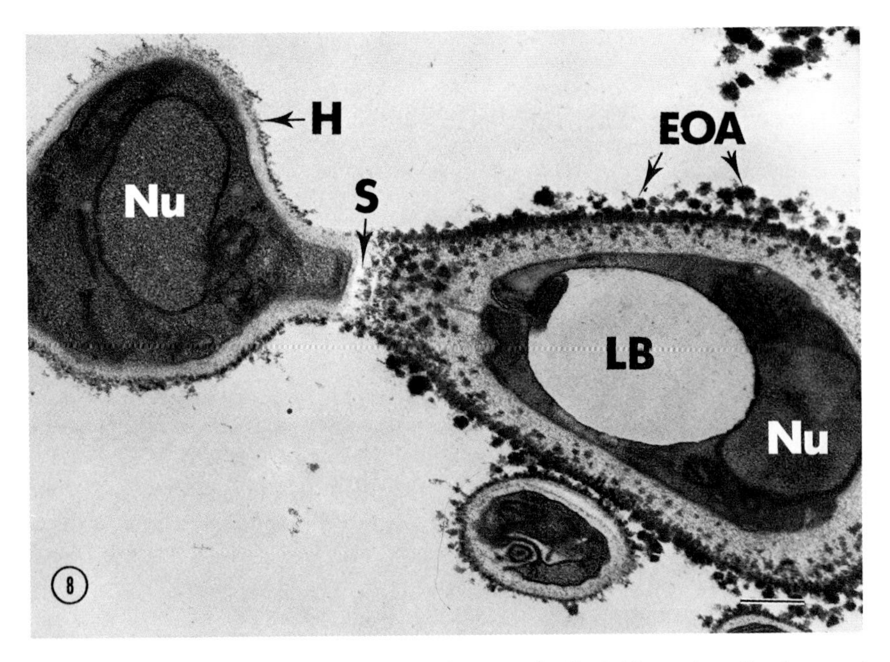

Figure 8. Cross section of a hypha (H) bearing a longitudinal thin section of a pigmented conidium of *S. schenckii* showing nuclei (Nu), septal area (S), lipid body (LB), and numerous electron-opaque aggregates (EOA) at the outer conidial wall. Potassium permanganate. Scale bar: 0.25 μm.

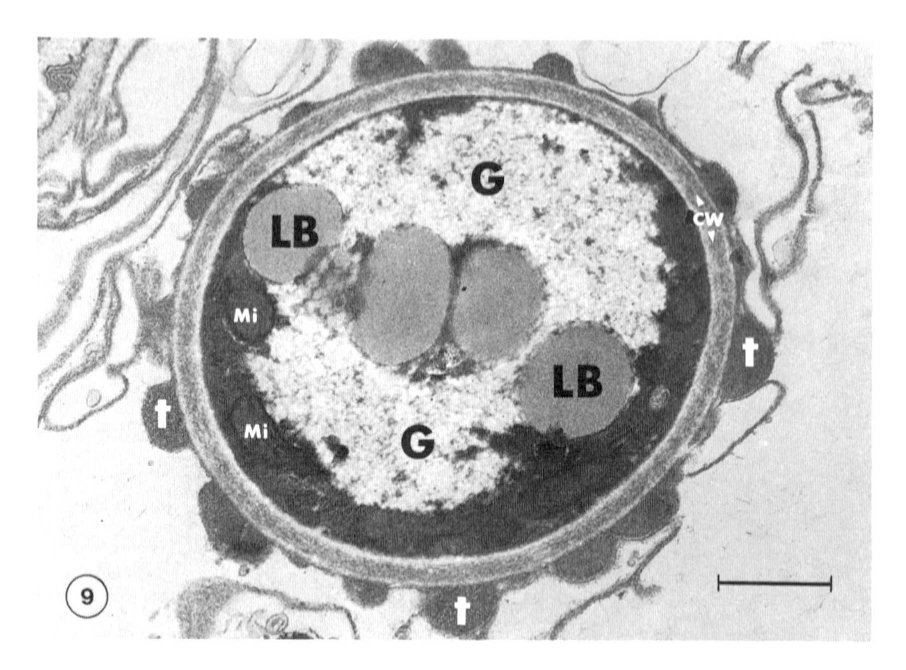

Figure 9. Thin section of a microconidium of *H. capsulatum* showing the cell wall (CW) proper with numerous tubercles (t), lipid bodies (LB), glycogenlike deposits (G), and mitochondria (Mi). Glutaraldehyde–osmium tetroxide. Scale bar: 0.5 μm.

Scanning electron microscopy has disclosed that conidia of *B. dermatitidis* may produce short, broad tubercles at the outer wall surface (Vermeil *et al.*, 1982).

The cytoplasmic organelles and inclusions consist of a nucleus, few mitochondria, profiles of smooth endoplasmic reticulum, ribosomes, scattered vacuoles, glycogenlike deposits, and lipid bodies. The conidia of *B. dermatitidis* are usually multinucleate. In the mature macroconidium of *H. capsulatum,* up to 95% of the cytoplasmic area may be filled with lipid droplets; the remainder is occupied by cytoplasmic and nuclear vestiges.

Ultrastructural aspects of various other types of reproductive cells of the pathogenic dimorphic fungi have been documented in some detail. Such studies include the adiaspore of *Chrysoporium parvum* (Kodousek *et al.*, 1972; Hejtmánek *et al.*, 1974), the chlamydospore of *C. albicans* (Cassone *et al.*, 1975), the arthrospore and spherule of *Coccidioides immitis* (Breslau *et al.*, 1961; Donnelly and Yunis, 1974; Sun *et al.*, 1979), and the ascospores of *Emmonsiella (Histoplasma) capsulata* (Glick and

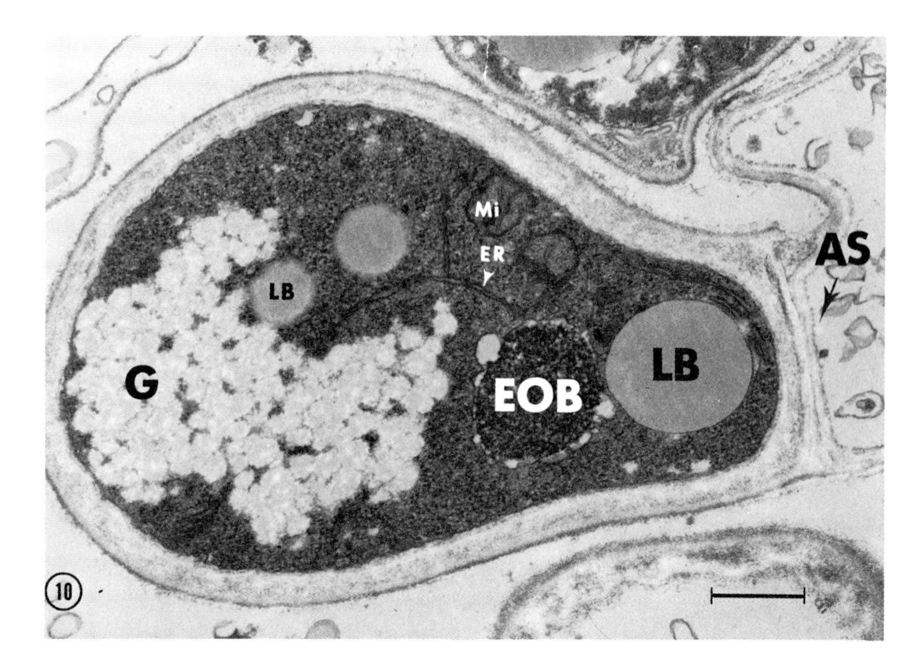

Figure 10. Thin section of a conidium of *B. dermatitidis* showing abscission scar (AS), lipid body (LB), mitochondrion (Mi), endoplasmic reticulum (ER), glycogenlike deposits (G), and an electron-opaque body (EOB). Glutaraldehyde–osmium tetroxide. Scale bar: 0.5 μm.

Kwon-Chung, 1973) and *Ajellomyces (Blastomyces) dermatitidis* (Garrison *et al.,* 1973). It is possible that arthrospores and chlamydospores may be capable of initiating phase transition under the appropriate environmental conditions.

3. ULTRASTRUCTURAL ASPECTS OF DIMORPHISM

3.1. Yeast-to-Hyphal Cell Transition

The fine structure of *in vitro* yeast-to-hyphal transition has been described in considerable detail for *P. brasiliensis* (Carbonell, 1969), *B. dermatitidis* and *H. capsulatum* (Garrison *et al.,* 1970), *S. schenckii* (Lane and Garrison, 1970), and *W. dermatitidis* (Oujezdsky *et al.,* 1973). In this sense, the ultrastructure of the germ tube and its formation by *C. albicans* have been discussed (Cassone *et al.,* 1973; Yamaguchi, 1974; Yamaguchi *et al.,* 1974).

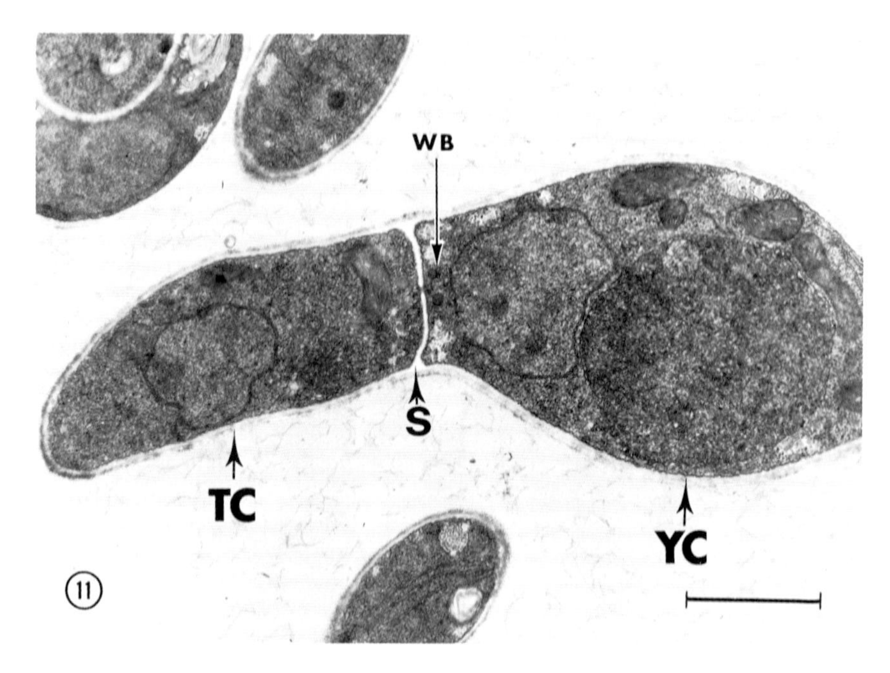

Figure 11. Yeast-to-hyphal cell transition by *H. capsulatum*. Note the parent yeast cell (YC), the elongate transitional or first hyphal cell (TC), and the Woronin bodies (WB) at the septum (S). Glutaraldehyde–osmium tetroxide. Scale bar: 1.0 μm. (Adapted from Garrison *et al.*, 1971.)

Generally, the transition process is regulated by conditions of the external cultural environment and occurs more or less rapidly after transfer of the yeast cell to an incubation temperature favoring hyphal growth. The formation of germ tubes by *C. albicans* blastospores seems to be influenced by nutritional factors in the medium.

Yeast cells do not convert at the same time, but the morphological changes brought about during the transition process are easily followed by electron microscopy of thin sections. The transition of *P. brasiliensis, B. dermatitidis, H. capsulatum,* and *S. schenckii* is initiated by formation of a budlike structure termed by some workers the transitional cell (Garrison *et al.*, 1971). It seems that the wall of this cell is related in its growth to an inner layer of the yeast cell wall. The transitional cell often contains abundant reserve material, ribosomes, and mitochondria. Occasionally, a complete septum with pore and Woronin bodies can be seen separating the parent yeast from the elongation (Figure 11). Transition at the ultrastructural level in most, if not all, pathogenic dimorphic fungi may be characterized by the presence of simple septa and associated Woronin bodies between the converting yeast and its first hyphal cell (Oujezdsky *et al.*, 1973).

In vitro yeast-to-hyphal transition by *W. dermatitidis* is a rather specialized event. Oujezdsky *et al.* (1973) showed that rapidly growing thin-walled yeast forms must first become thick-walled yeasts before phase transition occurs. Typically, the thick-walled yeast cell produces two to a number of moniliform hyphal cells that in turn often give rise to true hyphae. It seems that yeast cells of *W. dermatitidis* must first acquire sporelike characteristics by becoming thick-walled and by the accumulation of considerable endogenous reserves before they convert and produce hyphae.

Candida albicans is regarded as showing a true fungal dimorphism. The transition process starts when a blastospore produces a short filament (the germ tube) that can later evolve into a true mycelium. Germ-tube formation is accompanied by significant substructural changes in the wall of the blastospore (Cassone *et al.,* 1973). This wall is a multilayered structure having amorphous, granular, and fibrillar components of various electron opacities. Modifications of this substructural pattern occur with the induction of germ-tube formation. An electron-transparent layer forms from the inside of the blastospore wall that now contains materials of various shapes and dimensions. The transparent layer emerges through the wall proper to form the germ-tube initial. Degenerative changes of overlying wall structures likely result from mechanical and/or lytic changes. Later, these wall structures are reestablished as germ-tube elongation proceeds.

3.2. Hyphal-to-Yeast Cell Transition

A number of investigators have reported on aspects of hyphal-to-yeast transition as observed with the light microscope. Such studies have contributed valuable information about this phenomenon, which, in most species, has yet to be described in detail at the ultrastructural level.

The most comprehensive account of the morphological events associated with hyphal-to-yeast transition of *H. capsulatum* is that of Pine and Webster (1962). Static-slide culture and fixed-slide preparations were observed at various time intervals by light microscopy. Four types of events involving morphological changes of mycelial phase cells (hyphae and conidia) were described. These modes of ontogeny included: (1) the formation of yeast cells by budding of hyphal cells, (2) the probable conversion of hyphal cells by monilial chain formation, (3) the formation of stalked yeast cells arising in a manner similar to that observed for microconidial formation, and (4) the direct conversion of microconidia to yeast cells by polar and nonpolar budding. The origin of yeast cells from the microconidium has been confirmed and described in detail by means of electron microscopy (see Section 3.3).

Conant and Howell (1942) as well as Howard and Herndon (1961) employed light microscopy and von Tiegham and tissue-culture systems to study the development of yeast cells from hyphal-cell inocula of *B. dermatitidis*. Miyaji and Nishimura (1977) used both light and electron microscopy to study the transition of hyphae contained in agar blocks implanted into the mouse peritoneal cavity. Abou-Gabal and Fagerland (1981) described a cultural system in which hyphal-to-yeast transition seemed to be enhanced. All these studies propose that yeast cells of *B. dermatitidis* may arise either from hyphae via oidial cell formation or by budding of intercalary and terminal chlamydospores. Detailed, sequential ultrastructural analyses of these findings are not as yet available.

Attempts in our laboratory to define early ultrastructural changes

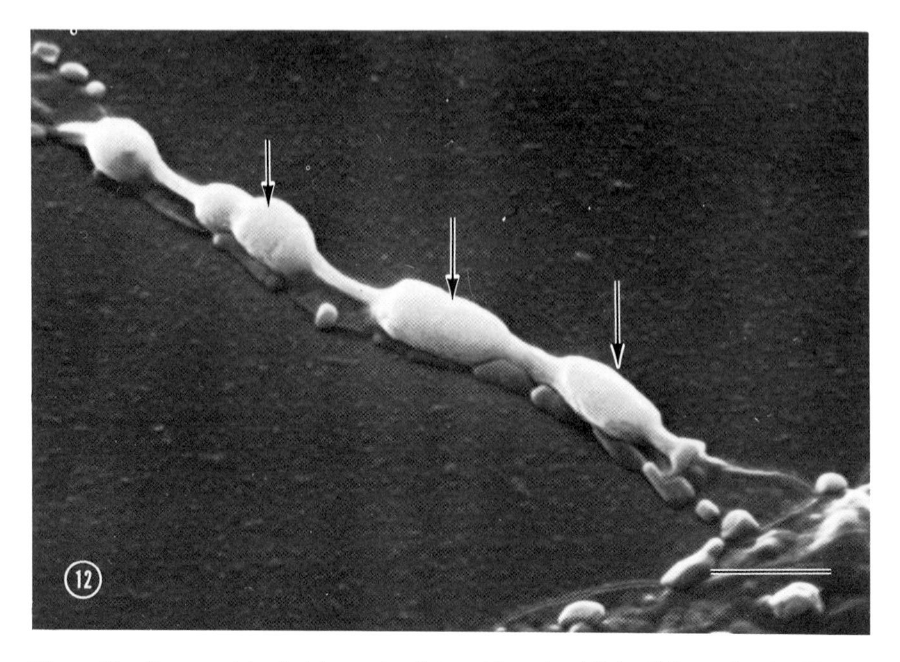

Figure 12. Presumed hyphal-to-yeast cell transition via oidial cell formation by *H. capsulatum* as seen by scanning electron microscopy. Note the ovate swellings (↓) contained within the collapsed mycelium. Scale bar: 3.0 μm.

characteristic of hyphal-to-yeast cell transition of *B. dermatitidis* and *H. capsulatum* have yielded only fragmentary information. Marked cellular degeneration and death of young hyphal cells occurs within 18–24 hr of incubation in an enriched liquid medium at 37°C. For most cells, such cultures represent a hostile environment. It seems that under these particular cultural conditions, only a few cells may be physiologically capable of initiating phase transition. If indeed this is more or less an isolated event, then its subsequent detection in thin section becomes technically difficult.

Observations of transition by hyphal-cell inocula using scanning electron microscopy have the advantage of visualizing much larger samples. On occasion, the mycelium of *H. capsulatum* has been seen to contain enlarged, round to ovate swellings thought to represent oidial yeast cells (Figure 12). Several swellings may occur, and the mycelium proper seems to be collapsed. Longitudinal thin sections of hyphal cells have been encountered that contain structures possibly representing early

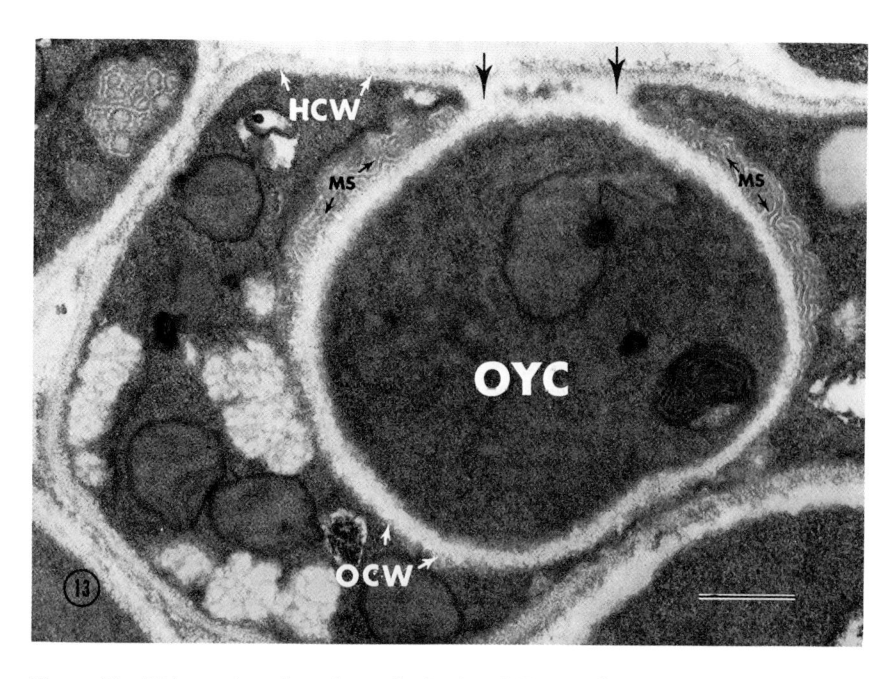

Figure 13. Thin section of portions of a hypha of *H. capsulatum* showing possible early oidial yeast cell (OYC) formation. Note the relationship of the hyphal cell wall (HCW) to oidial cell wall (OCW) as marked by the arrows and the delicate membrane systems (MS) at and along the periphery of the oidial cell wall. Glutaraldehyde–osmium tetroxide. Scale bar: 0.25 μm.

stages of phase transition via oidial cell formation (Figures 13–15). Cautious interpretations of these structures as oidial yeast primordia take into account the rather high incidence of intrahyphal hyphae formation by *H. capsulatum* (Garrison, 1983). It seems unlikely that these structures represent examples of intrahyphal hyphae, since their cell walls were always seen in intimate contact with the inner wall surfaces of the parent hyphal cells. Delicate membrane systems have been observed in close association with the wall of the oidial-like structures, suggesting their involvement in some manner with new wall formation (see Figure 13). These findings are provocative and merit further investigation.

Drouhet and Zapater (1954), as well as Carbonell and Rodriguez (1965), have investigated the transition process of *P. brasiliensis* by means of light microscopy. Certain aspects of the fine structure of mold-to-yeast transition of the fungus have been reported by Carbonell (1969). After 18-hr exposure of hyphal cells to cultural conditions favoring the yeast form, almost all the hyphae become nonviable in a manner quite

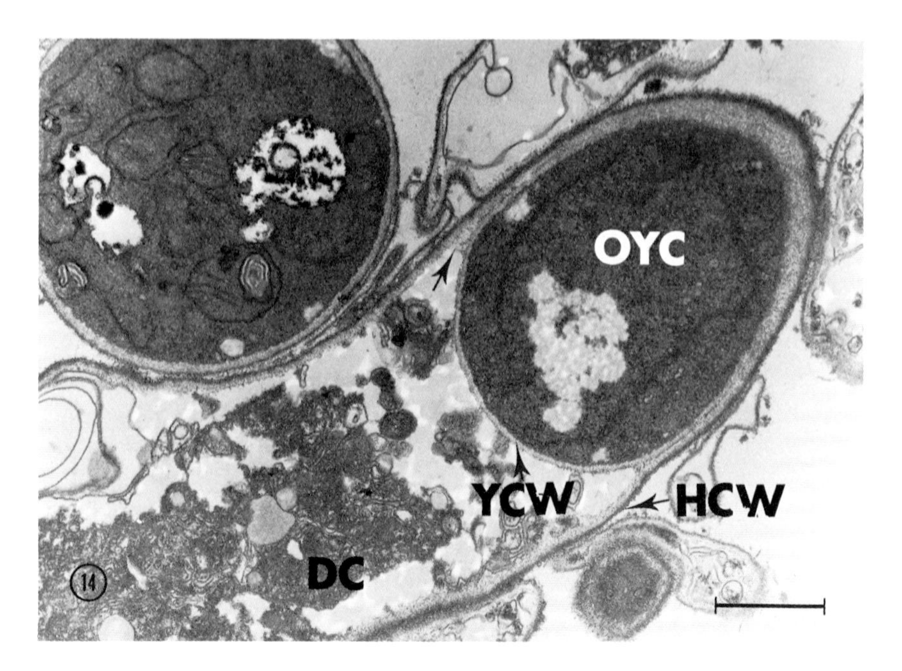

Figure 14. Longitudinal thin section of a hypha of *H. capsulatum* with a presumed oidial yeast cell (OYC) located at the apical region. Note the degenerate hyphal cytoplasm (DC) and the relationship of the hyphal cell wall (HCW) to the yeast cell wall (YCW) at the arrow. Glutaraldehyde–osmium tetroxide. Scale bar: 0.5 μm.

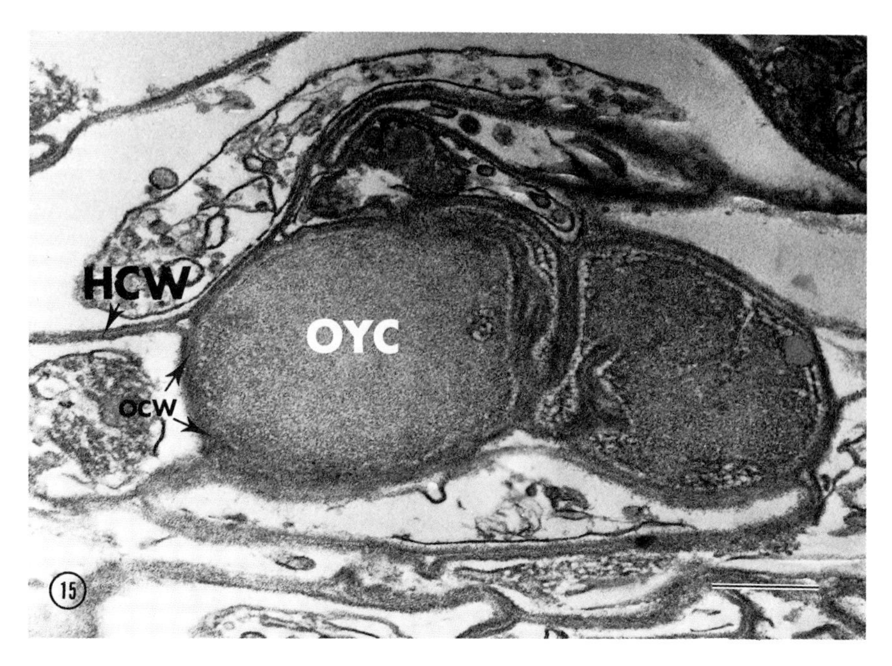

Figure 15. Presumed oidial yeast cells (OYC) contained within a degenerate hypha of *H. capsulatum*. Note the relationship of the hyphal cell wall (HCW) to the oidial cell wall (OCW). Glutaraldehyde–osmium tetroxide. Scale bar: 0.5 μm.

similar to that observed for *B. dermatitidis* and *H. capsulatum*. Electron microscopy of those hyphal cells thought to be undergoing phase transition revealed an increase in the diameter of the hypha at the interseptal spaces. The outer wall layers appear to rupture in places, leaving the innermost layers in direct contact with the cytoplasm. As the transition to yeast continues, the thickness of the cell wall and cracking of its outer layer(s) increase. After the interseptal spaces enlarge in diameter, they tend to separate and to become rounded in shape. Usually, hyphae with one or two interseptal spaces that are seemingly undergoing transition may be observed, but others are empty or contain various membranous vestiges. These findings might imply the transition to yeast growth via mechanisms of oidial-cell formation exclusively. At least in some strains of *P. brasiliensis,* we believe that transition may proceed additionally via a direct budding from the hypha, from swollen hyphal tips, or from intercalary chlamydospores.

Considerable information is available on the morphological events characteristic of mold-to-yeast transition in *S. schenckii*. Howard (1961) described the ontogenic relationship of the yeast cell of this fungus to its hyphal cell after light microscopy of tissue-culture systems inoculated with hyphal-cell suspensions. Two different modes of ontogeny were observed: (1) the formation of budding, club-shaped structures at hyphal tips or on lateral branches and (2) the formation of chains of oidia and subsequent fragmentation of the chains into their constituent yeast-phase elements. These modes of phase transition by *S. schenckii* have been documented at the ultrastructural level (Garrison *et al.*, 1975). A third mode of phase transition by this fungus involves the direct budding of yeast cells from conidia (see Section 3.3).

Many strains of *S. schenckii* readily undergo phase transition in an enriched medium at 37°C; the hyphal cell seems tolerant of these cultural conditions. The criterion for identifying early ultrastructural changes is the appearance of a conspicuous layer of microfibrils at and along the outer wall surface of the yeast-cell initial (see Section 2.1). The formation of yeast-cell primordia on lateral branches, at hyphal tips, and by oidial-cell production is depicted in Figures 16–18.

It seems that hyphal-to-yeast cell transition in certain species of the

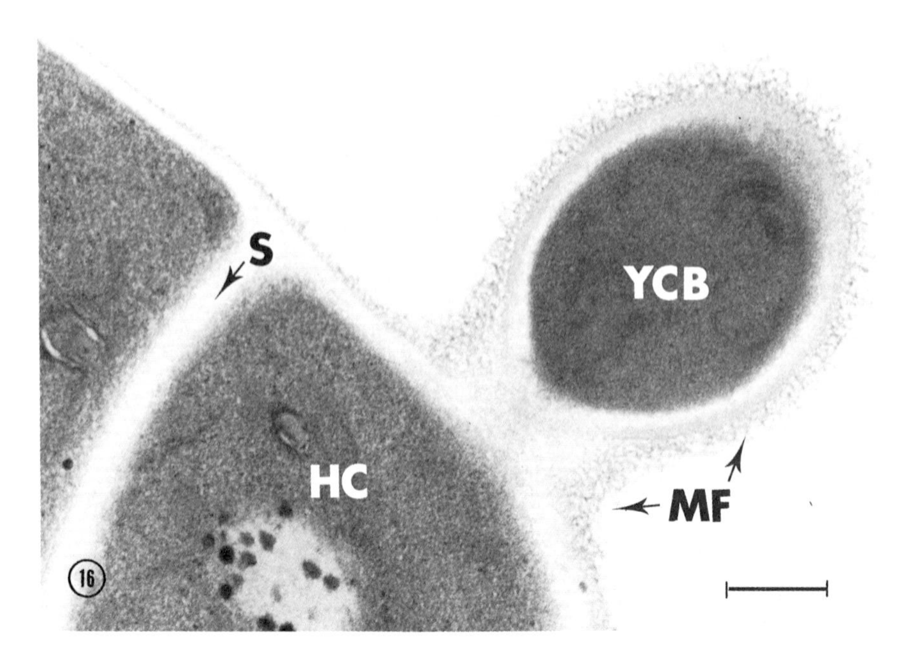

Figure 16. Hyphal (HC)-to-yeast cell transition of *S. schenckii* via lateral budding. Note the septum (S), the yeast cell bud (YCB), and the presence of numerous osmiophilic microfibrils (MF) in association with the wall of the yeast initial. Glutaraldehyde–osmium tetroxide. Scale bar: 0.25 μm.

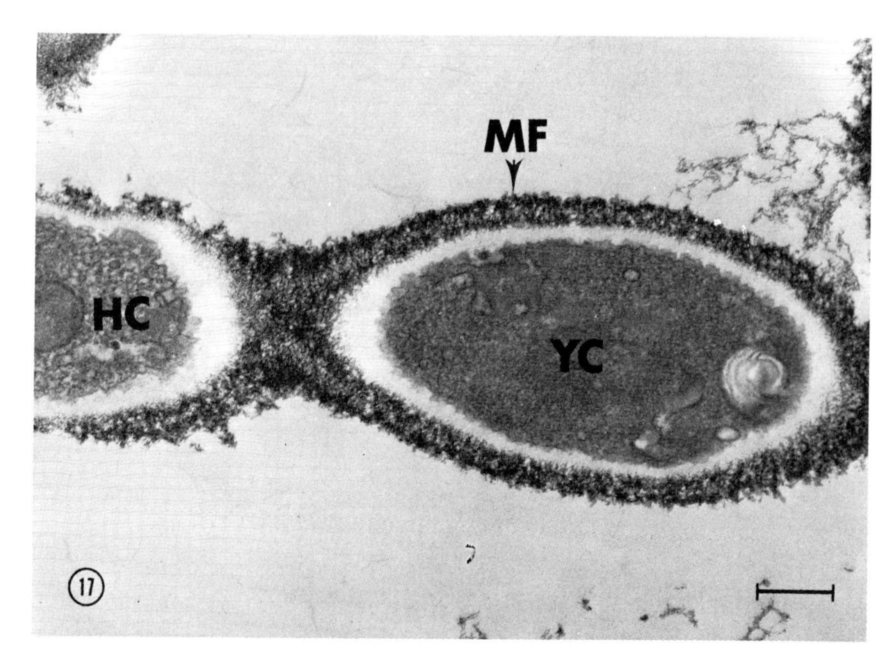

Figure 17. Hyphal (HC)-to-yeast cell (YC) transition of *S. schenckii* via terminal budding. The electron opacity of the microfibrils (MF) has been enhanced by staining with acidified dialyzed iron. Glutaraldehyde-dialyzed iron–osmium tetroxide. Scale bar: 0.25.

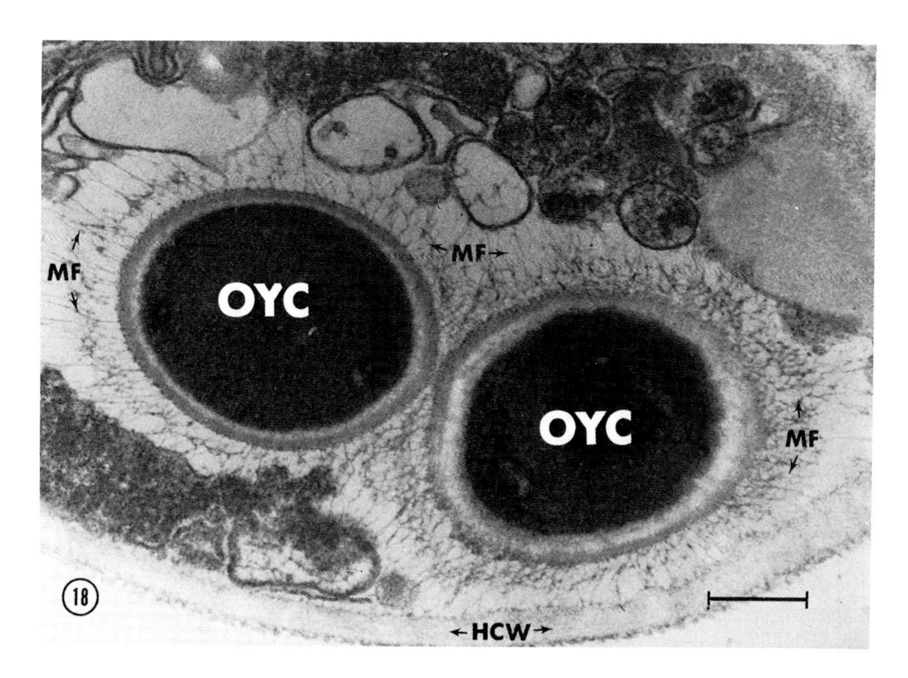

Figure 18. Oidial yeast cell (OYC) formation by *S. schenckii*. Note the microfibrils (MF) and the hyphal cell wall (HCW). Glutaraldehyde–osmium tetroxide. Scale bar: 0.25 μm.

pathogenic dimorphic fungi occurs by at least two general modes of morphogenesis: a direct budding from the hypha or oidial-cell formation within the hypha proper. An important but unresolved question is how the cell wall of the oidial yeast cell arises. It is possible that new wall materials are produced through synthetic activities associated with the plasma membrane and/or other cytomembranes of the parent hyphal cell.

A few other fungi of medical interest that are capable of undergoing dimorphic changes deserve mention. *Aspergillus parasiticus* is of interest by reason of its production of aflatoxin B_1, a potent hepatocarcinogen. Vegetative growth of this fungus is strongly influenced by the presence or absence of manganese ions in the medium (Detroy and Ciegler, 1971). When cultured in a manganese-deficient medium, the fungus grows as an enlarged, spherical, "yeastlike" structure that appears to be a stable, morphogenetic form. Electron microscopy of thin sections of these cells indicates that they possess hypertrophied, multilayered cell walls having profound changes in substructure, as illustrated in Figure 19 (Garrison and Boyd, 1974). These changes are most likely brought about by an incomplete or altered mechanism of cell-wall synthesis, which normally

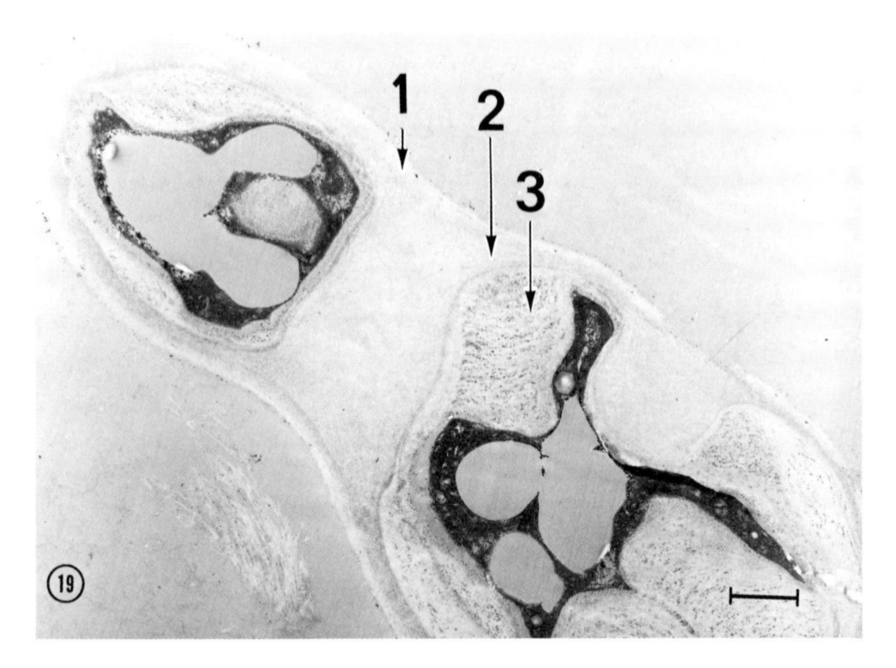

Figure 19. Nutritionally induced morphogenesis in *A. parasiticus*. Note the three distinct areas of the hypertrophied cell wall (1–3). Potassium permanganate. Scale bar: 1.0 μm. (Adapted from Garrison and Boyd, 1974.)

requires the presence of manganese ions. Other trace elements may well influence cell-wall synthesis in other fungi.

Penicillium marneffei is of interest to the medical mycologist since it seems at times to possess a pathogenic potential for man and animals in which the tissue form is distinctly yeastlike in appearance on light microscopy (Segretain, 1959). On histopathological sections of infected tissue, the pathological picture is that of a reticulosis and closely resembles similar parasitism by *H. capsulatum.* When the fungus is grown *in vitro* at 37°C on wort agar or in a liquid medium containing maltose and amino acids (Segretain, 1962), it undergoes a phase transiton to rounded, ovoid, or short bacillary elements (Figure 20). It is likely that other fungi may be induced to undergo changes in normal morphology as the consequence of unusual cultural conditions. Rippon *et al.* (1965) have described a type of induced morphogenesis by *Aspergillus sydowi* and *Penicillium lilacinum* obtained by growing the fungi in the presence of increasing concentrations of cysteine at 37°C. *In vitro* changes in morphology by the aforementioned fungi do not represent true mold–yeast dimorphism. The morphologically altered growth forms divide by cross

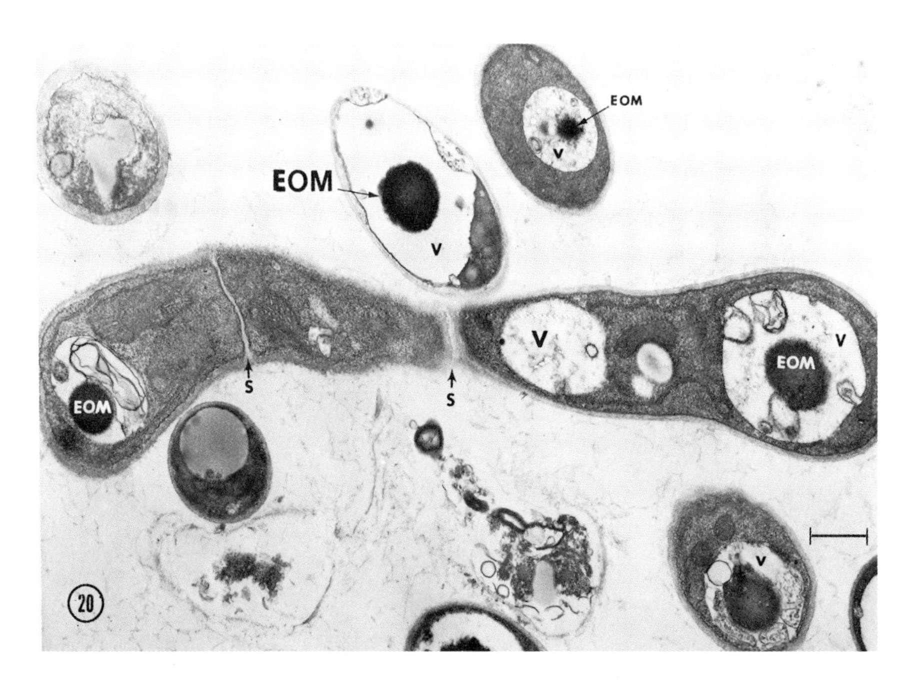

Figure 20. Arthrospore forms of *P. marneffei.* Note the transverse septa (S) and the vacuoles (V) containing electron-opaque material (EOM). Glutaraldehyde–osmium tetroxide. Scale bar: 1.0 μm. (Adapted from Garrison and Boyd, 1973.)

wall formation, and in this sense they more closely resemble arthrospores (Garrison and Boyd, 1973).

3.3. Conidial-to-Yeast Cell Transition

Conidia of certain of the pathogenic dimorphic fungi may readily undergo *in vitro* transition to the respective yeast growth form when they are placed in an enriched medium at 37°C. This fact has important epidemiological implications, and it is believed that the conidia of these fungi are the definitive natural infective units in the initiation of histoplasmosis, North American blastomycosis, and sporotrichosis.

3.3.1. *Histoplasma capsulatum*

This fungus may produce at least two types of conidia (Anderson and Marcus, 1968). These spores, termed micro- and macroconidia, are distinguished primarily on the basis of size. Procknow *et al.* (1960) described what was interpreted on light microscopy as a direct transition *in vivo* of the macroconidium to a spherulelike structure containing numerous yeast cells. This observation remains to be confirmed. In other light-microscopic studies, Dowding (1948), Pine and Webster (1962), and Goos (1964) reported that the microconidium of *H. capsulatum* may form yeast cells *in vitro.* This mode of yeast-cell ontogeny has since been described in fine-structural detail (Garrison and Boyd, 1978a).

Within 48-hr incubation in a cultural environment favoring yeast-phase growth, the microconidium undergoes rehydration, swelling, and at times a partial loss of portions of the outermost wall layers. The microconidium then germinates with the formation of a short germ tube the cell wall of which is a direct extension of an innermost layer of the parental conidial wall. One of two morphological events may then occur. In some germinants, the germ tube simply elongates to form hyphal filaments; in others, the germ tube undergoes a marked enlargement without further extension. This bulbous structure is termed the yeast mother cell. The wall of this intermediate structure is smooth and thin, whereas its cytoplasmic content is cytologically complex (Figure 21). Numerous mitochondria, lipid and carbohydrate reserves, and occasional membrane systems characterize the yeast mother cell. The formation of this specialized intermediate cell may not be a critical step in the transition process. We have observed that microconidia from some strains of *H. capsulatum* that are normally refractory to *in vitro* hyphal-to-yeast transition may indeed produce yeast mother cells under appropriate cultural conditions. However, these cells seem unable to continue the transition process further and instead degenerate and die.

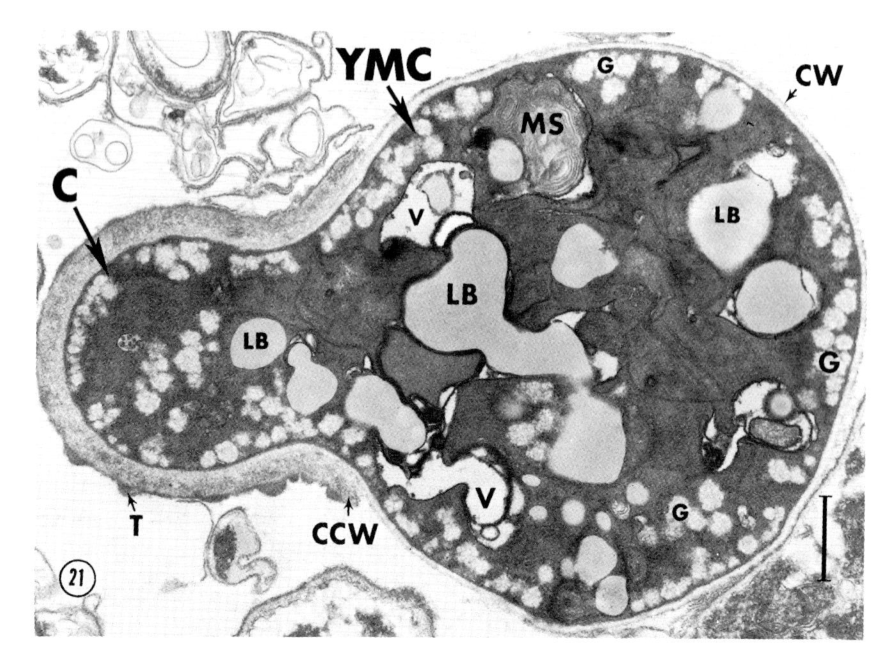

Figure 21. Microconidial (C)–yeast mother cell (YMC) complex of *H. capsulatum.* Note the ruptured conidial cell wall (CCW) with short tubercles (T), the thin yeast mother cell wall (CW), lipid bodies (LB), vacuoles (V), glycogenlike deposits (G), and a membrane system (MS). Glutaraldehyde–osmium tetroxide. Scale bar: 0.25 μm. (Adapted from Garrison and Boyd, 1978a.)

As the transition process continues, the yeast mother cell may give rise by a blastic action to single or multiple buds located at seemingly random sites along the cell-wall periphery (Figure 22). The wall of the bud initial arises from an innermost layer of the wall of the intermediate yeast mother cell. Its outermost wall surface is somewhat thickened and of increased electron opacity. A similar electron-opaque region has been noted for bud initials of hyphal and yeast cells of *P. brasiliensis* (Carbonell, 1972) and *W. dermatitidis* (Grove *et al.,* 1973). It is suggested that this area of increased electron opacity might result from the presence of lytic enzyme proteins or to enzymatic modifications of preexisting wall components. The yeast mother cell may also give rise to hyphal filaments the walls of which appear as direct extensions of the wall layers of the yeast mother cell. Formation of these two types of structures (yeast and hyphae) may occur simultaneously from the same yeast mother cell (Figure 23). On conclusion of the process, the yeast mother cell rapidly

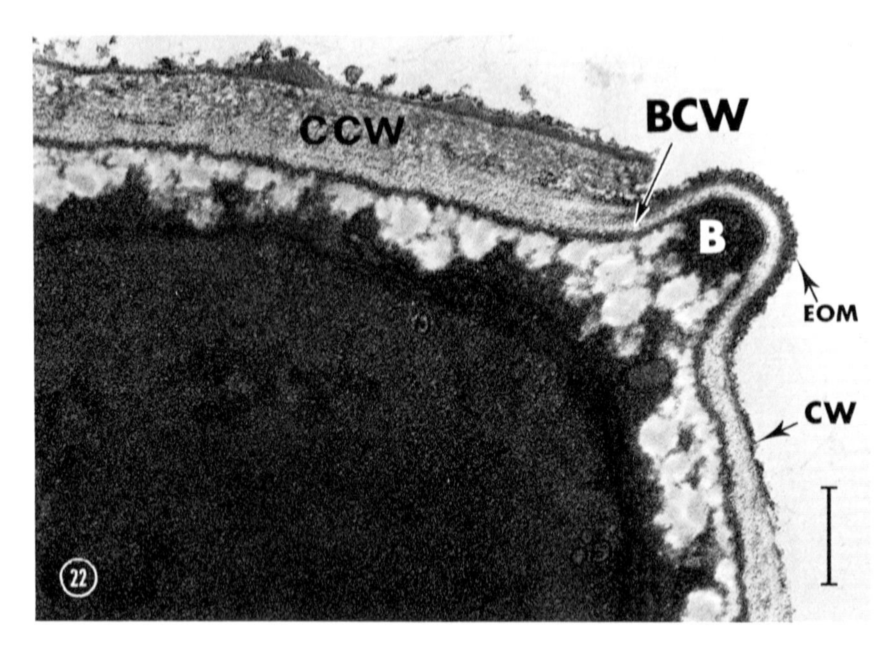

Figure 22. Bud initial (B) arising from the yeast mother cell of *H. capsulatum*. Note the origin of the bud cell wall (BCW) from an inermost layer of the yeast mother cell wall (CW), portions of the old conidial cell wall (CCW), and the electron-opaque material (EOM) at the outer wall surface of the bud initial. Glutaraldehyde–osmium tetroxide. Scale bar: 0.25 μm. (Adapted from Garrison and Boyd, 1978a.)

becomes degenerate and dies. Hyphal cells arising from the yeast mother cell may then undergo phase transition by alternate mechanisms.

The simultaneous formation of hyphal filaments and yeast mother cells has not been observed for germinating microconidia of *H. capsulatum*. It is suggested that individual microconidia may differ in their response to the transition stimuli. This concept deserves further study, since it implies that physiological differences may exist between microconidia. In a similar sense, the ability of the yeast mother cell to produce both hyphal filaments and ovate yeast-cell primordia simultaneously implies the presence of two different biochemical pathways that regulate the direction taken during budding or germination from the yeast mother cell.

Studies of conidial germination at 37°C indicate that the macroconidia of *H. capsulatum* do not form yeast mother cells or give rise to yeast cells directly (Pine and Webster, 1962; Garrison and Boyd, 1978a). It is

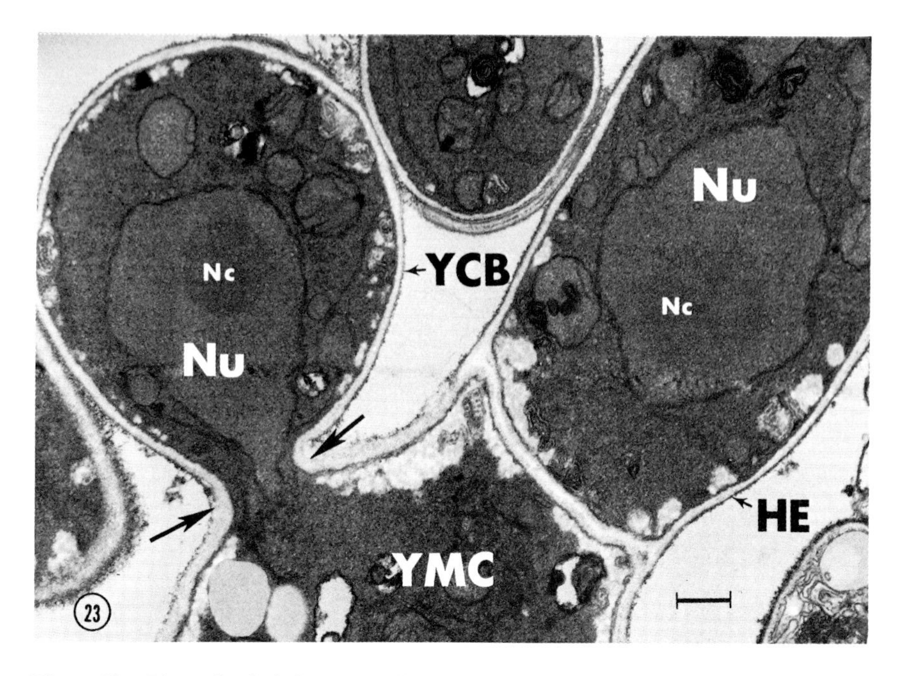

Figure 23. Linear hyphal element (HE) and ovate yeast-cell bud (YCB) arising simultaneously from the yeast mother cell (YMC) of *H. capsulatum*. Note the nuclei (Nu), the nucleoli (Nc), and the origin of the wall of the bud initial from an inner layer of the wall of the yeast mother cell as indicated by the arrows. Glutaraldehyde–osmium tetroxide. Scale bar: 0.25 μm. (Adapted from Garrison and Boyd, 1978a.)

believed that they simply germinate to form hyphal filaments that in turn may then undergo phase transition by one or more of the mechanisms described in Section 3.2.

3.3.2. *Blastomyces dermatitidis*

The fine structure of conidial-to-yeast cell transition has been reported for *B. dermatitidis* (Garrison and Boyd, 1978b). The sequence of morphological changes leading to yeast-cell formation by this fungus closely resembles that described for the microconidium of *H. capsulatum*.

Under appropriate cultural conditions, the conidium germinates to form an enlarged yeast mother cell that displays many of the usual fungal organelles (Figure 24). It is typically multinucleate. Scattered osmiophilic, globoid inclusions contained within vacuolar areas are characteristic features. The nature of these inclusions is unknown, but the presence of somewhat similar structures of varying sizes and shapes and of more

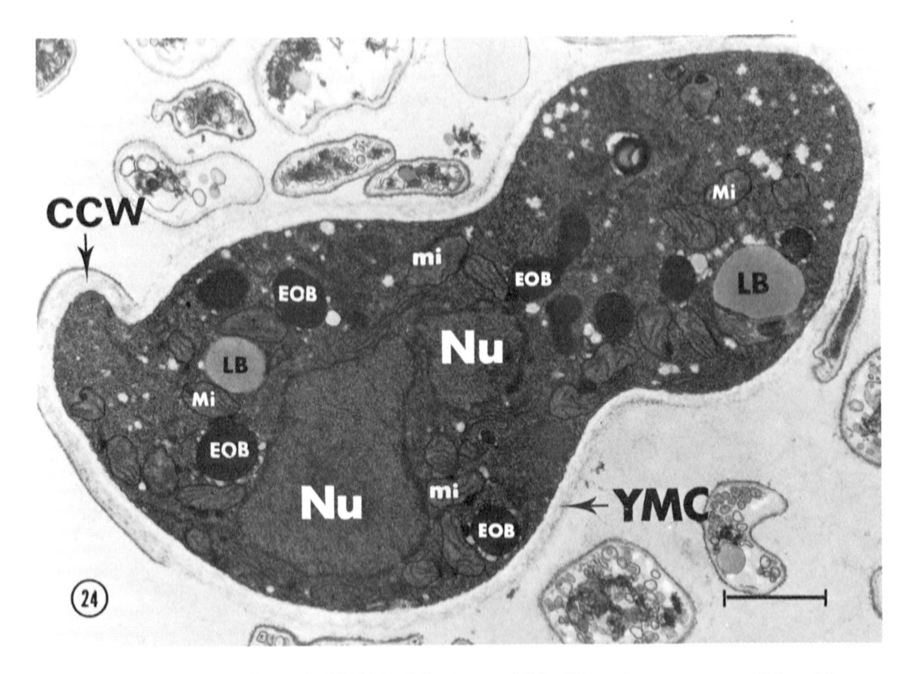

Figure 24. Yeast mother cell (YMC) of *B. dermatitidis.* Note the remnants of the old conidial cell wall (CCW), the multiple nuclei (Nu), lipid bodies (LB), mitochondria (Mi/mi), and the electron-opaque bodies (EOB). Glutaraldehyde–osmium tetroxide. Scale bar: 1.0 μm. (Adapted from Garrison and Boyd, 1978b.)

or less homogeneous textures has been reported from a number of pathogenic fungi (Garrison *et al.*, 1977; Garrison, 1983). Yeast-cell buds arise from the yeast mother cell by a blastic action through the cell wall. The simultaneous production of hyphal filaments and yeast-cell initials from the yeast mother cell of this fungus has not been observed.

3.3.3. *Sporothrix schenckii*

Weise (1931) reported that yeast cells could arise by direct budding from conidia of *S. schenckii.* We believe his observations fortuitous, since it is our opinion that light microscopy cannot distinguish with confidence true yeast-cell buds from morphologically similar secondary conidia. This mode of dimorphism by *S. schenckii* has now been described by means of the electron microscope (Garrison *et al.*, 1982).

Both hyaline and pigmented conidia germinate to form one or more germ tubes that subsequently elongate to become hyphal filaments. These hyphal cells may then give rise to yeast cells by budding or by the for-

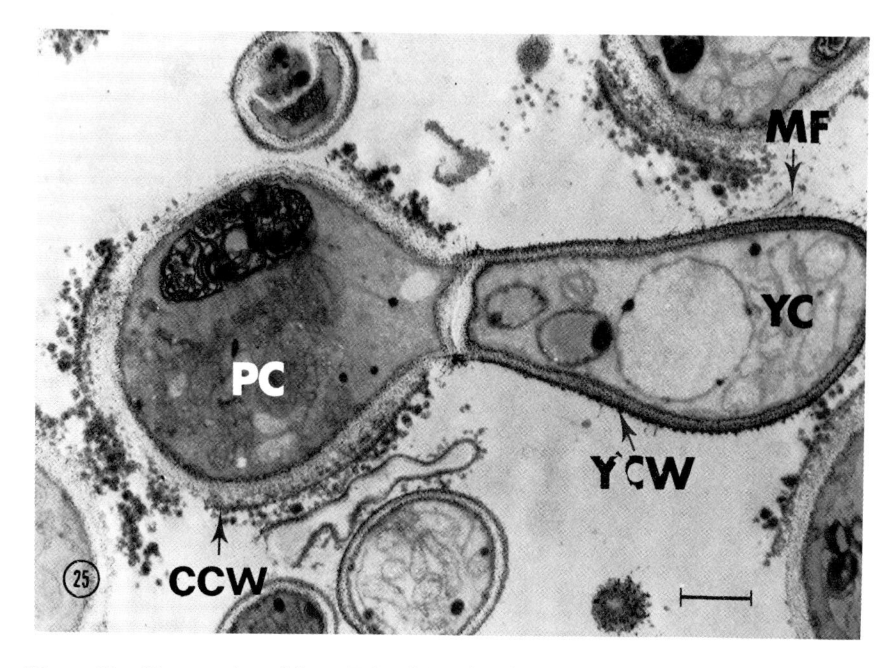

Figure 25. Pigmented conidium (PC) of *S. schenckii* giving rise to a yeast cell (YC) via direct budding. Note the electron-opaque aggregates at the ruptured conidial cell wall (CCW), the enhanced electron opacity of the yeast cell wall (YCW), and the microfibrils (MF). PATAg stain. Scale bar: 0.5 μm. (Adapted from Garrison *et al.*, 1982.)

mation of oidia within the hypha (see Section 3.1). Direct budding of the conidial cell may also occur with the formation of a yeast-cell initial but without evidence of an intermediate yeast mother cell. The yeast initial is characterized at the fine-structural level by the conspicuous layer of osmiophilic microfibrils at the wall surface, the electron opacity of which is enhanced after staining by the PATAg method (Figure 25). The wall of the bud initial arises from one or more inner layers of the parent conidium and consists of at least five layers of varying PATAg-staining intensities (Figure 26). Soon after germination, the conidium becomes degenerate.

The ability of the conidial germinant to form either hyphal filaments or yeast cells in an enriched medium at 37°C suggests the presence of two different mechanisms that regulate the direction of the germination process. The initial response of the conidium to its cultural environment at 37°C seems at first directed toward the rapid reestablishment of new hyphal growth. The formation of hyphal filaments is believed to precede the direct mode of yeast formation from the conidium.

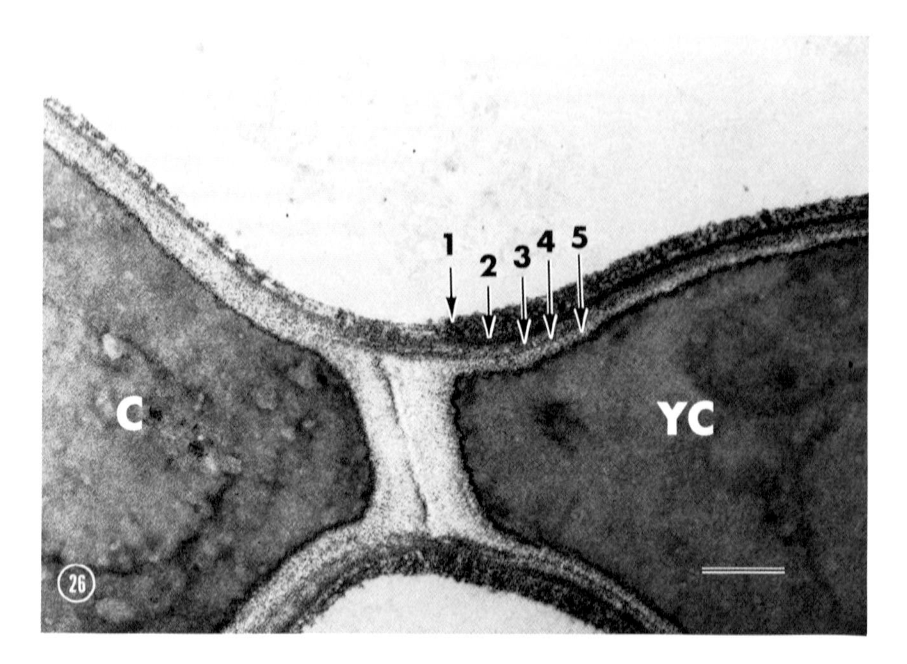

Figure 26. Portions of a hyaline conidium (C) and a yeast-cell (YC) bud of *S. schenckii.* Note the presence of at least five constitutive layers of the bud cell wall that differ in their PATAg-staining reactivity (1–5). PATAg stain. Scale bar: 0.25 μm. (Adapted from Garrison *et al.*, 1982.)

4. CONCLUDING REMARKS

Sequential ultrastructural changes that occur during transition from one growth phase to the other have been documented in some detail for certain of the pathogenic dimorphic fungi. In others, our knowledge of the mechanisms of morphological change is far from complete. It is evident that further studies are needed on the fine structure of hyphal-to-yeast cell transition. While much has been learned from studies at the ultrastructural level, we recognize the obvious limitations placed on strictly morphological documentations alone. Nevertheless, there is hardly any aspect of fungal biology associated with the phenomenon of dimorphism that could not benefit from companion fine-structural descriptions.

Future studies of fungal dimorphism by advanced techniques of electron microscopy are anticipated. The application of electron cytochemical localization of enzymes or cytochemical probes of substructural components is of potential value to a more complete understanding of morphogenesis as characterized by the dimorphic fungal pathogen. Indeed, the biochemical pathways that ultimately regulate mold–yeast–mold dimorphism may not be entirely synchronous in a given population of converting cells, which often seems to be the case. Thus, the observation at the fine-structural level of cytochemically demonstrable events associated with the converting cell systems may well provide insights not otherwise obtainable. It is obvious that methods that might achieve synchrony of the transition process would be of great value.

Dimorphism is the consequence of changes in morphology brought about by chemical pathway(s) within the fungal cytoplasm. It is reasonable to suppose that phase transition is a phenomenon more or less related to changes in cell-wall chemistry. Better and more sensitive methods are needed for the visualization of wall substructure as it undergoes alterations during critical stages of phase transition. Advances in cytochemical staining procedures that might take advantage of these chemical alterations may be forthcoming.

Future studies at the ultrastructural level might well take advantage of important technical developments in scanning transmission electron microscopy and high-voltage electron microscopy as these advanced instruments become more readily available to the fungal ultrastructuralist. Both these instruments have unique capabilities, and their application to study of fungal cytology and the phenomenon of fungal dimorphism is clearly of interest.

ACKNOWLEDGMENTS. The author wishes to thank Karen Boyd Grantham and Frank K. Mirikitani for their excellent technical assistance in the preparation of the electron micrographs used herein. This work was supported by the Veterans Administration Research Service.

REFERENCES

Abou-Gabal, M., and Fagerland, J., 1981, Electron microscopy of the tissue phase formation of *Blastomyces dermatitidis in vitro* and in naturally infected canine lung, *Mykosen* **24**:497–502.

Anderson, K. L., and Marcus, S., 1968, Sporulation characteristics of *Histoplasma capsulatum, Mycopathologia* **36**:179–185.

Bracker, C. E., 1967, Ultrastructure of fungi, *Annu. Rev. Phytopathol.* **5**:343–374.

Breslau, A. M., Hensley, T. J., and Erickson, J. O., 1961, Electron microscopy of cultured spherules of *Coccidioides immitis, J. Biophys. Biochem. Cytol.* **9**:627–637.

Carbonell, L. M., 1969, Ultrastructure of dimorphic transformation in *Paracoccidioides brasiliensis, J. Bacteriol.* **100**:1076–1082.

Carbonell, L. M., 1972, Ultrastructure of *Paracoccidioides brasiliensis,* in: Paracoccidioidomycosis, Proceedings of the First Pan American Symposium, World Health Organization Publication 254, Washington, D.C., p. 21.

Carbonell, L. M., and Rodriguez, J., 1965, Transformation of mycelial and yeast forms of *Paracoccidioides brasiliensis* in cultures and experimental inoculations, *J. Bacteriol.* **90**:504–510.

Cassone, A., Simonetti, N., and Strippoli, V., 1973, Ultrastructural changes in the wall during germ-tube formation from blastospores of *Candida albicans, J. Gen. Microbiol.* **77**:417–426.

Cassone, A., Simonetti, N., and Strippoli, V., 1975, Production, ultrastructure, and germination of *Candida albicans* chlamydospores, in: *Spores VI* (P. Gerhardt, R. N. Costilow, and H. L. Sadoff, eds.), American Society for Microbiology, Washington, D.C., pp. 172–178.

Cassone, A., Mattia, E., and Boldrini, L., 1978, Agglutination of blastospores of *Candida albicans* by concanavalin A and its relationship with the distribution of mannan polymers and the ultrastructure of the cell wall, *J. Gen. Microbiol.* **105**:263–273.

Conant, N. F., and Howell, A., 1942, The similarity of the fungus causing South American blastomycosis (paracoccidioidal granuloma) and North American blastomycosis (Gilchrist's disease), *J. Invest. Dermatol.* **5**:353–370.

Detroy, R. W., and Ciegler, A., 1971, Induction of yeastlike development in *Aspergillus parasiticus, J. Gen. Microbiol.* **65**:259–264.

Donnelly, W. H., and Yunis, E. J., 1974, The ultrastructure of *Coccidioides immitis, Arch. Pathol.* **98**:227–232.

Dowding, E. S., 1948, The spores of *Histoplasma, Can. J. Res. Sect. F.* **26**:265–273.

Drouhet, E., and Zapater, R. C., 1954, Phase levadure et phase filamentous de *Paracoccidioides brasiliensis:* Etude des noyaux, *Ann. Inst. Pasteur (Paris)* **87**:396–403.

Edwards, G. A., and Edwards, M. R., 1960, The intracellular membranes of *Blastomyces dermatitidis, Am. J. Bot.* **47**:622–632.

Edwards, M. R., Hazen, E. L., and Edwards, G. A., 1960, The micromorphology of the tuberculate spores of *Histoplasma capsulatum, Can. J. Microbiol.* **6**:65–70.

Garrison, R. G., 1981, Vegetative ultrastructure, in : *Yeast Cell Envelopes: Biochemistry, Biophysics, and Ultrastructure,* Vol. 2 (W. N. Arnold, ed.), CRC Press, Boca Raton, Florida, pp. 139–160.

Garrison, R. G., 1983, Ultrastructural cytology of the pathogenic fungi, in: *Fungi Pathogenic for Man and Animals,* Part A (D. H. Howard, ed.), Marcel Dekker, New York, pp. 229–321.

Garrison, R. G., and Arnold, W. N., 1983, Cytochemical localization of acid phosphatases in the dimorphic fungus *Sporothrix schenckii, Curr. Microbiol.* **9**:253–258.

Garrison, R. G., and Boyd, K. S., 1973, Dimorphism of *Penicillium marneffei* as observed by electron microscopy, *Can. J. Microbiol.* **19**:1305–1309.

Garrison, R. G., and Boyd, K. S., 1974, Ultrastructural studies of induced morphogenesis by *Aspergillus parasiticus, Sabouraudia* **12**:179–187.

Garrison, R. G., and Boyd, K. S., 1978a, Electron microscopy of yeastlike cell development from the microconidium of *Histoplasma capsulatum, J. Bacteriol.* **133**:345–353.

Garrison, R. G., and Boyd, K. S., 1978b, Role of the conidium in dimorphism of *Blastomyces dermatitidis, Mycopathologia* **64**:29–33.

Garrison, R. G., and Lane, J. W., 1973, Scanning-beam electron microscopy of the conidia of the brown and albino filamentous varieties of *Histoplasma capsulatum, Mycopathol. Mycol. Appl.* **49**:185–191.

Garrison, R. G., and Lane, J. W., 1974, The fine structure of the microconidium of *Blastomyces dermatitidis, Mycopathol. Mycol. Appl.* **52**:93–100.

Garrison, R. G., and Mirikitani, F. K., 1981, Electron cytochemical determination of periodic acid-reactive sites in *Histoplasma capsulatum, Microbios* **30**:19–25.

Garrison, R. G., and Mirikitani, F. K., 1983, Electron cytochemical demonstration of the capsule of yeast-like *Sporothrix schenckii, Sabouraudia* **21:**167–170.

Garrison, R. G., and Tally, J. F., 1981, Electron cytochemical evidence for lysosomal-like equivalents in *Histoplasma capsulatum, Mycopathologia* **73:**183–190.

Garrison, R. G., Lane, J. W., and Field, M. F., 1970, Ultrastructural changes during the yeastlike to mycelial phase conversion of *Blastomyces dermatitidis* and *Histoplasma capsulatum, J. Bacteriol.* **101:**628–635.

Garrison, R. G., Lane, J. W., and Johnson, D. R., 1971, Electron microscopy of the transitional cell of *Histoplasma capsulatum, Mycopathol. Mycol. Appl.* **44:**121–129.

Garrison, R. G., Lane, J. W., and Johnson, D. R., 1973, Ultrastructural studies on the cleistothecium of *Ajellomyces dermatitidis, Sabouraudia* **11:**131–136.

Garrison, R. G., Boyd, K. S., and Mariat, F., 1975, Ultrastructural studies of the mycelium-to-yeast transformation of *Sporothrix schenckii, J. Bacteriol.* **124:**959–968.

Garrison, R. G., Mariat, F., Boyd, K. S., and Fromentin, H., 1977, Ultrastructural observations of an unusual osmiophilic body in the hyphae of *Sporothrix schenckii* and *Ceratocystis stenoceras, Ann. Microbiol. (Inst. Pasteur)* **128B:**319–337.

Garrison, R. G., Mariat, F., Fromentin, H., and Mirikitani, F. K., 1982, Electron microscopic analysis of yeastlike cell formation from the conidia of *Sporothrix schenckii, Ann. Microbiol. (Inst. Pasteur)* **133B:**189–204.

Glick, A. D., and Kwon-Chung, K. J., 1973, Ultrastructural comparison of coils and ascospores of *Emmonsiella capsulata* and *Ajellomyces dermatitidis, Mycologia* **65:**216–220.

Goos, R. D., 1964, Germination of the macroconidium of *Histoplasma capsulatum, Mycologia* **56:**662–671.

Gow, N. A. R., Gooday, G. W., Newsam, R. J., and Gull, K., 1980, Ultrastructure of the septum in *Candida albicans, Curr. Microbiol.* **4:**357–359.

Greenhalgh, G. N., and Evans, L. V., 1971, Electron microscopy, in: *Methods in Microbiology,* Vol. 4 (C. Booth, ed.), Academic Press, New York, pp. 517–566.

Groove, S. N., Oujezdsky, K. B., and Szaniszlo, P. J., 1973, Budding in the dimorphic fungus *Phialophora dermatitidis, J. Bacteriol.* **81:**522–527.

Hejtmánek, M., Nečas, O., and Havelková, M., 1974, The ultrastructure of the spherules of *Emmonsia crescens* studied by the technique of freeze–etching, *Mycopathologia* **54:**79–83.

Howard, D. H., 1961, Dimorphism of *Sporotrichum schenckii, J. Bacteriol.* **81:**464–469.

Howard, D. H., and Herndon, R. L., 1961, Tissue cultures of mouse peritoneal exudates inoculated with *Blastomyces dermatitidis, J. Bacteriol.* **81:**522–527.

Kodousek, R., Hejtmánek, M., Havelková, M., and Strachová, Z., 1972, The ultrastructure of spherules of fungus *Emmonsia crescens*—a causative agent of adiaspiromycosis, *Beitr. Pathol.* **145:**83–88.

Kopp, F., 1975, Electron microscopy of yeasts, *Methods Cell Biol.* **11:**23–44.

Lane, J. W., and Garrison, R. G., 1970, Electron microscopy of yeast to mycelial phase conversion of *Sporotrichum schenckii, Can. J. Microbiol.* **16:**747–749.

Lane, J. W., Garrison, R. G., and Field, M. F., 1969, Ultrastructural studies on the yeastlike and mycelial phases of *Sporotrichum schenckii, J. Bacteriol.* **100:**1010–1019.

Mariat, F., Garrison, R. G., Boyd, K. S., Rouffaud, M. A., and Fromentin, H., 1978, Premières observations sur les macrospores pigmentees de *Sporothrix schenckii, C. R. Acad. Sci.* **286:**1429–1432.

Miyaji, M., and Nishimura, K., 1977, Investigation of dimorphism of *Blastomyces dermatitidis* by agar-implantation, *Mycopathololologia* **60:**73–78.

Nicot, J., and Mariat, F., 1973, Caractères morphologiques et position systèmatique de *Sporothrix schenckii,* agent de la sporotrichose humaine, *Mycopathol. Mycol. Appl.* **49:**53–65.

Oujezdsky, K. B., Grove, S. N., and Szaniszlo, P. J., 1973, Morphological and structural changes during the yeast-to-mold conversion of *Phialophora dermatitidis, J. Bacteriol.* **113**:468–477.

Persi, M. A., and Burnham, J. C., 1981, Use of tannic acid as a fixative–mordant to improve the ultrastructural appearance of *Candida albicans* blastospores, *Sabouraudia* **19**:1–8.

Pine, L., and Webster, R. E., 1962, Conversion in strains of *Histoplasma capsulatum, J. Bacteriol.* **83**:149–157.

Procknow, J. J., Page, M. I., and Loosli, C. G., 1960, Early pathogenesis of experimental histoplasmosis, *AMA Arch. Pathol.* **69**:413–426.

Rippon, J. W., Conway, T. P., and Domes, A. L., 1965, Pathogenic potential of *Aspergillus* and *Penicillium* species, *J. Infect. Dis.* **115**:27–32.

Segretain, G., 1959, *Penicillium marneffei* n. sp., agent d'une mycose du système réticulo-endothelial, *Mycopathol. Mycol. Appl.* **11**:327–353.

Segretain, G., 1962, Some new or infrequent fungous pathogens, in: *Fungi and Fungous Diseases* (G. Dalldorf, ed.), Charles C. Thomas, Springfield, Illinois, pp. 33–49.

Sun, S. H., Sekhon, S. S., and Huppert, M., 1979, Electron microscopic studies of saprobic and parasitic forms of *Coccidioides immitis, Sabouraudia* **17**:265–274.

Thiéry, J. P., 1967, Mise en évidence des polysaccharides sur coupes fines en microscopie électronique, *J. Microsc. (Paris),* **6**:987–1018.

Travassos, L. R., and Lloyd, K. O., 1980, *Sporothrix schenckii* and related species of Ceratocystis, *Microbiol. Rev.* **44**:683–721.

Travassos, L. R., Souza, W., Mendonca-Previato, L., and Lloyd, K. O., 1977, Location and biochemcal nature of surface components reacting with concanavalin A in different cell types of *Sporothrix schenckii, Exp. Mycol.* **1**:293–305.

Tronchin, G., Poulain, D., and Biguet, J., 1980, Localisation ultrastructurale de l'activité phosphatasique acide chez *Candida albicans, Biol. Cell.* **38**:147–152.

Tronchin, G., Poulain, D., Herbaut, J., and Biguet, J., 1981, Cytochemical and ultrastructural studies of *Candida albicans.* 2. Evidence for a cell wall coat using concanavalin A, *J. Ultrastruct. Res.* **75**:50–59.

Vermeil, C., Bouillard, C., Miegeville, M., Morin, O., and Marjolet, M., 1982, The echinulate conidia of *Blastomyces dermatitidis* Gilchrist and Stokes and the taxonomic status of this species, *Mykosen* **25**:251–253.

Weise, F. C., 1931, Sporotrichosis in Connecticut, *N. Engl. J. Med.* **205**:951–955.

Wilsenach, R., and Kessel, M., 1965, The role of lomasomes in wall formation in *Penicillium vermiculatum, J. Gen. Microbiol.* **40**:401–404.

Yamaguchi, H., 1974, Effect of biotin insufficiency on composition and ultrastructure of cell wall of *Candida albicans* in relation to its mycelial morphogenesis, *J. Gen. Appl. Microbiol.* **20**:217–228.

Yamaguchi, H., Kanda, Y., and Osumi, M., 1974, Dimorphism in *Candida albicans.* II. Comparison of fine structure of yeast-like and filamentous phase growth, *J. Gen. Appl. Microbiol.* **20**:101–110.

Part II

Fungi with Yeast Tissue Morphologies

Chapter 3

Blastomyces dermatitidis

Judith E. Domer

1. INTRODUCTION

The existence of two morphological entities of *Blastomyces dermatitidis*, the causative agent of blastomycosis (North American blastomycosis, Gilchrist's disease), was recognized by Gilchrist and Stokes (1898) soon after the disease was first described by Gilchrist (1896). Gilchrist and Stokes (1898) named the fungus and succeeded in culturing it at room temperature despite gross contamination of the cultures with pyogenic cocci. Ricketts (1901), however, was the first to publish detailed *in vitro* appearances of both yeast and mycelial forms, and it was he who suggested that temperature was a key factor in determining the type of growth observed. In an equally detailed and accurate presentation, Hamburger (1907) confirmed the importance of temperature in determining the morphological type and described how the "capsule" of the yeastlike cell ruptured, leaving "collarlike" projections through which a new bud was formed or a germ tube was initiated.

Both forms were well described in the early studies cited above, as well as in later studies (e.g., Stober, 1914; Michelson, 1928; DeMonbreun, 1935). Moreover, *in vitro* transition of the mycelium to the yeast form was reported by Ciferri and Redaelli (1935), but it was not until the 1940s that investigators began searching for clues to the maintenance of each form and to the regulation of the transition process itself. Initial studies involved physiology, specifically the growth requirements of each phase,

Judith E. Domer • Tulane University School of Medicine, New Orleans, Louisiana 70112.

and light microscopy. More recently, the emphasis has shifted to observations at the electron-microscopic (EM) level and to studies of cell-wall composition and structure. Some attention has been directed toward macromolecular composition as well, although there has not been a concerted effort to study any one aspect of metabolism in depth.

2. GROWTH REQUIREMENTS

Stewart and Meyer (1938) were among the first to investigate the growth requirements of *B. dermatitidis.* Their main objective, however, was to study *Coccidioides immitis,* and one strain of *B. dermatitidis* was included simply for comparative purposes. Cultures were incubated at 37°C in a basal medium consisting of salts, glucose, and arginine, and the authors concluded that *B. dermatitidis* had no vitamin requirements. Later, Levine and Ordal (1946) examined both the yeast and mycelial phases of *B. dermatitidis* incubated in a medium containing glucose, ammonium sulfate, and minimal salts. Both phases grew well in the absence of any additional nutrients, and it was concluded that temperature, as had been proposed much earlier (Ricketts, 1901; Hamburger, 1907), was indeed the key factor in determining form, with 35–37°C being optimum for the yeast phase and 31–33°C for the mycelial phase. Additionally, each phase grew over a wide range of pH, e.g., 4.5–7.5 for the mycelial phase and 5.5–8.5 for the yeast phase. Further studies (Salvin, 1949; Nickerson and Edwards, 1949; Area Lenao and Cury, 1950; Gilardi and Laffer, 1962) confirmed the studies of Levine and Ordal (1946) with both the yeast and mycelial forms.

Despite the accumulated evidence, there was a single study by Halliday and McCoy (1955) that indicated that *B. dermatitidis* requires biotin for growth. These investigators faulted previous workers for using cotton plugs or agar in their incubation systems, either of which can contain small quantities of biotin. On the basis of their studies, in which 6 strains of *B. dermatitidis* were incubated in liquid media with metal enclosures, they reported that biotin was a growth factor for the organism. Work by Gilardi and Laffer (1962), however, designed to test the same hypothesis, resulted in the opposite conclusion, viz., that *B. dermatitidis* had no growth requirements, because none of the 13 strains tested by them in synthetic liquid media with metal enclosures required amino acids or vitamins for growth. Halliday and McCoy (1955) are therefore in the minority, but there have been no additional studies to confirm or refute their work.

Nickerson and Edwards (1949), in addition to confirming the studies of Levine and Ordal (1946), coined the term *thermal dimorphism* to describe the temperature-dependent transition observed in *B. dermatitidis* and made several other observations. First, they determined that the glucose–ammonium sulfate–minimal salts medium that supported the growth of each individual phase also supported transition of one phase to the other. Second, they measured oxygen consumption in the absence of substrate and noted that the yeast phase consumed 5–6 times more O_2 than the mycelial phase. Unfortunately, the significance of this latter observation is still a mystery, but may simply be related to the relative quantities of a stored energy source, e.g., glycogen, or to increased rate of catabolic enzyme activity at the higher temperature.

In other studies, sugars or amino acids, which can serve as sources of carbon and/or nitrogen for growth of the organism, were determined, but since these do not bear directly on the phenomenon of dimorphism, they will not be discussed here. The reader interested in those data, however, is directed to a review by Gilardi (1965).

3. MICROSCOPY

The light-microscopic appearances of the yeast and mycelial forms of *B. dermatitidis* had been described in the early 1900s, but it was not until much later that the specifics of subcellular structure became known. DeLamater (1948, 1949), using fixed preparations, was the first to describe the multinucleate character of both forms, and Bakerspigel (1957) confirmed this observation using living cells and noted that there were no differences in staining characteristics between yeast and mycelial nuclei. Further, he observed that nuclear division within a given compartment, i.e., yeast cell or hyphal cell, was not synchronous. The first EM study of *B. dermatitidis*, limited to the yeast phase, was published in 1960 (Edwards and Edwards, 1960). The usual eukaryotic organelles, such as nuclei and mitochondria, were shown, in addition to endoplasmic reticulum, a plasma membrane, and cell wall. Further, the observations suggested that the membranes of the cell all seemed to be interconnected, allowing, presumably, for maximum communication among the various compartments of the cell. The membrane interconnections have not been confirmed by others, however. A thin section of a yeast cell in which the various organelles can be seen appears in Figure 1.

Carbonell and Rodriquez (1968) presented the first thorough study of the ultrastructure of the mycelial phase. Structures similar to those described for the yeast phase were noted, including multiple nuclei, well-developed mitochondria, ribosomes, and endoplasmic reticulum,

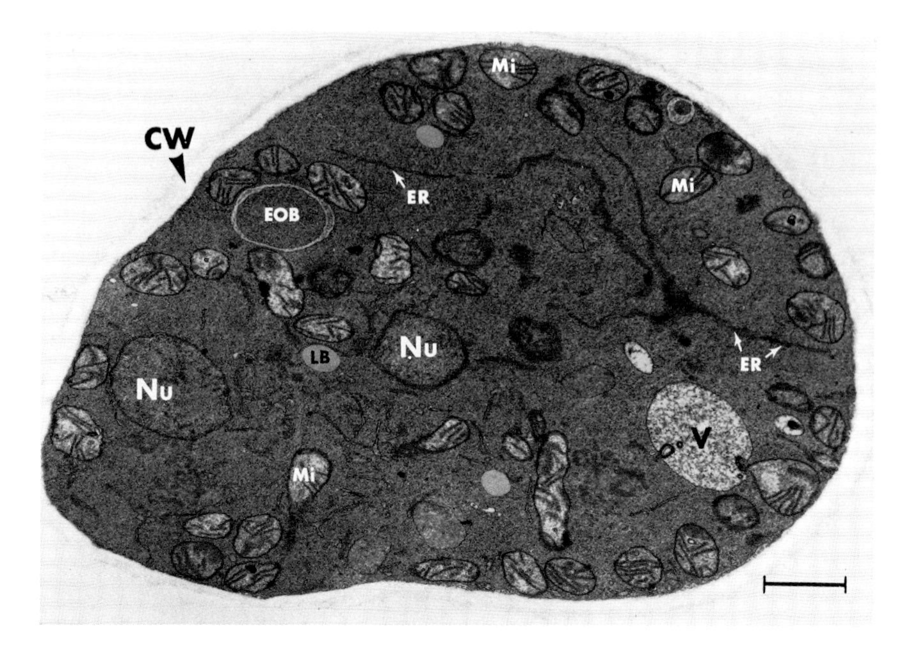

Figure 1. *Blastomyces dermatitidis* yeast cell. Note the poorly contrasted cell wall (CW), electron-opaque body (EOB), lipid body (LB), numerous mitochondria (Mi), profiles of endoplasmic reticulum (ER), multiple nuclei (Nu), and vacuole (V). Glutaraldehyde–osmium tetroxide. Scale bar: 1.0 μm. (Micrograph courtesy of Robert G. Garrison.)

although the last was scarce. In addition, they described extensive lamellated intracytoplasmic membrane systems (ICMS), an observation confirmed later by Garrison *et al.* (1970b). Glycogen granules were often concentrated in the vicinity of the ICMS, but they were not actually in contact with the membranes. The function of the ICMS is unknown, but one theory is that they participate in some unknown manner in cell division, especially as it relates to septum formation. Electron-dense bodies, similar to those described as Woronin bodies in other fungi, were found associated with the septal pores. The cell wall of the mycelial phase was thinner than that of the yeast phase, and the texture appeared to be different (Carbonell, 1969). A thin section showing the ultrastructural detail of the mycelial phase, including the septal area but excluding the nucleus, is shown in Figure 2. Self-parasitism, i.e., hyphae growing within other hyphae or even within yeast, has been described for *B. dermatitidis* as well (Carbonell and Rodriquez, 1968; Lane and Garrison, 1970), but its link to dimorphism, or perhaps survival, is unknown.

Microscopic studies of the transition process, as opposed to studies involving each established phase, have been limited and, in the case of mycelial-to-yeast transition, controversial. Two schools of thought have evolved concerning the process. One hypothesis, supported by the studies of Conant and Howell (1942), Howard and Herndon (1960), and Miyaji and Nishimura (1977), is that the hyphal cells themselves undergo a series of changes and transform into yeast cells. Conant and Howell (1942), observing transition in van Tiegham cell cultures, stated that small fragments of hyphae could be seen concentrating their cytoplasmic contents into one or two cells from which yeast cells that budded were formed. Howard and Herndon (1960), using a tissue-culture system of mouse peritoneal exudate cells, noted that within 24 hr of inoculation, fragments of mycelium could be seen concentrating cytoplasmic organelles and granules into discrete units resembling oidia that seemed to form in alternate hyphal cells. At 48–72 hr after inoculation of the tissue culture, the "oidia" broke apart, releasing single cells that in turn reproduced by budding. Miyaji and Nishimura (1977) described a similar phe-

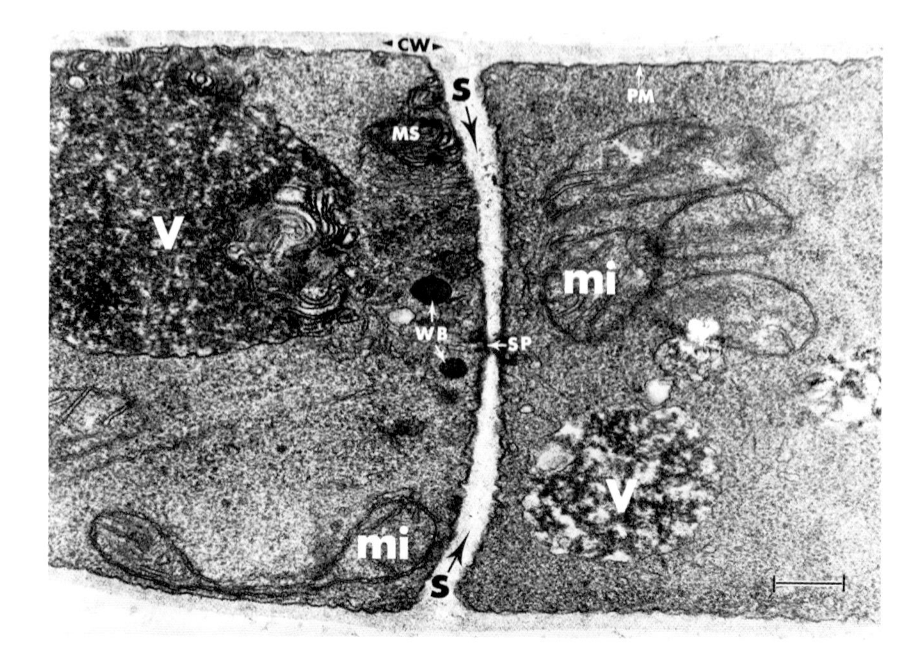

Figure 2. *Blastomyces dermatitidis* hyphal cell. Note the typical ascomycetous septum (S) with septal pore (SP) and associated Woronin bodies (WB), mitochondria (mi), intracytoplasmic membrane system (MS), plasma membrane (PM), vacuoles (V) containing amorphous electron-opaque material, and cell wall (CW). Glutaraldehyde–osmium tetroxide. Scale bar: 0.15 μm. (Micrograph courtesy of Robert G. Garrison.)

nomenon in mycelial fragments incorporated into agar blocks that had been implanted into the peritoneal cavities of mice. They referred to the rounded cells as chlamydospores. The chlamydospores were either terminal or intercalary and became the yeast mother cell.

In contrast to the aforecited observations, Garrison and Boyd (1978) presented evidence that conidia only were capable of becoming yeast mother cells; thus, the second hypothesis was proposed. They incubated *B. dermatitidis* in a shaking apparatus for 14 days at 25°C to obtain suspensions containing both short hyphal elements and conidia. When the suspensions were reincubated at 37°C and observed by EM, the hyphae degenerated within 24 hr, whereas the conidia underwent changes consistent with a mycelial-to-yeast transition. The conidia first germinated, then the germ tubes became yeast mother cells, which presumably then budded. The conidia, in contrast to early observations, were multinucleate, contained the usual other cytoplasmic organelles, and had walls that appeared to have four layers, of which only the innermost became

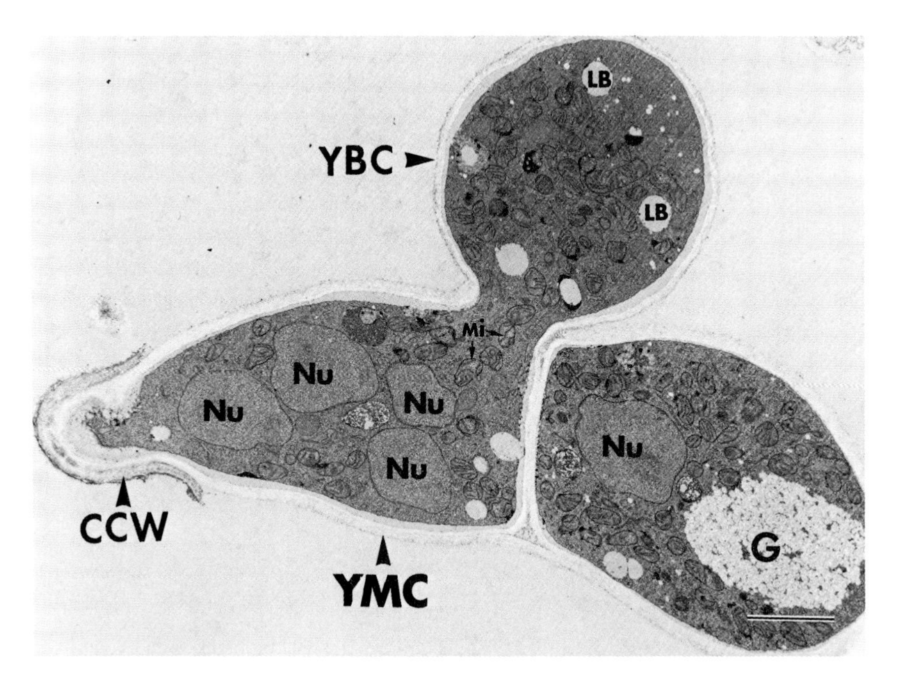

Figure 3. Conidial–yeast mother cell complex showing remnants of the conidial cell wall (CCW), yeast mother cell (YMC), and yeast bud cell (YBC). Note the scattered mitochondria (Mi), glycogenlike deposit (G), lipid bodies (LB), and multiple nuclei (Nu). Glutaraldehyde–osmium tetroxide. Scale bar: 2.0 μm. (From Garrison and Boyd, 1978.)

the wall of the germ tube. Yeast mother cells could be detected within 32 hr and free, budding yeast cells within 48 hr. A photomicrograph showing the conidial–yeast mother cell complex is presented in Figure 3. The remnants of the conidial cell wall as well as the newly formed yeast cell are clearly visible.

It is less likely that controversy will arise regarding the transition of yeast cells to hyphae, since the yeast cell is the only entity capable of undergoing change. Garrison *et al.* (1970b) have studied transition in this direction at the EM level. Within 6–8 hr of transfer from 37 to 25°C, large discrete ICMS associated with the cell membrane could be observed. Within 12–18 hr, there was a significant increase in the number of mitochondria, septa had been formed in enlarged cells giving rise to intermediate or transitional forms, and Woroninlike bodies could be detected on either side of the septa. In addition to the large ICMS, smaller systems scattered throughout the cytoplasm were noted in the intermediate cell. True hyphal cells could be observed between 18 and 24 hr.

4. CELL WALLS

Since the most obvious difference between yeasts and hyphal cells is shape, and since the chemistry and architecture of the cell wall may be a crucial determinant of that shape, considerably more effort has been devoted to cell-wall studies of *B. dermatitidis* than to any other aspect of the fungus. The basic composition of the wall, regardless of form, is glucose, mannose, galactose, *N*-acetylglucosamine, readily extracted and tightly bound lipids, and amino acids (Kanetsuna, 1967; Kanetsuna *et al.*, 1969; Odds *et al.*, 1971; Domer, 1971; Cox and Best, 1972; Roy and Landau, 1972a,b; Massoudnia and Scheer, 1982). The percentages of the various components determined by selected investigators are collated in Table I. None of the studies involved the same strains of *B. dermatitidis*, with the exception of Kanetsuna *et al.* (1969) and Kanetsuna and Carbonell (1971).

From the data presented in Table I, it is obvious that the predominant neutral sugar is glucose and the only amino sugar present is *N*-acetylglucosamine. While it is clear that the yeast form contains more total amino sugar than the mycelial form, differences between the yeast and mycelial forms with respect to total monosaccharide concentration are variable. As will be emphasized later, however, the major difference between the two forms with respect to glucose is the manner in which the monomers are linked to form glucan (Kanetsuna and Carbonell, 1971).

It is also clear from the data in Table I that major differences exist

Table I
Chemical Composition of Cell Walls of Yeast and Mycelial Phases of *B. dermatitidis* (Expressed as Percentages of Unextracted Cell Walls with the Exceptions Noted)

	Yeast						Mycelia				
	Kanetsuna *et al.* (1969)	Roy and Landau (1972a)	Kanetsuna and Carbonell (1971)	Domer (1971)	Domer and Hamilton (1971)	Odds *et al.*, (1971)	Kanetsuna *et al.* (1969)	Roy and Landau (1972a)	Kanetsuna and Carbonell (1971)	Domer (1971)	Domer and Hamilton (1971)
Lipids[a]											
R-E	1	—	—	—	2	—	2	—	—	—	1
PC	—	—	—	—	16[b]	—	—	—	—	—	29[b]
PE	—	—	—	—	11[b]	—	—	—	—	—	13[b]
TG	—	—	—	—	73[b]	—	—	—	—		58[b]
Bound	4	—	—	—	—	—	7	—	—	—	—
Neutral sugars											
Glu	47	58[c]	36a[b]	35	—	—	44	52[c]	51	22	—
(α1-3)	—	—	95[b]	—	—	—	—	—	60[b]	—	—
(β1-3)	—	—	5[b]	—	—	—	—	—	40[b]	—	—
Man	—	—	Trace	1	—	—	—	—	2	4	—
Gal	—	—	Trace	—	—	—	—	—	1	—	—
Amino sugars											
GLcNAc	48	28[c]	37	32	—	33	14	17[c]	23	28	—

Total P	1	—	1	—	—	—	1	—	1	—	—
Total N	5	—	4	—	—	—	5	—	4	—	—
Amino acids[d]											
Total	7	5[c]	8	—	—	—	27	19[c]	11	—	—
Lys	6	3	—	—	—	—	10	6	—	—	—
His	5	2	—	—	—	—	3	2	—	—	—
Arg	1	2	—	—	—	—	5	5	—	—	—
Asp	8	5	—	—	—	—	15	14	—	—	—
Thr	2	2	—	—	—	—	20	6	—	—	—
Ser	3	2	—	—	—	—	15	6	—	—	—
Glu	5	4	—	—	—	—	23	18	—	—	—
Pro	3	3	—	—	—	—	30	12	—	—	—
Gly	5	3	—	—	—	—	53	12	—	—	—
Ala	3	3	—	—	—	—	17	12	—	—	—
Val	2	3	—	—	—	—	12	10	—	—	—
Meth	1	1	—	—	—	—	2	2	—	—	—
Ile	1	2	—	—	—	—	12	8	—	—	—
Leu	1	3	—	—	—	—	14	12	—	—	—
Tyr	—	2	—	—	—	—	—	4	—	—	—
Phe	1	2	—	—	—	—	7	5	—	—	—

[a](R-E) Readily extracted; (PC) phosphatidylcholine; (PE) phosphatidylethanolamine; (TG) triglycerides.
[b]Expressed as relative percentage within a given class of compounds.
[c]Expressed as relative percentage of alkali-resistant fraction, which was 54% of the yeast wall and 70% of the mycelial wall.
[d]All individual amino acids expressed as M/100 mg cell wall.

in the amino acid composition of the two forms, not only in total concentration, but also in the relative percentages of amino acids within the unextracted cell wall (Kanetsuna *et al.,* 1969) or the alkali-resistant component (Roy and Landau, 1972a). Regardless of preparation, mycelial cell walls had more total amino acids than yeast walls. All amino acids, with the exception of histidine, arginine, methionine, and phenylalanine, were elevated in the unextracted mycelial wall (Kanetsuna *et al.,* 1969). Except for threonine and serine, the same amino acids were also present in relatively high concentrations in the alkali-resistant fraction (Roy and Landau, 1972a). Determinations of sulfhydryl content of the alkali-resistant fraction of yeast and hyphal walls (Roy and Landau, 1972a) revealed that the mycelial fraction had higher levels than the yeast fraction. The authors hypothesized, therefore, that an enzyme-catalyzing disulfide reduction was not necessarily active during budding, as had been suggested earlier for *Candida albicans* and *Saccharomyces cerevisiae* (Nickerson and Falcone, 1956). Roy and Landau (1972a) assumed that the amino acids in the wall were present as proteins, and therefore investigated protein profiles by sodium dodecyl sulfate–polyacrylamide gel electrophoresis (SDS-PAGE) of the alkali-soluble wall fractions. Yeast and mycelial extracts were again quite different. The yeast extract had four demonstrable proteins, whereas the mycelial form had only one. The one protein in the mycelial extract migrated parallel to one of the proteins in the yeast extract, but nothing was done to ascertain that the proteins were the same.

The arrangement of the monomeric units into polymers in the wall has been defined by alkali solubility, infrared spectra, optical rotations, and enzymatic analyses. *N*-Acetylglucosamine is present as the polymer chitin (Blank, 1954; Kanetsuna *et al.,* 1969; Domer, 1971; Odds *et al.,* 1971; Davis et al., 1977), and glucose is present as either α- or β-glucan (Kanetsuna and Carbonell, 1971; Domer, 1971; Davis *et al.,* 1977). The glucan linkages, in fact, provide one of the striking differences between the yeast and mycelial walls. Ninety-five percent of glucan of the yeast wall is α1-3 linked, whereas only 60% of the mycelial wall has that specific linkage (Kanetsuna and Carbonell, 1971; Davis *et al.,* 1977). The remaining glucan linkages are β1-3. The premise that more β1-3-glucan is present in the mycelial wall than in the yeast wall is supported by the studies of Domer (1971) as well, in that a chitinase-β-glucanase preparation released both glucose and *N*-acetylglucosamine from the mycelial wall of *B. dermatitidis,* but only *N*-acetylglucosamine from the yeast wall. Mannose and galactose are also present in the wall in small quantities, regardless of phase, but both are in somewhat higher concentration in the mycelial phase. It is difficult to determine how the galactomannan might be arranged in the wall, but Azuma *et al.* (1974) have extracted a galactomannan from mycelial cells of *B. dermatitidis* that was equivalent to 0.5–1% of the dry weight of the cell. A similar extraction of yeast cells did not yield a galactomannan.

In addition to analyzing for the basic wall constituents and attempting to determine their linkages into polymers, information can be acquired by investigating the effects of solubilizing agents, in particular alkaline agents, on the intact wall. Sodium or potassium hydroxide and ethylenediamine have been used as such agents. Regardless of the agent, in two of three studies, more of the mycelial wall than of the yeast wall was resistant to alkaline extraction (Roy and Landau, 1972b; Domer, 1971; Kanetsuna and Carbonell, 1971). Moreover, the alkali-resistant portion of the wall retained all the chitin (Domer, 1971; Kanetsuna and Carbonell, 1971; Kanetsuna, 1981) and some of the protein (Kanetsuna and Carbonell, 1971). The alkali-soluble material could be fractionated further into ammonium-sulfate-precipitable and -soluble components. Practically all the alkali-soluble material of the mycelial phase was precipitable with ammonium sulfate. Further, SDS-PAGE indicated that this material contained only a single protein as stated above (Roy and Landau, 1972a). In contrast, the alkali-soluble preparation of the yeast form separated equally into ammonium-sulfate-percipitable and -soluble fractions, each of which had two proteins demonstrable by electrophoresis.

Other attempts have been made to correlate morphology, as determined by EM, with chemical composition. For example, Odds *et al.* (1971) looked at the effect of a chitinase–glucanase complex on the cell wall of the yeast form of *Histoplasma capsulatum* and *B. dermatitidis.* The isolated cell wall of *B. dermatitidis* was much more extensively degraded than that of *H. capsulatum,* whereas the reverse was true if whole cells were treated with the enzyme. The authors used this information to suggest that the outer layer of the yeast wall of *B. dermatitidis* is α-glucan and therefore, in the intact cell, protects the chitin from attack by chitinase in the absence of α-glucanase. Only after the chitin layer is exposed by disruption of the cell is it susceptible to attack by chitinase. On the other hand, the *H. capsulatum* wall, which does not contain α-glucan but does contain β-glucan and chitin, would be equally susceptible in the intact cell or in the isolated state because the enzyme preparation contains both β-glucanase and chitinase. More recently, Kanetsuna (1981) published an ultrastructural study of the cell walls of *Paracoccidioides brasiliensis, B. dermatitidis,* and *H. capsulatum* chemotype II in which whole cells or isolated cell walls were treated with sodium hydroxide, β1-3-glucanase, and pronase. Microfibrils remaining after all these treatments were presumed to be chitin, since chemical analyses of the residue revealed predominantly amino sugar. In the yeast form, microfibrils were tightly interwoven and randomly oriented, whereas in the mycelial form, there were large fragments that contained the microfibrils lying in a longitudinal orientation. Interestingly, the residue of the yeast-form wall retained its shape, but the mycelial wall was obviously extensively degraded.

There have been essentially no studies investigating cell-wall synthetic activities in *B. dermatitidis*. In a study published by Davis *et al.* (1977), however, both yeast and mycelial forms of *B. dermatitidis* were found to be producing high levels of β1-3-glucanase constituitively in addition to several glycosidases. This finding was surprising in that the yeast wall contains only small quantities of β-glucan. Perhaps the yeast wall contains such small quantities of β-glucan because the enzyme is present and more active at 37°C than at lower temperatures.

Although it has not been stressed above, a comparison of the data available on the cell wall of *B. dermatitidis* with that of *P. brasiliensis* reveals that the two walls are quite similar and that the walls of *H. capsulatum* chemotype II share some of the similarities as well. On the basis of these similarities, Carbonell (1969) proposed a model for the conversion of the yeast to the mycelial form. This model with more recent modifications is discussed in Chapter 5 in conjunction with *P. brasiliensis.*

5. METABOLIC CONSIDERATIONS

The search for metabolic parameters associated with or responsible for the visual changes observed in dimorphism began relatively early—e.g., Nickerson and Edwards (1949) published their study, which included oxygen consumption, in 1949—but the data obtained in subsequent studies have not strengthened the hypothesis summarized below and first proposed by Nickerson (1948). In fact, the accumulated literature represents a series of studies that provide anecdotal information that to date does not fit together coherently.

The original hypothesis of Nickerson (1948) was that yeast–mycelial dimorphism could be considered an uncoupling of cell division from growth and that the maintenance of the yeast form was dependent on the maintenance of -SH groups on the surface of the yeast cell. Although this hypothesis may have some validity for *C. albicans* (see Chapter 7) or *H. capsulatum* (see Chapter 4), it does not appear to be important in the dimorphism of *B. dermatitidis*. Garrison *et al.* (1970a), for example, compared the uptake of low-molecular-weight sulfur-containing compounds, including L-cystine, in *H. capsulatum, Sporothrix schenckii,* and *B. dermatitidis.* They noted that the uptake of L-cystine by the latter two fungi, in either phase, was considerably less than that of the yeast form of *H. capsulatum* and that unlike the suppressive effects by L-cystine observed on the mycelial form of *H. capsulatum,* the respiratory activities of *B. dermatitidis* and *S. schenckii* were affected. Somewhat later, however, Bawdon and Garrison (1974), examining the uptake of L-cystine and L-leucine by yeast and mycelial forms, did find that the uptake was somewhat greater in the mycelial form, as is the case with *H. capsulatum.* At low concentrations, these two amino acids entered both types of cells by a permease-type system. At high concentrations, simple diffusion appeared to be a factor as well. There was a requirement for energy because the uptake and incorporation of both amino acids was prevented by 2,4-dinitrophenyl or sodium azide.

Since Nickerson (1948) had stated that RNA content of *B. dermatitidis* was much lower in the mycelial than in yeast forms, Taylor (1961) analyzed both RNA and DNA as well as nitrogen content in both forms over a period of 35 days. The RNA content of the yeast phase increased approximately 2-fold between 6 and 10 days of incubation, but immediately thereafter dropped to pre-6-day levels and remained there for the duration of the experiment. Although a growth curve was not presented, it would be logical to consider that the abrupt increase represented synthetic activities occurring during the logarithmic growth of the organism. The RNA content of the mycelia was considerably less than that of the yeasts at any observation point, and there was little variation in the amount present from point to point. The uniformity of RNA content of the mycelial phase may simply reflect a slow and more uniform metabolic rate as might be expected with apical extension rather than budding. The DNA content was the same in both cultures and the level uniform throughout the observation period. Nitrogen levels were initially high in the yeast phase, but dropped with age, whereas those of the mycelial phase were consistently low.

In addition to the studies discussed above, there are several unrelated studies that contain data documenting differences between yeast and mycelial forms of *B. dermatitidis.* First, Roy and Landau (1971) compared the isoenzyme patterns of malate dehydrogenase of cytoplasmic or mitochondrial origin from both yeasts and mycelia and found that the yeasts had six different bands of activity demonstrable in the gels, four in the cytoplasm, and two in the mitochondria, while the mycelia had only two bands in the cytoplasm and two in the mitochondria. None of the mycelial bands appeared to correspond to the yeast bands, but the cytoplasmic and mitochondrial enzymes of the mycelial phase migrated similar distances. In a second study, Domer and Hamilton (1971) analyzed yeast and mycelial forms for lipid content extracted with chloroform–methanol. Extracts of the cytoplasm or cell sap were compared with cell-wall extracts. Two strains of *B. dermatitidis* were examined, and in general, the mycelial-phase cell saps contained about one half the amount of lipid of their respective yeast cell saps. The cell sap of one of the yeast forms contained approximately 12% readily extracted lipid, but the other contained only about 5%. All extracts contained phosphatidylethanolamine, phosphatidylcholine, phosphatidylserine, triglycerides, diglycerides, sterols, sterol esters, and free fatty acids. The mycelial phase, cell sap or cell walls, contained slightly less triglyceride and relatively more phospholipid than the yeast-phase extracts. The major fatty acids, as determined either in the total extract or in the individual phospholipids or neutral lipids, were oleic (18:1) and linoleic (18:2) acids. Together, they accounted for 75–80% of the total fatty acids. In general, mycelial-phase extracts, whether cell sap or cell wall, had slightly less oleic and more linoleic acid than the corresponding yeast-phase preparations. Finally, cell walls had less linoleic acid than cell sap, although the levels of oleic acid in each were similar.

In the final studies, Massoudnia and Scheer (1982) and Zahraee *et al.* (1982) determined the influence of growth medium on ultrastructure and chemical composition, respectively, of both phases of *B. dermatitidis.* Ultrastructure varied considerably from medium to medium, presumably because some of the media were not ideal for optimal growth of the organism. Since most of the media were complex, however, attempts to correlate ultrastructural changes with specific media ingredients were not possible. Chemical analyses of the whole cells for total carbohydrate, total protein, and total readily extractable or bound lipid revealed only minor differences that seemed unrelated to medium or phase. In contrast, when the bound lipids (i.e., those lipids extracted with 10% KOH in 95% methanol after a preliminary extraction with chloroform–methanol) from whole cells were examined for specific fatty acids, differences were noted between yeast and mycelial cells that had been incubated in brain–heart infusion broth or in the medium of Levine and Ordal (1946) modified by the addition of peptone. There were no significant differences in the fatty acid composition of the bound lipids of cell walls, regardless of phase or medium. There was one major difference between whole-cell and cell-wall extracts; viz., cell-wall extracts contained significant amounts of saturated long-chain fatty acids, C20:0, C22:0, and C24:0, whereas the longest-chain fatty acid detected in whole-cell extracts was C18:2. The authors provided no explanation for this discrepancy. Comparison of the data just presented with the lipid studies of Domer and

Hamilton (1971) described above is difficult because the latter investigators looked only at the fatty acids in the chloroform–methanol extract. It is interesting to note, however, that Domer and Hamilton found no C20:0 or larger fatty acids in any of their extracts from *B. dermatitidis.*

6. SUMMARY

Clearly, temperature appears to be the most important determinant of form in *B. dermatitidis,* and the most striking differences between the two forms have been demonstrated at the level of the cell wall and the ICMS observed by EM. Many questions remain unanswered, however. Can both hyphal cells and conidia transform into yeast mother cells as the intermediate step between mycelia and yeasts? How important are the striking differences noted in the cell-wall composition and architecture of the yeast vs. mycelial forms? Are the cell-wall differences simply the result of temperature-induced activation or suppression of cell-wall degradative and synthetic enzymes, or is there a much more fundamental metabolic change responsible for the initiation of morphogenesis? What role do the ICMS play in the transition of the yeast to the mycelial form? Answers to these and other questions will come primarily from detailed studies of metabolic pathways and cell-wall synthetic mechanisms, as well as from expanded light- and electron-microscopic studies of purified conidia and hyphal cells.

REFERENCES

Area Leao, A. E. de, and Cury, A., 1950, Deficiencias vitaminicas de cogumelos pathogenicos, *Mycopathol. Mycol. Appl.* **5:**65–90.

Azuma, I., Kanetsuna, F., Tanaka, Y., Yamamura, Y., and Carbonell, L. M., 1974, Chemical and immunological properties of galactomannans obtained from *Histoplasma duboisii, Histoplasma capsulatum, Paracoccidioides brasiliensis* and *Blastomyces dermatitidis, Mycopathol. Mycol. Appl.* **54:**111–125.

Bakerspigel, A., 1957, The structure and mode of division of the nuclei in the yeast cells and mycelium of *Blastomyces dermatitidis, Can. J. Microbiol.* **3:**923–936.

Bawdon, R. E., and Garrison, R. G., 1974, The uptake and incorporation of leucine and cystine by the mycelial and yeastlike phases of *Blastomyces dermatitidis, Mycopathol. Mycol. Appl.* **54:**421–433.

Blank, F., 1954, On the cell walls of dimorphic fungi causing systemic infections, *Can. J. Microbiol.* **1:**1–5.

Carbonell, L. M., 1969, Ultrastructure of dimorphic transformation in *Paracoccidioides brasiliensis, J. Bacteriol.* **100:**1076–1082.

Carbonell, L. M., and Rodriguez, J., 1968, Mycelial phase of *Paracoccidioides brasiliensis* and Blastomyces dermatitidis: An electron microscope study, *J. Bacteriol.* **96:**533–543.

Ciferri, R., and Redaelli, P., 1935, Prima contribuzione allo studio delle cosidette blastomicosi americane, *Atti Ist. Bot. Univ. Pavia* **6**:55–105.

Conant, N. F., and Howell, A., 1942, The similarity of the fungi causing South American blastomycosis (paracoccidioidal granuloma) and North American blastomycosis (Gilchrist's disease), *J. Invest. Dermatol.* **5**:353–370.

Cox, R. A., and Best, G. K., 1972, Cell wall composition of two strains of *Blastomyces dermatitidis* exhibiting differences in virulence for mice, *Infect. Immun.* **5**:449–453.

Davis, T. E., Jr., Domer, J. E., and Li, Y.-T., 1977, Cell wall studies of *Histoplasma capsulatum* and *Blastomyces dermatitidis, Infect. Immun.* **15**:978–987.

DeLamater, E. D., 1948, The nuclear cytology of *Blastomyces dermatitidis, Mycologia* **40**:430–444.

DeLamater, E. D., 1949, Rough–smooth variation in *Blastomyces dermatitidis* Gilchrist and Stokes 1898, *J. Invest. Dermatol.* **12**:101–110.

DeMonbreun, W. A., 1935, Experimental chronic cutaneous blastomycosis in monkeys, *Arch. Dermatol. Syphilol.* **31**:831–854.

Domer, J. E., 1971, Monosaccharide and chitin content of cell walls of *Histoplasma capsulatum* and *Blastomyces dermatitidis, J. Bacteriol.* **107**:870–877.

Domer, J. E., and Hamilton, J. G., 1971, The readily extracted lipids of *Histoplasma capsulatum* and *Blastomyces dermatitidis, Biochim. Biophys. Acta* **231**:465–478.

Edwards, G. A., and Edwards, M. R., 1960, The intracellular membranes of *Blastomyces dermatitidis, Am. J. Bot.* **47**:622–632.

Garrison, R. G., and Boyd, K. S., 1978, Role of the conidium in dimorphism of *Blastomyces dermatitidis, Mycopathologia* **64**:29–33.

Garrison, R. G., Dodd, H. T., and Hamilton, J. W., 1970a, The uptake of low molecular weight sulfur-containing compounds by *Histoplasma capsulatum* and related dimorphic fungi, *Mycopathol. Mycol. Appl.* **40**:171–180.

Garrison, R. G., Lane, J. W., and Field, M. F., 1970b, Ultrastructural changes during the yeastlike to mycelial-phase conversion of *Blastomyces dermatitidis* and *Histoplasma capsulatum, J. Bacteriol.* **101**:628–635.

Gilardi, G. L., 1965, Nutrition of systemic and subcutaneous pathogenic fungi, *Bacteriol. Rev.* **29**:406–424.

Gilardi, G. L., and Laffer, N. C., 1962, Nutritional studies on the yeast phase of *Blastomyces dermatitidis* and *B. brasiliensis, J. Bacteriol.* **83**:219–227.

Gilchrist, T. C., 1896, A case of blastomycetic dermatitis in man, *Johns Hopkins Hosp. Rep.* **1**:269–290.

Gilchrist, T. C., and Stokes, W. R., 1898, A case of pseudolupus vulgaris caused by a *Blastomyces, J. Exp. Med.* **3**:53–78.

Halliday, W. J., and McCoy, E., 1955, Biotin as a growth requirement for *Blastomyces dermatitidis, J. Bacteriol.* **70**:464–468.

Hamburger, W. W., 1907, A comparative study of four strains of organisms isolated from four cases of generalized blastomycosis, *J. Infect. Dis.* **4**:201–209.

Howard, D. H., and Herndon, R. L., 1960, Tissue cultures of mouse peritoneal exudates inoculated with *Blastomyces dermatitidis, J. Bacteriol.* **80**:522–527.

Kanetsuna, F., 1967, Estudio bioquimico del *Paracoccidioides brasiliensis, Acta Cient. Venezolana* **3**:308–317.

Kanetsuna, F., 1981, Ultrastructural studies on the dimorphism of *Paracoccidioides brasiliensis, Blastomyces dermatitidis* and *Histoplasma capsulatum, Sabouraudia* **19**:275–286.

Kanetsuna, F., and Carbonell, L. M., 1971, Cell wall composition of the yeastlike and mycelial forms of *Blastomyces dermatitidis, J. Bacteriol.* **106**:946–948.

Kanetsuna, F., Carbonell, L. M., Moreno, R. E., and Rodrigeuz, J., 1969, Cell wall composition of the yeast and mycelial forms of *Paracoccidioides brasiliensis, J. Bacteriol.* **97:**1036–1041.

Lane, J. W., and Garrison, R. G., 1970, Electronmicroscropy of self-parasitism by *Histoplasma capsulatum* and *Blastomyces dermatitidis, Mycopathol. Mycol. Appl.* **40:**271–276.

Levine, S., and Ordal, Z. J., 1946, Factors influencing the morphology of *Blastomyces dermatitidis, J. Bacteriol.* **52:**687–694.

Massoudnia, A., and Scheer, E. R., 1982, The influence of medium on the chemical composition of *Blastomyces dermatitidis, Curr. Microbiol.* **7:**25–28.

Michelson, I. D., 1928, Blastomycosis: A pathologic and bacteriologic study, *J. Am. Med. Assoc.* **91:**1871–1876.

Miyaji, M., and Nishimura, K., 1977, Investigation of dimorphism of *Blastomyces dermatitidis* by agar-implantation, *Mycopathologia* **60:**73–78.

Nickerson, W. J., 1948, Enzymatic control of cell division in microorganisms, *Nature (London)* **162:**241–245.

Nickerson, W. J., and Edwards, G. A., 1949, Studies on the physiological bases of morphogenesis in fungi. I. The respiratory metabolism of dimorphic pathogenic fungi, *J. Gen. Physiol.* **33:**41–55.

Nickerson, W. J., and Falcone, G., 1956, Identification of protein disulfide reductase as a cellular division enzyme in yeasts, *Science* **124:**722–723.

Odds, F. C., Kaufman, L., McLaughlin, D., Callaway, C., and Blumer, S. O., 1971, Effect of chitinase complex on the antigenicity and chemistry of yeast-form cell walls and other fractions of *Histoplasma capsulatum and Blastomyces dermatitidis, Sabouraudia* **12:**138–149.

Ricketts, H. T., 1901, Oidiomycosis of skin and its fungi, *J. Med. Res.* **6:**373–546.

Roy, I., and Landau, J. W., 1971, Polymorphism of malate dehydrogenase in cytoplasmic and mitochondrial fractions of *Blastomyces dermatitidis, Sabouraudia* **9:**39–42.

Roy, I., and Landau, J. W., 1972a, Protein constituents of cell walls of the dimorphic phases of *Blastomyces dermatitidis, Can. J. Microbiol.* **18:**473–478.

Roy, I., and Landau, J. W., 1972b, Composition of the alkali resistant cell wall material of dimorphic *Blastomyces dermatitidis, Sabouraudia* **10:**107–112.

Salvin, S. B., 1949, Phase-determining factors in *Blastomyces dermatitidis, Mycologia* **41:**311–319.

Stewart, R. A., and Meyer, K. F., 1938, Studies in the metabolism of *Coccidioides immitis* (Stiles), *J. Infect. Dis.* **63:**196–205.

Stober, A. M., 1914, Systemic blastomycosis: A report of its pathological, bacteriological and clinical features, *Arch. Intern. Med.* **13:**509–556.

Taylor, J. J., 1961, Nucleic acids and dimorphism in *Blastomyces, Exp. Cell Res.* **24:**155–158.

Zahraee, M. H., Wilson, T. E., and Scheer, E. R., 1982, The effect of growth media upon the ultrastructure of *Blastomyces dermatitidis, Can. J. Microbiol.* **28:**211–218.

Chapter 4

Studies on Phase Transitions in the Dimorphic Pathogen *Histoplasma capsulatum*

G. S. Kobayashi, G. Medoff, B. Maresca, M. Sacco, and B. V. Kumar

1. INTRODUCTION

Histoplasma capsulatum, the etiological agent of histoplasmosis, is a dimorphic pathogenic fungus. The disease histoplasmosis occurs in many different parts of the world, but has a particularly high prevalence in temperate and subtropical zones such as the Ohio and Mississippi river valleys of the United States, South and Central America, parts of the Mediterranean basin, and West Africa (P. Q. Edwards and Billings, 1971). The epidemiology of *H. capsulatum* and problems related to human infection have been extensively studied (Sweany, 1960; Ajello *et al.*, 1971; Schwarz, 1981). The nature of dimorphism in *H. capsulatum* has also received a great deal of interest ever since the fungus was observed in tissue and

G. S. Kobayashi • Divisions of Infectious Diseases, Dermatology, and Laboratory Medicine, Washington University School of Medicine, St. Louis, Missouri 63110. **G. Medoff and B. V. Kumar** • Division of Infectious Diseases, Washington University School of Medicine, St. Louis, Missouri 63110. **B. Maresca and M. Sacco** • International Institute of Genetics and Biophysics, CNR, 10 Naples, Italy.

cultured *in vitro* and discovered to have a saprophytic hyphal phase and a parasitic yeast phase (DeMonbreun, 1934).

This chapter will not be a comprehensive review of studies on *H. capsulatum*. There have been several excellent reviews of the growth requirements of this organism (Gilardi, 1965), antigenic studies and chemistry of the cell wall (Pine, 1977), physiological studies (Boguslawski and Stetler, 1979), and the epidemiology and clinical syndromes of histoplasmosis (Goodwin *et al.*, 1981; Wheat *et al.*, 1982). We will limit our discussion to those studies concerned with the phase transitions of *H. capsulatum* and cover only those aspects of the physiology, molecular biology, and morphology that appear to be involved in these processes.

Mycelia are found in soil and never in infected tissue; in contrast, the yeast phase is the only form present in tissue. This implies that each growth phase is an adaptation to two critically different environments. Which phase grows may conceivably be simply determined, for example, by the temperature difference between soil and body, or may involve a more complicated set of environmental factors, such as pH, nutrients available, oxidation–reduction potential, serum factors, or cell interactions. An important notion related to the specificity of each of the two phases for markedly different environments is that the growth and multiplication of the yeast or tissue-specific phase may be involved in virulence. In other words, a reversible differentiation occurs between two markedly different vegetative phases of the organism, and one of the phase transitions may promote pathogenicity. The relative ease with which the phase transitions can be reversibly accomplished in culture implies that the regulatory mechanisms of morphogenesis can be studied.

A sexual phase of *H. capsulatum* has been described by Kwon-Chung (1972) and named *Emmonsiella capsulata*. *Emmonsiella capsulata* is heterothallic, and when suitable mating pairs, (+) and (−), are seeded onto sporulation media (Kwon-Chung, 1973), cleistothecia, morphologically consistent with those of fungi in the family Gymnoascaceae of the Ascomycetes, are produced. In a survey of mating types, Kwon-Chung *et al.* (1974) found an equal distribution of (+) and (−) types in 939 soil isolates, but in 184 isolates from clinical material tested, the frequency of (−) mating types was 7 times higher than that of (+). More important, the discovery of a sexual phase and two mating types provided an opportunity to analyze the genetics of an important systemic fungal pathogen; unfortunately, the system is very difficult to control, and little progress has been made.

2. EXPERIMENTAL STUDIES ON DIMORPHISM

2.1. Morphological Studies

The mycelial phase of *H. capsulatum* consists of thin-walled septate hyphal elements. The ultrastructure of freeze-substituted hyphal tip cells of *H. capsulatum* (Figure 1) is similar to that reported for *Giberella acuminata* (Howard and Aist, 1979; Howard, 1981) and *Laetisaria arvalis* (Hoch and Howard, 1980). Hyphal elements of *H. capsulatum* are narrow

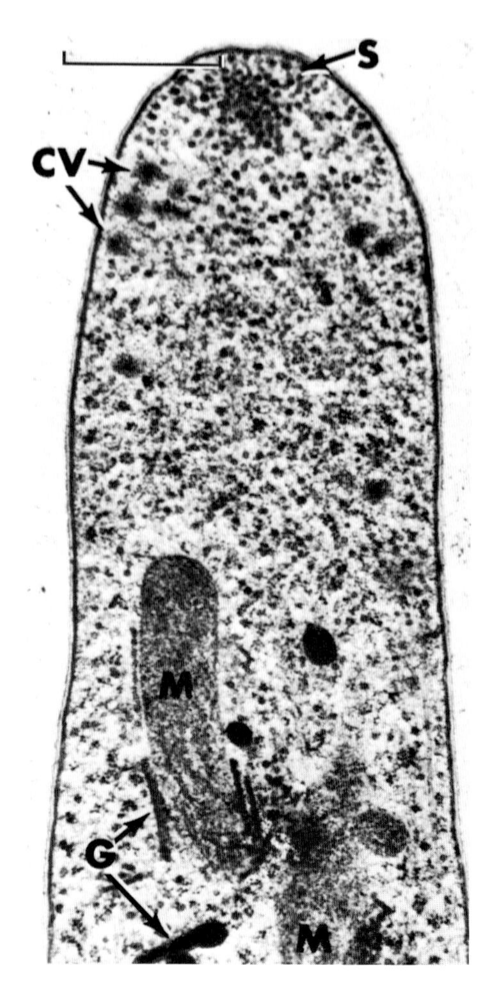

Figure 1. Apical portion of freeze-substituted mycelial tip cell showing Spitzenkorper (S), mitochondria (M), coated vesicles (CV), and Golgi-equivalents (G). Scale bar: 1.0 μm. (Courtesy of K. L. O'Donnell.)

(1.25–2.0 μm in diameter) and possess a bilaminate wall that is approximately 20 nm thick. Tip cells are either uni- or binucleate. Nuclei typically undergo synchronous mitotic division in binucleate cells. A Spitzenkorper at the cell apex is unique in being composed primarily of microvesicles (28–42 nm in diameter). Coated vesicles [filasomes *sensu* Howard (1981)] that measure 110–150 nm in diameter are numerous in the region subtending the Spitzenkorper and along the lateral cell wall, and these appear to fuse with the plasmalemma. Multivesicular bodies also aggregate in the subapical region. Mitochondria, rough endoplasmic reticulum, and microtubules are generally oriented with their long axis parallel to the lateral cell wall. Golgilike endomembrane cisternae are conspicuous and are composed of either an electron-dense, tubular cisterna or a completely fenestrated sheet that is typically wrapped around a mitochondrion. Septa are ascomycetous in possessing a narrow central pore (100 nm in diameter) that may become occluded with a Woronin body (Figure 2).

On gross examination, mycelial-phase cultures of *H. capsulatum* exhibit a wide range of morphological variation, particularly on primary isolation. Berliner (1968) characterized four distinct groups after examining 36 recent isolates from sources that included humans, bats, guinea pig, soil, and water. The predominant colonial morphologies were albino (A) or brown (B) forms, both of which were phentotypically stable and could be maintained *in vitro* on Sabouraud's medium. The type B isolates exhibited a flat, sparse growth, and the colonies developed a tan to brown diffusible pigment within a week. Microscopically, hyphae were narrow and pigmented. Abundant tuberculate macroconidia and relatively few microconidia were present. Type A colonies grew rapidly and produced

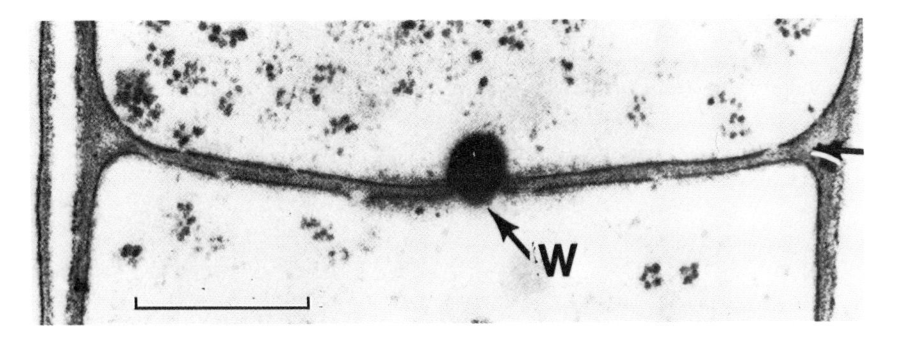

Figure 2. Simple septum (unlabeled arrow) with central pore occluded by Woronin body (W). Scale bar: 0.5 μm. (Courtesy of K. L. O'Donnell.)

little or no pigment even after 1 month in culture. Microscopically, the aerial hyphae were coarse and broad. Smooth-walled macroconidia or smooth-walled or spiny microconidia, or both, were present in abundance. The A type colonies gradually became non-spore-bearing on repeated passage in culture. If care was not taken to separate these two colonial morphologies, the A type eventually predominated because of its rapidly growing characteristic. For this reason, many isolates of *H. capsulatum* in laboratory stock culture collections are A-type organisms.

The yeast phase consists of round to oval budding yeast cells having an average diameter of 2–4 μm (Garrison and Boyd, 1978; M. R. Edwards *et al.*, 1959). The laminated yeast cell wall has an average thickness of 90 nm and encloses a cytosolic matrix containing a membrane-bound nucleus, well-defined endoplasmic reticulum, and mitochondria. The ultrastructure of conventionally fixed yeast cells of *H. capsulatum* (Figure 3) is generally similar to that of *Saccharomyces cerevisiae,* but does not display a conspicuous vacuole (Byers and Goetsch, 1974, 1975). Yeast cells of *H. capsulatum* are small ($\approx 2.5 \times 4$ μm) and possess a two-layered cell wall (100 nm thick). Cells are typically uninucleate and contain the same complement of organelles as in the mycelium, with the exception that Golgilike cisternae have never been demonstrated in conventionally fixed yeasts. Electron-dense polyphosphate granules are conspicuous in cells grown in GYE medium. The ultrastructure of mitosis is ascomycetous in that the intranuclear spindle is set up in the parent cell (Byers and Goetsch, 1974, 1975; Morris, 1980). Subsequent spindle elongation at anaphase–telophase is across the parent–sibling cell isthmus. Karyokinesis and cytokinesis are closely coordinated temporally and spatially. Following nuclear division, a nonperforate, bilaminate septum develops at the isthmus separating the parent and sibling cells. Subsequent abscission is through the septum.

Studies on the yeast phase of type A and B colonies showed no morphological differences at 37°C, but when these yeasts were converted back to the mycelial phase at 25°C, they maintained their phenotypic identities. In further comparative studies on the yeast phase of A and B isolates, Reca and Campbell (1967) found their growth rates to be identical, as was their ability to reduce tetrazolium (Reca, 1968). Daniels *et al.* (1968) showed that the yeast phase of B forms was more pathogenic for rabbits than was that of A forms. In similar kinds of studies, Tewari and Berkhout (1972) showed that the B forms were more virulent for mice than the A form. The reason for the difference between the A and B forms of *H. capsulatum* is unknown, as are the reasons for the gradual conversion of B colonies to A colonies.

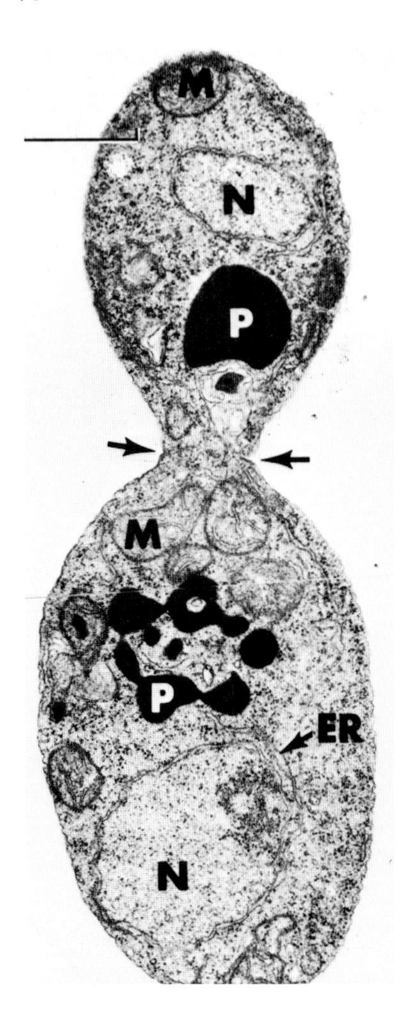

Figure 3. Yeastlike cell with uninucleate (N) parent and bud. Mitochondria (M), endoplasmic reticulum (ER), and polyphosphate granules (P) are conspicuous. Unmarked arrows indicate septal initials. Glutaraldehyde–osmium fixation. Scale bar: 1.0 μm. (Courtesy of K. L. O'Donnell.)

On the basis of some elegant time-lapse photomicrographic studies on the morphological transition, Pine and Webster (1962) were able to describe three mechanisms by which hyphal cells of *H. capsulatum* could convert to the yeast phase. These events involved (1) enlargement of contiguous hyphal cells to form chains of monilial or yeastlike cells, (2) spontaneous budding of an unswollen hyphal cell to form a yeast, and (3) development of yeast cells from a stalk directly connected to an unswollen hyphal cell. In related studies concerning attempts to block the mycelial-to-yeast transition with actinomycin D, Cheung *et al.* (1975) observed similar mechanisms of yeast development. Pine and Webster (1962) also described the direct conversion of microconidia to yeast cells by polar and nonpolar budding. While other workers (Garrison and Boyd, 1978) have described the morphological changes that occur during the mycelium-to-yeast transition, this work has been difficult to interpret because the observations have been made on fixed specimens sampled from unsynchronized cultures.

Preliminary ultrastructural studies of the hyphal-to-yeast transition suggest that enlarged parent yeast cells can be derived from either terminal or intercalary hyphal cells (O'Donnell, unpublished observations). At present, detailed studies on the ultrastructural changes that occur during the hyphal-to-yeast transition are lacking, and whereas Szaniszlo *et al.* (1983) have suggested that most details are probably similar to those associated with microconidial germination at 37°C (Garrison and Boyd, 1978), a direct comparison has not yet been made.

2.2. Growth Requirements of the Two Phases: Cysteine Metabolism

Most of the early studies to determine the growth requirements of the mycelial and yeast phases were reviewed by Gilardi (1965). It is evident that the mycelial-phase growth requirements are relatively uncomplicated compared to those of the yeast. Mycelia can be grown by incubating the cultures at 25°C with glucose as the sole carbon source and ammonia as the inorganic source of nitrogen. The yeast phase, on the other hand, appears to be more fastidious and requires cysteine and certain growth factors such as biotin, thiamine, or thioctic acid.

Salvin (1947) was probably the first to document specific nutritional differences between yeast and mycelia when he showed that the yeast phase of certain strains had a specific requirement for biotin, whereas this requirement was not present in the mycelial phase. The biotin requirement was expressed in the yeast phase only when cysteine was the sole nitrogen source. More important than the finding of a need for biotin was Salvin's discovery (Salvin, 1949) that the addition of cysteine or cystine to a glucose salts medium was necessary to maintain the yeast phase.

Scherr (1957), and later Pine and Peacock (1958), showed that in addition to a temperature of 37°C, sulfhydryl-containing compounds must be present in the medium for the initiation of yeast development. Once formed, the yeast phase could be maintained at temperatures lower than 37°C provided high concentrations of cysteine were maintained in the medium. Scherr (1957) speculated that at least two factors governed the mycelia-to-yeast transition. The first dealt with a nutritional requirement for sulfhydryl-containing compounds because *H. capsulatum* lacked the ability to reduce sulfur-containing compounds at 37°C. The second raised the possibility that sulfhydryl compounds regulated the oxidation–reduction potential of the growth environment necessary for yeast development. Experiments in support of the latter point were provided by Rippon (1968), who was able to show conversion of mycelia to yeast when he electrolytically lowered the oxidation–reduction potential of the medium. This work is difficult to interpret because the medium was complex (i.e., brain–heart infusion broth). However, McVeigh and Houston (1972) showed later that in a defined medium, mycelia exposed to a low oxidation–reduction potential at 37°C for 18–24 hr will transform to the yeast phase. They further pointed out that while the transition was induced at reduced oxygen levels in the absence of sulfur-containing compounds, both were needed for the maintenance of the yeast morphology. McVeigh and Houston (1972) showed that under most conditions of culture of yeasts at 37°C, the requirement for cysteine was specific. This conclusion was supported by the finding that cysteine could not be replaced in the medium by glutathione. Others have concluded that cysteine stimulates the growth of the yeast phase by providing sulfhydryl groups to the medium (Salvin, 1949; Scherr, 1957; McVeigh and Houston, 1972).

Therefore, it is clear from the literature on this subject that cysteine is required for growth of the yeast phase. In fact, Stetler and Boguslawski (1979) analyzed the growth requirements of several strains of *H. capsulatum* and were able to conclude that the cysteine requirement of yeast was due to the absence of an active form of sulfite reductase, normally needed for cysteine biosynthesis. The role of cysteine, however, is much less clear. As we have described, the conclusions in the literature are not consistent, and it is unknown whether cysteine satisfies a nutritional requirement for growth of the yeast phase or whether it functions as well to provide sulfhydryl groups required for the mycelial-to-yeast transition.

Garrison *et al.* (1970) attempted to analyze this question by comparing uptake of cysteine and cystine into yeast and mycelia. These workers equated stimulation of respiration by cysteine and cystine to uptake into the cell. They observed that cysteine and cystine stimulated respiration in yeast and not mycelia and therefore concluded that uptake occurred in the former and not the latter. Unfortunately, this conclusion was incorrect. Maresca *et al.* (1977) have shown that cystine and cysteine can stimulate respiration in *H. capsulatum* and therefore confirmed the observations, but not the conclusion, of Garrison *et al.* (1970). Cysteine and cystine do indeed stimulate respiration in yeast, but not in mycelia. However, in contrast to the inference of Garrison *et al.* (1970), the effect on respiration cannot be equated to uptake. Using direct measurements of uptake, Maresca *et al.* (1978) showed that cysteine and cystine were taken up equally well by both phases of *H. capsulatum.*

Subsequent publications have clarified this issue. The cysteine-stimulated respiration is due to a cytosolic cysteine oxidase found in yeast-phase cells and absent in mycelia. The oxidase has been purified and characterized by Kumar *et al.* (1983). It is an iron-containing dioxygenase with a molecular weight of about 10,500; the product of the oxidation is cysteine sulfinic acid. Cystine also works in this system because it is first reduced to cysteine by a membrane-bound cystine reductase, which is also present in the yeast phase and absent in mycelia (Maresca *et al.*, 1978). The work on the cysteine oxidase revealed that cysteine also has a second effect on oxygen consumption that is quite separate from the function of the oxidase. This second role of cysteine involves the mitochondrial respiratory pathways (Maresca *et al.*, 1981).

2.3. Role of Cysteine in Regulating Morphogenesis and Mitochondrial Activity

When the transition from the mycelial to the yeast phase is induced by a temperature shift from 25 to 37°C, the earliest and most striking metabolic changes that have been detected occur in cell respiration and in the response of respiration to added cysteine. To study these changes in detail, it was necessary first to characterize the respiration pathways in both phases of *H. capsulatum.*

Repiration in *H. capsulatum,* as in *Neurospora* and other fungi studied (Lambowitz and Slayman, 1971), proceeds through two terminal oxidase systems (Maresca *et al.*, 1979); one is the standard cytochrome system, which can be inhibited by antimycin and cyanide; the other is an unidentified alternate oxidase that is insensitive to these inhibitors, but can be specifically inhibited by salicylhydroxamic acid (SHAM). The alternate oxidase is induced by inhibition of the cytochrome oxidative pathway or by the so-called "poky mutants," which have defects in the cytochrome system. Unlike the other systems studied thus far, however, the alternate oxidase of *H. capsulatum* is constitutive. We could find no differences between yeast and mycelia in regard to the responses of the two oxidase systems to the inhibitors cyanide and SHAM. However, cytochrome respiration (SHAM-resistant) in the yeast phase is completely sensitive to antimycin, but in mycelia this respiratory pathway is only partially sensitive, with a maximum inhibition of only 50% (Figure 4). This point will be discussed in more detail later in this section.

We have been able to distinguish three distinct stages in the transi-

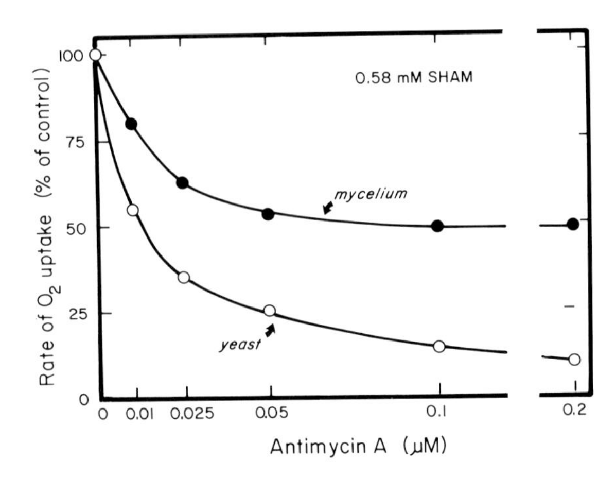

Figure 4. Effect of antimycin A on SHAM-resistant respiration of yeast (○) and mycelial (●) phases of *H. capsulatum*. (From Maresca *et al.*, 1979.)

tion following the temperature shift from 25 to 37°C (Figure 5) (Maresca *et al.*, 1981). Stage 1, encompassing the first 24–40 hr, is characterized by a progressive decrease in cellular respiration rate of the mycelia and in the intracellular concentrations of cysteine and other amino acids. In stage 2, the cells are essentially dormant and have no spontaneous respiration. This dormant stage lasts 4–6 days, at which time the cells enter stage 3, characterized by a progressive return of the rate of cell respiration to normal. Yeast cells are seen after the initiation of stage 3.

In the absence of cysteine, cells could progress up to stage 2 of the transition, but cysteine or other sulfhydryl-containing compounds such as glutathione are required to complete the transition and permit cells to progress from stage 2 to stage 3.

It is important to note that the requirement for cysteine or other sulfhydryl compounds to complete the mycelial-to-yeast transition is *different* from the yeast requirement for cysteine. Yeasts appear to have a nutritional need for cysteine that cannot be satisfied by other sulfhydryl-containing compounds. In contrast, in stage 2 cells, cysteine or other sulfhydryl-containing compounds act by affecting mitochondrial respiration in stage 2 cells. These cells have no spontaneous respiration, and mitochondria isolated from these cells show no respiration when incubated with standard substrates. Both cellular and mitochondrial respiration are partially restored by the addition of cysteine or other sulfhydryl-containing compounds.

In a study of the mycelial-to-yeast transition in progress, we found

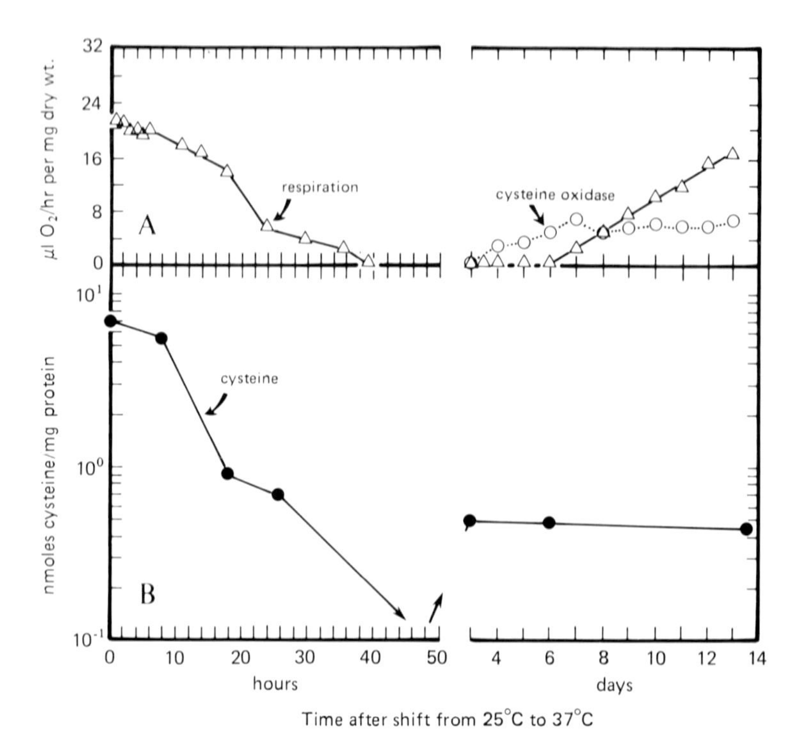

Figure 5. Respiration (△), cysteine levels of (●), and cysteine oxidase (○) activities during the mycelial-to-yeast phase transition. (A) Oxygen uptake in mycelia (dry weight) shifted to 37°C. Respiration was measured in both buffer and fresh medium, with essentially identical results. (B) Level of cysteine in mycelia incubated at 37°C. Recoveries of cysteine were 85–92% as determined by addition of radioactive cysteine just before cell breakage. (From Maresca *et al.*, 1981.)

that the activities of the cytochrome system and the alternate oxidase decrease in parallel during stage 1 of the transition. Our preliminary findings indicate that the decrease in activity of the cytochrome system is correlated with a striking decrease in the concentrations of cytochromes *b*, *c*, and aa_3, assayed spectrophotometrically.

The cysteine-restored respiration in both stage 2 cells and mitochondria is resistant to antimycin, even in the presence of 0.5 mM SHAM, which should force respiration through the cytochrome system. These results suggest that cysteine-stimulated respiration proceeds via shunt pathways in which cysteine can shuttle electrons around the site of the antimycin block. This result is relevant to our earlier statement that cytochrome respiration in yeast is completely sensitive to antimycin, but it is only partially sensitive in the mycelial phase. This implies that the shunt pathways are active in mycelia and inactive in yeast. This pattern of activity of the shunt pathways *in vivo* can be correlated with intracellular levels of cysteine, which are high in mycelia, where the shunt pathways are active, and low in yeast, where the shunt pathways are inactive. In addition, the inactivation of the shunt pathways can be correlated with the measured decline in intracellular cysteine that occurs during stage 1 of the mycelial-to-yeast transition (Figure 5).

Our previous work (Maresca *et al.*, 1981) has shown that cysteine or other sulfhydryl-containing compounds are required for transforming cells to recover from stage 2 of the transition and that increasing the level of cysteine or other sulfhydryl groups in the medium decreases the length of the dormant period in stage 2. The requirement for extracellular cysteine or other sulfhydryl groups to progress beyond stage 2 of the transition may be explained in part by the reactivation of the shunt pathways that restore respiration, thereby providing energy to the transforming cells.

When cells enter stage 3 and spontaneous respiration returns, the transition to yeast is completed. At this point, the shunt pathways do not operate spontaneously, probably because of the low intracellular levels of cysteine. Cysteine is required for growth of the yeast phase, but as we have already stated, this requirement is quite different from the one during the transition. This requirement for cysteine by yeast cells is quite specific and cannot be satisfied by other sulfhydryl-containing compounds or other amino acids. Cysteine is probably metabolized in the yeast phase to satisfy a nutritional requirement, and the cysteine oxidase that appears late in stage 2 may be involved in this process.

Therefore, this study indicates that cysteine has at least two functions in *H. capsulatum.* One is required to complete the mycelial-to-yeast transition; the sulfhydryl groups are crucial to this function, but can be provided by other thiol compounds. The second is to supply a nutrient to yeast cells.

2.4. RNA and Protein Synthesis

When RNA synthesis in both phases of *H. capsulatum* was measured by the amount of radioactive guanine incorporated into trichloroacetic acid (TCA) precipitates of cells, Cheung *et al.* (1974) found that the total RNA synthesized over an 8-hr period was 12 times higher for mycelia than for yeast cells. However, measurements of RNA synthesis in this organism by radioactive guanine incorporation are difficult to interpret. One reason radioactive experiments have been difficult to perform with

H. capsulatum is that few nucleotide precursors are incorporated. Even for guanine incorporation, the specific activity of RNA formed by actively growing yeasts was much lower than that formed in mycelia, so that uptake of this metabolite probably differed for the two growing phases.

The differences in RNA synthesis between the two phases were much smaller when a direct chemical method was used by Cheung *et al.* (1974). Mycelia at 25°C made about twice as much total RNA as yeasts growing at 37°C, but there are also problems with the direct chemical determination of RNA. The heavy sugar contamination from cell-wall material makes the conventional orcinol reaction unusable. Instead, RNA has to be estimated by a modification of the Schmidt–Thannhauser procedure (Fleck and Munro, 1962), a method with some inherent inaccuracies. Despite the problem, it is probable that this latter method is a better measure of RNA synthesis in *H. capsulatum* than the radioactive method.

Cheung *et al.* (1974) also fractionated the RNA of both phases on acrylamide gels and showed that radioactive guanine was incorporated into the large ribosomal RNA molecules (25 S and 18 S) of both yeast and mycelial phases; the gels also showed that yeast and mycelial phases had indistinguishable ribosomal RNA patterns.

Gates and Brownstein (1980) examined polyacrylamide gel electrophoresis patterns of ribosomal RNA from both phases under denaturing conditions and found that the mycelial 17 S RNA was slightly smaller than the yeast 17 S RNA. However, these differences in the RNA species of the two strains appeared to be relatively minor.

The most dramatic changes in RNA synthesis occurred in stages 1 and 2 during the mycelial-to-yeast transition (Maresca *et al.,* 1981). In the first 24–40 hr after the 25 to 37° temperature shift, coincident with the fall in respiration, RNA and protein synthesis decreased to nondetectable levels. During most of stage 2, the transforming cells were not making RNA; synthesis restarted about 1–2 days after respiration resumed in stage 3 of the transition. Up to the present, there has been no careful characterization of the pattern of fall and resumption of RNA synthesis. It is not known whether all species change at the same rate or whether there are specific RNAs that are made later or earlier in the transition.

When partially purified extracts from the yeast and mycelial phases were examined for RNA polymerase activity (Boguslawski *et al.,* 1974), yeast cells were found to contain three distinct species of RNA polymerases, but mycelial cells had only one, with very low activity. Further purification of the mycelial enzymes, however, resulted in three species of RNA polymerases. The recovery of three RNA polymerases from each phase of *H. capsulatum* is in agreement with work on other eukaryotes (Kumar *et al.*, 1980). A number of the properties of these polymerases were also comparable to those from other eukaryotes. For example, the number of protein subunits observed in dissociating electrophoretic gels, the elution profiles from column chromatography, and the salt and metal ion requirements of the enzymes were similar to those of enzymes from other eukaroytes. The RNA polymerases from both phases were also similar to those of other eukaryotes in regard to the number of enzymes that were inhibited by α-amanitin (Figure 6); one of the enzymes was very sensitive, one was intermediate, and one was resistant. However, the pattern of sensitivity differed from that described for *Saccharomyces cerevisiae* or other eukaryotes. In both phases of *H. capsulatum*, RNA polymerase II was most resistant to α-amanitin and polymerase III was most sensitive, whereas in higher eukaryotes, RNA polymerase II was most sensitive and polymerase I was most resistant. In *S. cerevisiae*, enzyme III was most resistant and enzyme II was most sensitive.

A most unexpected finding during the purification and characterization of the RNA polymerases was the difference between corresponding enzymes of the two phases. The mycelial enzymes were 6- to 10-fold more resistant to α-amanitin at every level of purification than the yeast-phase enzymes. A direct comparison of the subunits of corresponding enzymes showed one or two subunit differences in each. In addition, there were also minor differences in ion and salt requirements and subunit structure. In subsequent work, specific antisera generated to the RNA polymerases have been used to determine the level of antigenic differences between enzymes of the two phases. Kumar *et al.* (1982) found that rabbit antisera directed against RNA polymerase III from the yeast phase detected major

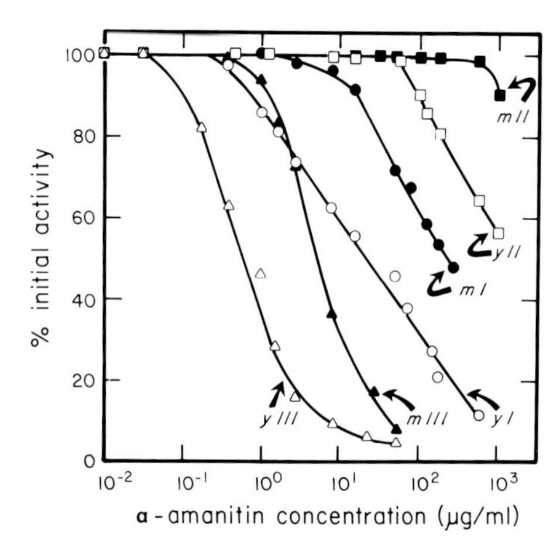

Figure 6. α-Amanitin sensitivity of RNA polymerases. Equal quantities (2–4 units) of yeast- and mycelial-phase enzymes were assayed in the presence of specified concentrations of α-amanitin at room temperature for 60 min. The percentage of the initial activity is plotted against α-amanitin concentration for each enzyme. Yeast- and mycelial-phase enzymes are designated by "y" and "m," respectively. (From Kumar *et al.*, 1980.)

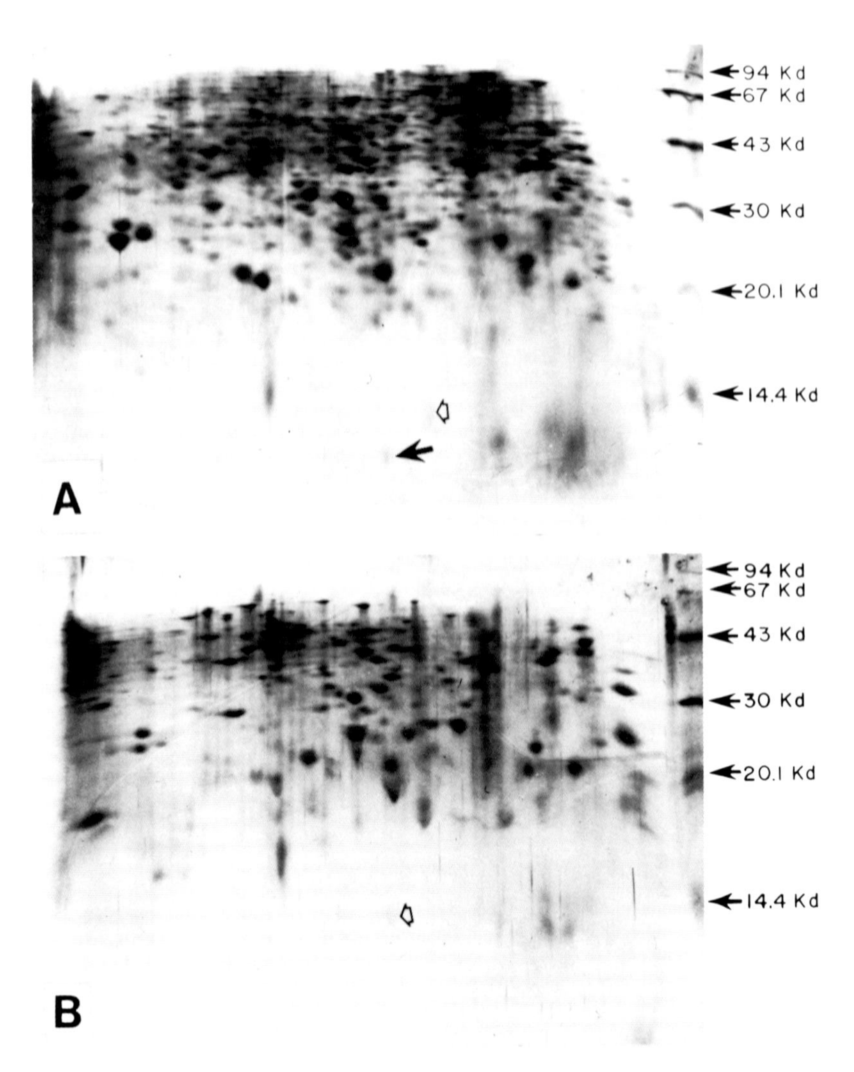

Figure 7. Two-dimensional gel electrophoresis of the cytoplasmic fractions of yeast (A) and mycelia (B). Cytoplasmic fractions of yeast- and mycelial-phase cells of *H. capsulatum* were mixed with ^{125}I-labeled cysteine oxidase purified from the yeast phase and subjected to two-dimensional electrophoresis as described in the text. After the electrophoresis, the gels were stained with silver nitrate and subjected to autoradiography as described in the text. The large dark arrow in (A) indicates the position of the radioactive spot obtained with ^{125}I-labeled oxidase. The arrows in (A) and (B) indicate the other spots subjected to tryptic mapping. (From Kumar *et al.*, 1983.)

antigenic differences between yeast polymerase III and its corresponding enzyme in the mycelial phase.

The fate of the RNA polymerases during the transition has not yet been studied. It may be possible to study changes in each of the enzymes when specific antisera become available.

Differences have been detected in the pattern of protein spots in the gels from the two phases (Figure 7) when cytoplasmic fractions from both yeast and mycelial cells were compared using two-dimensional electrophoresis, but these have not been further quantitated. Only a few of the proteins unique to each phase have been characterized. We have already made reference to the cysteine oxidase that Kumar *et al.* (1983) have purified and characterized from the cytoplasm of the yeast phase of *H. capsulatum* and the differences in the RNA polymerases. Immunological techniques have detected differences in protein antigens between the two phases. Using antisera generated to each of the phases and cross-absorbed to the opposite phase, Kumar has estimated that about 5% of the labeled proteins are unique to each phase (unpublished observations).

Protein synthesis follows the same pattern as respiration and RNA synthesis during the mycelial-to-yeast transition; it falls to nondetectable levels in stages 1 and 2 and resumes in stage 3. In preliminary observations, Yuckenberg *et al.* (unpublished) have found that despite the fall of overall protein synthesis, unique proteins are made at an increased level during stage 1.

2.5. Cyclic AMP Levels

The level of cyclic AMP (cAMP) is about 5 times higher in the mycelial phase than in the yeast phase (Maresca *et al.*, 1977). The most striking change in cAMP levels occurs during the yeast-to-mycelial transition (Medoff *et al.*, 1981). Intracellular cAMP increases at the same rate in control cultures and in yeast incubated at 25°C for the first 72 hr. However, after 72 hr, when morphological evidence of transition is apparent, and most cells are extending germ tubes, the intracellular cAMP concentration in the transforming cells begins to increase compared with that of controls. During the next stages of the transition, when hyphae undergo elongation and branching, the cAMP concentration in both controls and transforming cells continues to rise, but the levels reached by differentiating cells are about 2-fold greater than those in yeast controls at 37°C.

The change in extracellular levels of cAMP during the yeast-to-mycelial transition is even more striking. In transforming cultures at 25°C, substantial quantities of cAMP are detected in the medium between 48 and 72 hr after the temperature switch, coincident with the first morphological signs of phase transition. During the remainder of the transition from yeast to mycelium, the extracellular cAMP increases dramatically, reaching levels 5 times greater than those in yeast controls.

The finding that the morphological changes during the yeast-to-mycelial transformation are accompanied by dramatic increases in intracellular and extracellular cAMP suggests that cAMP has an important regulatory role in this process. This hypothesis is supported by our finding that even at 37°C, the yeast-to-mycelial transition could be induced by cAMP and agents that raise the intracellular levels of cAMP (theophylline, acetylsalicylic acid, prostaglandin E, and nerve growth factor) (Sacco *et al.*, 1981). The mechanism of the cAMP effect and how it influences other changes during the yeast-to-mycelial transition are all unknown.

Changes in intracellular cAMP levels during the mycelial-to-yeast transition are more difficult to interpret; levels fall in both control and transforming cultures. However, the levels fall much more sharply in transforming cultures, particularly during the 5-day period after the temperature shift from 25 to 37°C. Later in the transition, when buds begin to emerge on hyphal surfaces, the cAMP content of the transforming cells begins to rise to levels characteristic of yeast cells.

The mycelial-to-yeast transition is a more complex process, quite different from the reverse transition. First, it takes much longer than the yeast-to-mycelial transition; second, it occurs in discrete stages with the complex changes in RNA and protein synthesis and respiration we have already noted. Therefore, it is difficult to interpret the changes in cAMP. They may be a result of the marked changes in metabolism of the cells, or they may signify a role for cAMP in this phase transition.

3. DISCUSSION OF DIMORPHISM

It is clear from the experimental data discussed in the earlier sections of this review that in addition to changes in morphology, the phase transitions of *H. capsulatum* appear to involve alterations in many aspects of the metabolic processes of the cell. This is particularly true of the mycelial-to-yeast transition. The most immediate effect of increasing the temperature from 25 to 37°C is a marked decline in the level of cytochromes that results in cessation of respiration. RNA and protein synthesis then fall to nondetectable levels, most likely because of the absence of respiration and the resultant fall in ATP concentrations and a winding down of the metabolic processes of the cell. The reason for the dramatic change in cytochrome levels and the cessation of respiration is unclear, but it certainly dominates cell metabolism in stage 1.

It has been known for quite some time that cysteine and other sulfhydryl-containing compounds are necessary to complete the mycelial-to-yeast transition and are also required for growth of the yeast phase. Now it seems that sulfhydryls have two functions. In their presence, shunt pathways are initiated that bypass the block in the cytochromes and alternate oxidase that occurs in stage 1. The shunt pathways maintain a level of ATP that keeps the cell viable through stages 1 and 2 of the transition until normal respiration resumes. Cysteine is also required for growth by the yeast phase.

In stage 3, an adaptation to the new environmental conditions (increased temperature) has occurred because cytochrome levels return to normal and spontaneous respiration begins. This is a critical point in the phase transition, and insight into what this adaptation may be is central to an understanding of what is happening. There is then a return of all the normal metabolic processes, and the yeast begins to grow and divide. The nature of the adaptation that completes the transition is unknown, but for several reasons, we believe it likely that it occurs at the level of the cell membrane. Important support for this notion is that *p*-chloromercuriphenylsulfonic acid, a sulfhydryl blocking agent that binds to cell membranes and is not taken up by the cell, irreversibly blocks the mycelial-to-yeast transition at a point between stages 2 and 3 (Maresca *et al.*, 1977). Therefore, we believe that a careful examination of the lipids and proteins of the cell membrane of transforming cultures might give important clues about what is happening during the latter part of the phase transition.

Two other changes in the cell support the importance of cysteine in the mycelial-to-yeast-phase transition. Within the first 24 hr after the temperature shift, an enzyme activity that reduces cystine to cysteine is induced (Maresca *et al.*, 1978). This cystine reductase likely functions to keep the level of cysteine high in the cell so that the shunt pathways can remain active. Later in the transition, just before stage 3 begins, the cysteine oxidase appears (Maresca *et al.*, 1981). The function of this enzyme is less apparent. It may provide a metabolic product of cysteine that is important to the maintenance of the yeast phase, or it may also function to keep intracellular levels of cysteine low to turn off the shunt pathways in stage 3 and to keep them from operating in the yeast phase. This would be important in the yeast because the shunt pathways are relatively inefficient in regard to the generation of ATP, since it bypasses site II phosphorylation (Sacco et al., unpublished observations). Since the yeast phase is found in macrophages, an intracellular environment rich in TCA-cycle intermediates, it would be to the advantage of the yeast cell to have an efficient system of generating ATP. It is also interesting that the yeast cell requires cysteine and a highly reduced environment; both conditions appear to be present in the intracellular environment of macrophages where yeasts are found in the infected hosts. On the other hand, mycelia are found in soil fertilized by bird excreta. This is a nutritionally enriched environment, and under these conditions, the operation of the shunt pathways may be advantageous to permit rapid utilization of glycolytic substrates. Although this analysis is highly speculative, it is consistent with the experimental results and the different ecological niches of the two phases.

The available data on the yeast-to-mycelial transition are relatively meager. It is obvious, however, that this transition is not a mirror image of the mycelial-to-yeast transition. The changes appear to be quite different, and it is likely that it is a different process with unique regulatory factors. It appears that one of the control mechanisms in this transition is cAMP. This conclusion is supported by the striking differences in levels between the two phases and the finding that cAMP and hormones that raise cAMP levels can induce the yeast-to-mycelial transition at 37°C. Changes in respiration and in RNA and protein synthesis are not as striking as in the mycelial-to-yeast transition and actually probably only reflect the fall in the temperature of incubation and the level of metabolism of the cell.

Obviously, our understanding of dimorphism in *H. capsulatum* is incomplete. However, we have come a long way over the past few years, and the clues that are available at present will undoubtedly generate further experiments and questions. We have no doubt that over the next few years, there will be a much greater understanding of the regulation of both transitions. It would be helpful if mutants defective in the ability to undergo the transition could be selected. In initial efforts, only two sets of mutants of *H. capsulatum* have been generated (Maresca *et al.*, 1978; Jacobson and Harrell, 1981, 1982), and unfortunately these appear to be unrelated to the phase transitions. Further effort is necessary. It would also be helpful to be able to do experiments with synchronized cultures. Body *et al.* (unpublished results) have observed that cultures of *H. capsulatum* can be synchronized, but the method is tedious and the efficiency is poor. Further effort in this area is also warranted.

Histoplasma capsulatum is a pathogen and must be handled carefully in the laboratory. It grows slowly with doubling times that vary from 8 to 24 hr, and the phase transitions are slow, requiring 3–14 days. However, we believe it is worthwhile to study *H. capsulatum* and try to establish it as a model system of a differentiation process. Unlike sporulation, this differentiation system involves two vegetative phases that are quite different in form as well as in metabolic processes. One of the triggers for the transition is a temperature change that has intrinsic interest because of its relationship to the so-called SOS phenomenon (Little and Mount, 1982) and heat shock (Ashburner and Bonner, 1979). It is also apparent from our work that changes in the cell membrane, cAMP levels, and oxidation–reduction potential of the cell are likely involved. Other triggers will probably become apparent with subsequent work. Despite the complexity of the system, we believe we now have the biochemical and genetic tools to work out the relationships among the regulatory factors and to try to determine mechanisms. We believe it is worth the effort because it is rare to find a differentiation system that is so intrinsically interesting and that is also involved in the pathogenesis of an important human disease.

ACKNOWLEDGMENTS. Portions of these studies were supported by Public Health Service Grants AI 10622, AI 00459, and AI 07015 from the National Institutes of Health and by a grant from the John A. Hartford Foundation, Inc. We wish to thank Dr. Kerry L. O'Donnell for the electron photomicrographs used in this chapter and for his description of the fine structure of the yeast and mycelial phases of *H. capsulatum.* We are also grateful to Dr. David Schlessinger and Dr. Alan Lambowitz for helpful discussions.

REFERENCES

Ajello, L., Chick, E. W., and Furcolow, M. L., 1971, *Histoplasmosis, Proceedings of the Second National Conference,* Charles C Thomas, Springfield, Illinois.

Ashburner, M., and Bonner, J., 1979, The induction of gene activity in *Drosophila* by heat shock, *Cell* **17:**241–254.

Berliner, M. D., 1968, Primary subcultures of *Histoplasma capsulatum:* Macro- and micromorphology of the mycelial phase, *Sabouraudia* **6:**111–118.

Boguslawski, G., and Stetler, D. A., 1979, Aspects of physiology of *Histoplasma capsulatum* (a review), *Mycopathologia* **67:**17–24.

Boguslawski, G., Schlessinger, D., Medoff, G., and Kobayashi, G. S., 1974, Ribonucleic acid polymerases of the yeast phase of *Histoplasma capsulatum, J. Bacteriol.* **118:**481–485.

Buguslawski, G., Akagi, J. M., and Ward, L. G., 1976, Possible role for cysteine biosynthesis in conversion from mycelial to yeast form of *Histoplasma capsulatum, Nature (London)* **261:**336–338.

Byers, B., and Goetsch, L., 1974, Duplication of spindle plaques and integration of the yeast cell cycle, *Cold Spring Harbor Symp. Quant. Biol.* **38:**123–131.

Byers, B., and Goetsch, L., 1975, Behavior of spindles and spindle plaques in the cell cycle and conjugation of *Saccharomyces cerevisiae, J. Bacteriol.* **124:**511–523.

Cheung, S. C., Kobayashi, G. S., Schlessinger, D., and Medoff, G., 1974, RNA metabolism during morphogenesis in *Histoplasma capsulatum, J. Gen. Microbiol.* **82**:301–307.

Cheung, S. C., Medoff, G., Schlessinger, D., and Kobayashi, G. S., 1975, Response of yeast and myeclial phases of *Histoplasma capsulatum* to amphotericin B and actinomycin D, *Antimicrob. Agents Chemother.* **8**:498–503.

Daniels, L. S., Berliner, M. D., and Campbell, C. C., 1968, Varying virulence in rabbits infected with different filamentous types of *Histoplasma capsulatum, J. Bacteriol.* **96**:1535–1539.

DeMonbreun, W. A., 1934, The cultivation and cultural characteristics of Darlings' *Histoplasma capsulatum, Am. J. Trop. Med. Hyg.* **14**:93–125.

Edwards, M. R., Hazen, E. L., and Edwards, G. A., 1959, The fine structure of the yeast-like cells of *Histoplasma capsulatum* in culture, *J. Gen. Microbiol.* **20**:496–593.

Edwards, P. Q., and Billings, E. L., 1971, Worldwide pattern of skin sensitivity to histoplasmin, *Am. J. Trop. Med. Hyg.* **20**:228–319.

Fleck, A., and Munro, H. N., 1962, The precision of ultraviolet absorption measurements in the Schmidt–Thannhauser procedure for nucleic acid estimation, *Biochim. Biophys. Acta* **55**:571–583.

Garrison, R. G., and Boyd, K. S., 1978, Electron microscopy of yeast-like cell development from the microconidium of *Histoplasma capsulatum, J. Bacteriol.* **133**:345–353.

Garrison, R. G., Dodd, H. T., and Hamilton, J. W., 1970, The uptake of low molecular weight sulfur-containing compounds by *Histoplasma capsulatum* and related dimorphic fungi, *Mycopathologia* **40**:171–180.

Gates, D. W., and Brownstein, B. H., 1980, Ribosomal RNA from the yeast and mycelial phases of *Histoplasma capsulatum, Exp. Mycol.* **4**:231–238.

Gilardi, G. L., 1965, Nutrition of systemic and subcutaneous pathogenic fungi, *Bacteriol. Rev.* **29**:406–424.

Goodwin, R. A., Loyd, J. E., and DesPres, R. M., 1981, Histoplasmosis in normal hosts, *Medicine* **60**:231–266.

Hoch, H. C., and Howard, R. J., 1980, Ultrastructure of freeze-substituted hyphae of the Basidiomycete *Laetisaria arvalis, Protoplasma* **103**:281–297.

Howard, R. J., 1981, Ultrastructural analysis of hyphal tip cell growth in fungi: Spitzenkorper, cytoskeleton and endomembranes after freeze-substitution, *J. Cell Sci.* **48**:89–103.

Howard, R. J., and Aist, J. R., 1979, Hyphal tip cell ultrastructure of the fungus *Fusarium:* Improved preservation by freeze-substitution, *J. Ultrastruct. Res.* **66**:224–234.

Jacobson, E. S., and Harrell, A. C., 1981, Selenocystine-resistant mutants of *Histoplasma capsulatum, Mycopathologia* **73**:177–181.

Jacobson, E. S., and Harrell, A. C., 1982, A prototrophic strain of *Histoplasma capsulatum, Mycopathologia* **77**:65–68.

Kumar, B. V., McMillian, R. A., Medoff, G., Gutwein, M., and Kobayashi, G. S., 1980, Comparison of the ribonucleic acid polymerases from both phases of *Histoplasma capsulatum, Biochemistry* **19**:1080–1087.

Kumar, B. V., Medoff, G., Painter, A., and Kobayashi, G. S., 1982, Antigenic differences between corresponding DNA-dependent RNA polymerases from both phases of *Histoplasma capsulatum, Exp. Mycol.* **6**:90–94.

Kumar, B. V., Maresca, B., Sacco, M., Goewert, R., Kobayashi, G. S., and Medoff, G., 1983, Purification and characterization of a cysteine dioxygenase from the yeast phase of *Histoplasma capsulatum, Biochemistry* **22**:762–768.

Kwon-Chung, K. J., 1972, Sexual stage of *Histoplasma capsulatum, Science* **175**:326.

Kwon-Chung, K. J., 1973, Studies on *Emmonsiella capsulata.* I. Heterothallism and development of ascocarp, *Mycologia* **65**:109–121.

Kwon-Chung, K. J., Weeks, R. J., and Larsh, H. W., 1974, Studies on *Emmonsiella capsulata (Histoplasma capsulatum).* II. Distribution of the 2 mating types in 13 endemic states of the U.S., *Am. J. Epidemiol.* **99**:44–49.

Lambowitz, A. M., and Slayman, C. W., 1971, Cyanide-resistant respiration in *Neurospora crassa, J. Bacteriol.* **108**:1087–1096.

Little, J. W., and Mount, D. W., 1982, The SOS regulatory system of *Escherichia coli, Cell* **29**:11–22.

Maresca, B., Medoff, G., Schlessinger, D., Kobayashi, G. S., and Medoff, J., 1977, Regulation of dimorphism in the pathogenic fungus *Histoplasma capsulatum, Nature (London)* **266**:447–448.

Maresca, B., Jacobson, E., Medoff, G., and Kobayashi, G. S., 1978, Cystine reductase in the dimorphic fungus *Histoplasma capsulatum, J. Bacteriol.* **135**:987–992.

Maresca, B., Lambowitz, A. M., Kobayashi, G. S., and Medoff, G., 1979, Respiration in the yeast and mycelial phases of *Histoplasma capsulatum, J. Bacteriol.* **138**:647–649.

Maresca, B., Lambowitz, A. M., Kumar, B. V., Grant, G., Kobayashi, G. S., and Medoff, G., 1981, Role of cysteine in regulating morphogenesis and mitochondrial activity in the dimorphic fungus *Histoplasma capsulatum, Proc. Natl. Acad. Sci. U.S.A.* **78**:4596–4600.

McVeigh, I., and Houston, W. E., 1972, Factors affecting mycelial to yeast phase conversion and growth of the yeast phase of *Histoplasma capsulatum, Mycopathol. Mycol.* **47**:135–151.

Medoff, J., Jacobson, E., and Medoff, G., 1981, Regulation of dimorphism in *Histoplasma capsulatum* by cyclic adenosine 3′,5′-monophosphate, *J. Bacteriol.* **145**:1452–1455.

Morris, N. R., 1980, Chromosome structure and the molecular biology of mitosis in eukaryotic micro-organisms, in: *The Eukaryotic Microbe* (G. W. Gooday, D. Llloyd, and A. P. J. Trinci, eds.), Cambridge University Press, Cambridge, pp. 41–76.

Pine, L., 1977, *Histoplasma* antigens: Their production, purification and uses, *Contrib. Microbiol. Immunol.* **3**:138–168.

Pine, L., and Peacock, C. L., 1958, Studies on the growth of *Histoplasma capsulatum, J. Bacteriol.* **75**:167–174.

Pine, L., and Webster, R. E., 1962, Conversion in strains of *Histoplasma capsulatum, J. Bacteriol.* **83**:149–157.

Reca, M. E., 1968, Reduction of a tetrazolium salt in determining growth activity of yeast-phase *Histoplasma capsulatum, Appl. Microbiol.* **16**:236–238.

Reca, M. E., and Campbell, C. C., 1967, Growth curves with yeast phase of *Histoplasma capsulatum, Sabouraudia* **5**:267–273.

Rippon, J. W., 1968, Monitored environment system to control cell growth, morphology, and metabolic rate in fungi by oxidation–reduction potentials, *Appl. Microbiol.* **16**:114–121.

Sacco, M., Maresca, B., Kumar, B. V., Kobayashi, G. S., and Medoff, G., 1981, Temperature- and cyclic nucleotide-induced phase transitions of *Histoplasma capsulatum, J. Bacteriol.* **146**:117–120.

Salvin, S. B., 1947, Cultural studies on the yeast-like phase of *Histoplasma capsulatum* Darling, *J. Bacteriol.* **54**:655–660.

Salvin, S. B., 1949, Cysteine and related compounds in the growth of the yeast-like phase of *Histoplasma capsulatum, J. Infect. Dis.* **84**:275–283.

Scherr, G. H., 1957, Studies on the dimorphism of *Histoplasma capsulatum, Exp. Cell Res.* **12**:92–107.

Schwarz, J., 1981, *Histoplasmosis,* Praeger, New York.

Stetler, D. A., and Boguslawski, G., 1979, Cysteine biosynthesis in the fungus, *Histoplasma capsulatum*, *Sabouraudia* **17**:23–34.

Sweany, H. C., 1960, *Histoplasmosis*, Charles C Thomas, Springfield, Illinois.

Szaniszlo, P. J., Jacobs, C. W., and Geis, P. A., 1983, Dimorphism: Morphological and biochemical aspects, in: *Fungi Pathogenic for Humans and Animals, Part A, Biology* (D. H. Howard, ed.), Marcel Dekker, New York, pp. 323–436.

Tewari, R. P., and Berkhout, F. J., 1972, Comparative pathogenicity of albino and brown types of *Histoplasma capsulatum* for mice, *J. Infect. Dis.* **125**:504–508.

Wheat, L. J., Slama, T. G., Norton, J. A., Kohler, R. B., Eitzen, H. E., French, M. L. V., and Sathapatayavongs, B., 1982, Risk factors for disseminated or fatal histoplasmosis: Analysis of a large urban outbreak, *Ann. Intern. Med.* **96**:159–163.

Chapter 5

Paracoccidioides brasiliensis

Felipe San-Blas and Gioconda San-Blas

1. INTRODUCTION

Although it has been nearly 80 years since the dimorphic nature of *Paracoccidiodes brasiliensis* was first described by Lutz (1908), our knowledge of the biological events that take place in this process has been acquired very slowly, and even today many important questions remain unanswered. The emphasis of research on dimorphism has been mostly on the terminal effects, mainly changes in cell-wall structure and composition; the nature of the primary reactions leading to the manifestation of these terminal effects is still unknown.

It was not until 1931 that *in vitro* transition from the mycelial (M) to the yeast (Y) form was first reported (Negroni, 1931). Since then, it has been satisfactorily demonstrated that the dimorphic transition of *P. brasiliensis* depends exclusively on the temperature of incubation (Nickerson and Edwards, 1949) and is independent of the nature and composition of the culture media and other external parameters (Inlow, 1979). The ability of several auxotrophic mutants to undergo phase transition on minimal media that did not allow growth (F. San-Blas and Centeno, 1977) confirms that temperature is the only factor responsible for inducing dimorphism in *P. brasiliensis.*

Paracoccidioides brasiliensis is a pleomorphic organism that depends on the temperature of incubation for the expression of its morphology (Figure 1). *In vitro* at 37°C and in infected tissues, *P. brasiliensis*

Felipe San-Blas and Gioconda San-Blas • Department of Microbiology and Cellular Biology, Venezuelan Institute of Scientific Investigations (I.V.I.C.), Caracas 1010A, Venezuela.

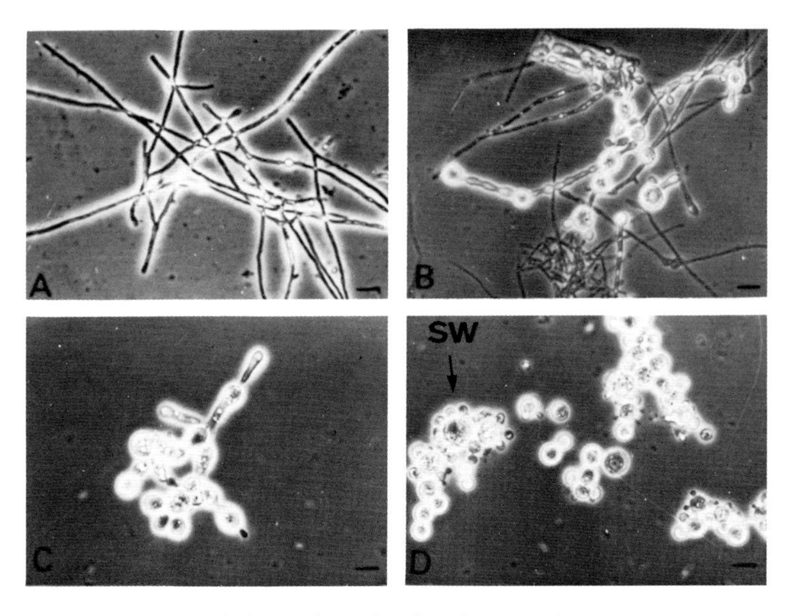

Figure 1. Morphology of dimorphism of *P. brasiliensis* strain IVIC Pb73. (A) Mycelial form; (B) initiation of transition to the Y form; (C) late stage of transition to the Y form. Both (B) and (C) represent transitional forms. (D) Typical Y cells. Note the ship's-wheel cell (sw): Scale bar: 10 μm. (From Hallak *et al.*, 1982.)

grows in the form of spherical or oval cells that vary in size from a few nanometers in young, recently separated buds to 10–30 μm or more in a mature yeast cell (Furtado *et al.,* 1967; Carbonell, 1972). Yeast cells are multinucleate (Emmons, 1959) and cenocytic and multiply by polar or multipolar budding. Multiple budding occurs synchronously on the surface of a mature cell (Ciferri and Redaelli, 1936). Buds are connected to the mother cell by narrow necks, giving the whole structure the appearance of a ship's-wheel (Figure 1D). This ship's-wheel structure is the most important taxonomic and diagnostic characteristic of *P. brasiliensis.* The yeast cell wall varies in thickness (150–300 nm) with the age of the cell and is composed of an outer, thin, electron-dense layer and an inner, broad, electron-lucent layer. The hyphal wall is thinner and more homogeneous and consists of a single electron-dense layer with an average thickness of 100 nm, depending on the region of the hypha (Carbonell and Pollak, 1968; Carbonell and Rodriguez, 1968).

The mycelial form of *P. brasiliensis* grows slowly at room temperature. Microscopic observations show septate, slender, and freely branching hyphae, 1–3 μm in width (Figure 1A). In nutrient-deficient media and in old cultures, the presence of structures similar to chlamydospores, arthroconidia, and aleurioconidia, none of them unique to *P. brasiliensis*, has been reported (Restrepo, 1970). However, not enough physiological or ultrastructural evidence has been produced to demonstrate conclusively the sporogeneous nature of these structures, that classification as spores having been based mainly on observations with the light microscope.

2. MORPHOLOGY OF DIMORPHISM

Hyphae of *P. brasiliensis* give rise to the Y form by rounding up of the space between two septa and by swelling of the tip of the hyphae or of spores resulting from hyphal fragmentation. The number of intercalary and terminal swellings increases during the first hours of transition, forming certain types of aggregates that have been named transitional forms (Figure 1B, C) (Carbonell, 1969). These forms occur during the early stages of transformation in either direction (M ⇆ Y), and also when cultures are grown at intermediate temperatures (Inlow, 1979). Microscopically, they cover a wide range of different morphologies: pseudohyphae, chains, and groups of Y-like structures. Typical hyphae or Y cells are not formed during these intermediate stages (Inlow, 1979). The morphology of the transitional forms may be explained by assuming that the biochemical systems responsible for the morphology of both Y and M forms are expressed simultaneously during this stage. The Y structures become free by degradation of the hyphal segments. Budding occurs not only in the free Y cells, but also in the Y structures that are forming part of the transitional forms. The morphological events occurring during Y → M transition have also been studied with the light and electron microscopes (Carbonell, 1969; Inlow, 1979). Sequential observations on this transition (Inlow, 1979) showed that the first indication of hyphal formation occurs 2 hr after the change of temperature from 37 to 22°C. Initiation of Y → M transition is characterized by the formation of a mycelial bud (Figure 2) that elongates as the process continues and while new buds keep appearing. The elongated buds, which may be considered germ tubes, have larger diameters than typical hyphae (Carbonell, 1969). The morphology of the mycelial bud suggests that its formation originates as a consequence of deformation of the yeast cell rather than by initiation of apical growth. This suggestion is supported by the fact that during the first 18 hr of transition, true branching does not occur, although in some cases pseudobranching at the base of mycelial buds occurs (Figure 3). Possibly, branching is a specialized activity of true hyphae, whereas the pseudoramifications may be more related to the ability of yeast to give rise to

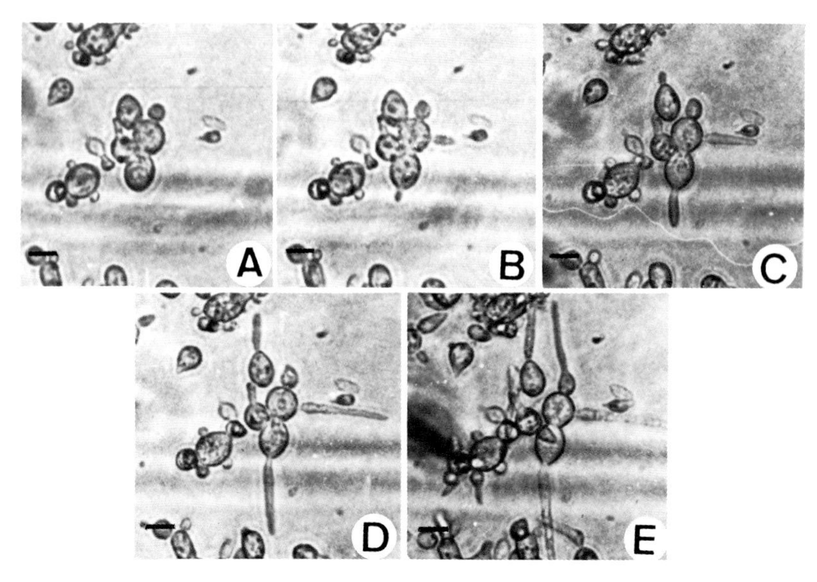

Figure 2. Transition of Y cells to the M form. A drop of a Y-cell suspension was placed on Mycosel agar (BBL) on a Neubauer chamber, covered with a coverslip, incubated in a moist chamber at 37°C for 18 hr, and transferred to 22°C. Times after incubation at 22°C: (A) 2 hr, (B) 4 hr, (C) 6 hr, (D) 8 hr, (E) 18 hr. Scale bar: 10 μm. (From F. San-Blas *et al.*, 1980.)

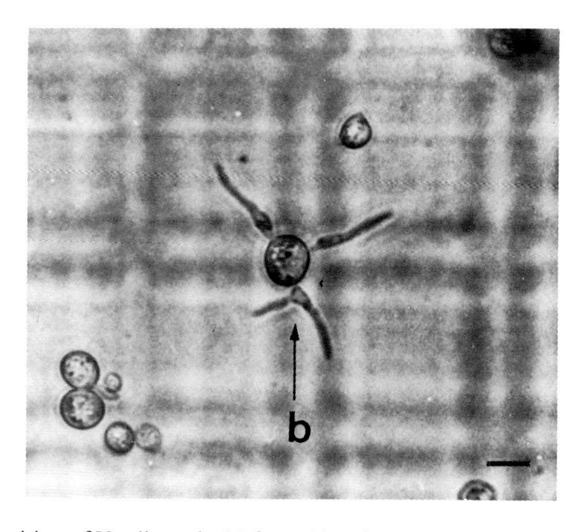

Figure 3. Transition of Y cells to the M form 6 hr after the change of temperature to 22°C. Notice elongation of the mycelial buds and pseudoramification in one of the buds (b). Scale bar: 10 μm. (From Inlow, 1979.)

several hyphae. The formation of the mycelial bud and its elongation could represent the first morphological step in transition, that is, the interval between the inhibition of growth of the Y form and the rearrangement of the cell system for initiation of mycelial growth.

When exponentially growing populations of the Y form of *P. brasiliensis* are induced to undergo M-form transition at 22°C, growth as measured by optical density stops for about 12 hr (Figure 4). During this interval, the morphological modifications shown in Figure 2 occur. Normal growth of the Y form resumes immediately if the cultures are shifted back to 37°C. This behavior suggests inhibition, rather than inactivation, of the enzymatic systems involved and represents a possible time lag in which the enzymes responsible for transition are either synthesized *de novo* or activated from zymogenic states preexisting in the Y cells.

3. BIOCHEMISTRY OF DIMORPHISM

One of the first studies done to relate dimorphism in *P. brasiliensis* to any biochemical function was carried out by Nickerson and Edwards

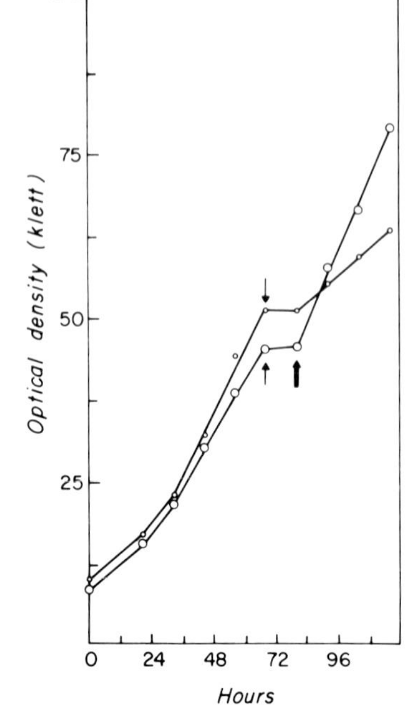

Figure 4. Influence of temperature on the growth of *P. brasiliensis*. Cultures in 0.2% glucose, 0.2% bactopeptone (Difco), and 10 μg/ml thiamine-HC1 were incubated at 37°C on a reciprocating shaker for 72 hr. The temperature was then shifted to 22°C (light arrows). One of the cultures (small circles) was kept at this temperature, while the other (large circles) was shifted back (heavy arrow) to 37°C. (From F. San-Blas *et al.*, 1980.)

(1949). Their results showed a higher endogenous respiration in the Y form than in the M form and an exogenous glucose oxidation in yeasts not observed in mycelia. Because of the high endogenous respiration of both forms, comparative studies of glucose metabolism were not carried out. Kanetsuna and Carbonell (1966) used cell-free extracts to study the enzymes involved in the process of glycolysis, the citric acid cycle, and the hexose monophosphate shunt. Enzymes associated with these metabolic pathways (Table I) were identified in both the Y and the M form. However, their activities differed, being between 1.1 and 4.5 times higher in the Y form, except in the case of glucose-6-phosphate and malic dehydrogenases, which were higher in the mycelial phase. The latter enzyme was studied further to identify possible differences between yeast and mycelial enzymes (Kanetsuna, 1972). After partial purification, both Y and M malic dehydrogenases behaved similarly, having an optimum pH between 6.5 and 7.5, similar Michaelis constants (K_m for NADH: 2.5×10^{-5} M; K_m for oxaloacetate: 5.6×10^{-5} M), and the same sensitivity to inhibitors. The reported differences between yeast and mycelial enzymatic activities, though important as an explanation for the higher endogenous respiration of the Y-like form, did not provide a tool to furnish a hypothesis for explaining the thermal dimorphism exhibited by this fungus.

Biochemical studies of yeast and mycelial cell walls were carried out by Kanetsuna *et al.* (1969, 1972). Alkaline extraction of cell walls produced three fractions: an alkali-insoluble fraction 1, an alkali-soluble, acid-insoluble fraction 2, and an alkali- and acid-soluble fraction 3. Analyses of these fractions indicated that the main constituents in both phases were lipids, carbohydrates, and proteins (Table II) (Kanetsuna *et al.*, 1969).

Yeast lipids were analyzed in detail (Kanetsuna, 1972). Four fractions were obtained: acetone-soluble lipids, phosphatides, and two fractions of associated lipids. The main fatty acids were oleic, palmitic, and linoleic acids. The main phosphatides were phosphatidylcholine, phosphatidylethanolamine, phosphatidylserine, and phosphatidylinositol.

Protein levels in mycelial preparations, though variable, were consistently higher than in yeast preparations, the latter having a cysteine/cystine content 12 times lower (Kanetsuna *et al.*, 1969, 1972).

No significant differences are observed in the total hexose content in each phase (Table II). However, the nature of these polysaccharides is not the same in both. Glucosamine as chitin is found in both forms. Glucose in the yeast cell wall is the main neutral sugar in fractions 1 and 2 and polymerized as an alkali-soluble, α1-3-glucan (95%) and an alkali-insoluble β1-3-glucan (5%) (Kanetsuna *et al.*, 1969). Traces of galactose and mannose are found in fraction 3.

Table I
Specific Enzymatic Activities in *P. brasiliensis*

Enzyme	Y/M ratio
Aconitase	2.4
Aldolase	1.1
Enolase	1.9
Fumarase	1.6
Glucose-6-phosphate dehydrogenase	0.8
Glyceraldehyde-3-phosphate dehydrogenase	4.5
Hexokinase	1.5
Isocitrate dehydrogenase	2.1
Malic dehydrogenase	0.5
Phosphofructokinase	1.6
Phosphoglucoisomerase	1.2
Phosphoglucomutase	1.7
6-Phosphogluconate dehydrogenase	1.2
Phosphoglyceromutase	1.8
Phosphorylase	1.2
Pyruvate kinase	2.2
Succinic dehydrogenase	1.9

Table II
Chemical Analyses of *P. brasiliensis* Strain Pb9 Cell Walls[a]

	Percentages	
	Y form	M form
Cell wall		
Hexoses	38.4	37.9
Amino sugars	43.4	13.3
Amino acids	10.1	32.9
Lipids	11.0	7.9
Fraction 1 (alkali-insoluble)		
Percentage of fraction in cell wall	40.0	83.0
Hexoses	19.0	42.8
Amino sugars	44.0	25.1
Amino acids	20.6	18.2
Fraction 2 (alkali-soluble, acid-insoluble)		
Percentage of fraction in cell wall	45.0	0.4
Hexoses	100.0	—
Amino sugars	0.0	—
Amino acids	0.0	—
Fraction 3 (alkali- and acid-soluble)		
Percentage of fraction in cell wall	5.0	16.6
Hexoses	29.8	35.1
Amino sugars	1.0	0.5
Amino acids	31.7	21.4

[a]From Kanetsuna *et al.* (1969, 1972).

The main neutral hexose in the mycelial cell wall is also glucose, which is polymerized into a singly branched homopolysaccharide consisting predominantly of two β1-3-glucan chains joined through β1-6 linkages (Figure 5). Galactomannan in the mycelial cell wall was determined by methylation analysis to consist of a main chain of mannose linked through 1-6 linkages, to which galactofuranosyl residues are joined as nonreducing ends of the molecule (Figure 5) (Azuma *et al.,* 1974). Some glucose in undetermined positions was also detected in the galactomannan. Molar ratios for glucose/galactose/mannose were 1.0:12.3:16.5. From these results, Azume *et al.* (1974) concluded that *P. brasiliensis* galactomannan is similar to the galactomannans of *Blastomyces dermatitidis* and *Histoplasma capsulatum.* They also found that these polysaccharides are antigenic and induce delayed responses in hamsters and humans. These galactomannans show cross-reactivity due to similarities in their structures; therefore, their potential use in clinical diagnosis is seriously limited.

The use of radioactive precursors of DNA, RNA, and proteins to study the role of these macromolecules in the process of dimorphism in *P. brasiliensis* has shown that exogenous [^{3}H]thymidine is not incorporated into DNA by this fungus (F. San-Blas *et al.,* 1980). This result may suggest that *P. brasiliensis,* like some other fungi, lacks the enzyme thymidine kinase (Grivell and Jackson 1968). The incorporation of [^{3}H]leucine into proteins in *P. brasiliensis* lacks reproducibility, whereas [^{3}H]uridine goes on for some 30 hr (Figure 6). This period of time corresponds to the duration of the exponential growth phase of the Y form. Immediately after the temperature is shifted from 37 to 22°C, uridine incorporation halts during the following 8 hr. This interval corresponds to the time in which mycelial buds are formed during the early stages of transition to the M form (see Figure 2). If one assumes that this fall in uridine incorporation is a consequence of the inhibition of RNA synthesis, it follows that initiation of the Y → M transition may not require *de novo* protein synthesis.

The role of macromolecular synthesis in the process of dimorphism in *P. brasiliensis* has also been studied with the use of inhibitors of these functions. Sublethal concentrations (up to 200 μg/ml) of mitomycin C, an inhibitor of DNA synthesis, do not affect dimorphism. Typical hyphae are produced by the Y form in the presence of this antibiotic. Due to the multinucleate nature of the Y form, it would be expected that new synthesis of DNA should not be necessary as a requisite for apical growth. Sublethal concentrations of inhibitors of proteins (pactomycin, 10^{-5} M; anisomycin, 0.5 μg/ml) and RNA synthesis (actinomycin D, 50 μg/ml) (Figure 6) affect the late stages of the morphogenesis of dimorphism in

α-Glucan

β-Glucan

Galactomannan

Figure 5. Cell-wall polysaccharides from *P. brasiliensis.* α1-3-Glucan and β1-3-glucan have sugars in the pyranose form; galactomannan is structured by mannopyranosyl and galactofuranosyl residues. (From Kanetsuna *et al.*, 1972.)

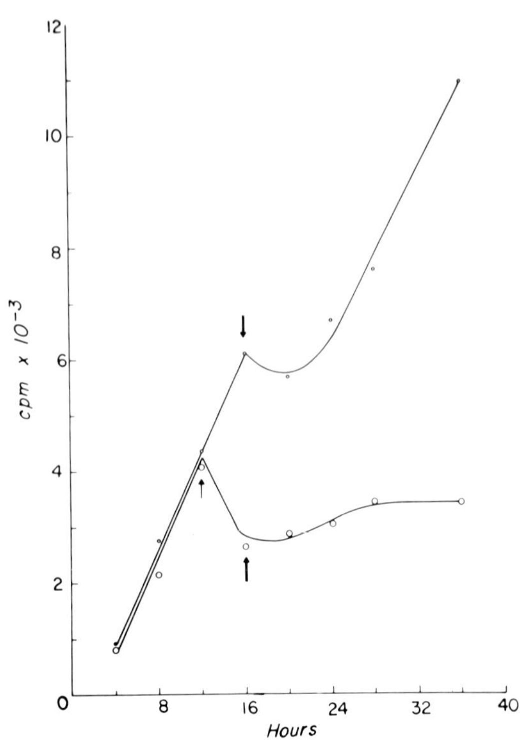

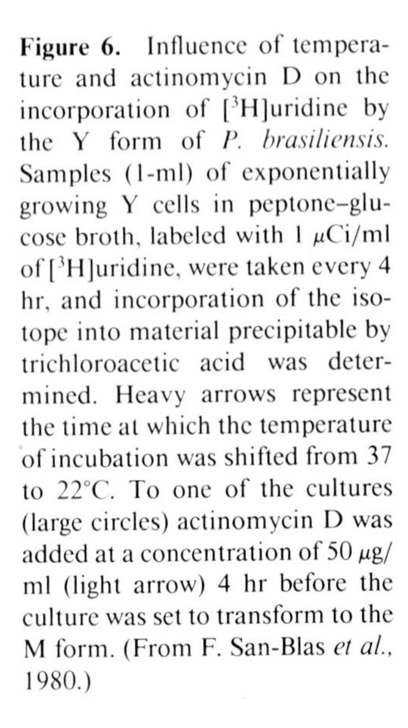

Figure 6. Influence of temperature and actinomycin D on the incorporation of [^{3}H]uridine by the Y form of *P. brasiliensis.* Samples (1-ml) of exponentially growing Y cells in peptone–glucose broth, labeled with 1 μCi/ml of [^{3}H]uridine, were taken every 4 hr, and incorporation of the isotope into material precipitable by trichloroacetic acid was determined. Heavy arrows represent the time at which the temperature of incubation was shifted from 37 to 22°C. To one of the cultures (large circles) actinomycin D was added at a concentration of 50 μg/ml (light arrow) 4 hr before the culture was set to transform to the M form. (From F. San-Blas *et al.*, 1980.)

either direction (Y ⇆ M). In the Y → M transition, the formation of typical hyphae is completely inhibited. However, even in the presence of these inhibitors, Y cells are able to elongate, producing pseudohyphae or elongated mycelial buds characteristic of the early stages of transition (Figure 7A). On the other hand, when typical hyphae are incubated at 37°C in the presence of any of these antibiotics, they swell and produce yeast structures, although the latter are not able to proceed further than this stage (Figure 7B). These observations strongly suggest that initiation of transition in both directions does not require RNA or protein synthesis and that the enzymatic system for the earlier steps of transition may be already present, though in an inactive form. Once the temperature changes, enzymatic activation proceeds, allowing for reassumption of RNA and protein syntheses. This, in turn, leads to complete transition to either typical hyphae or isolated multipolar budding yeast cells.

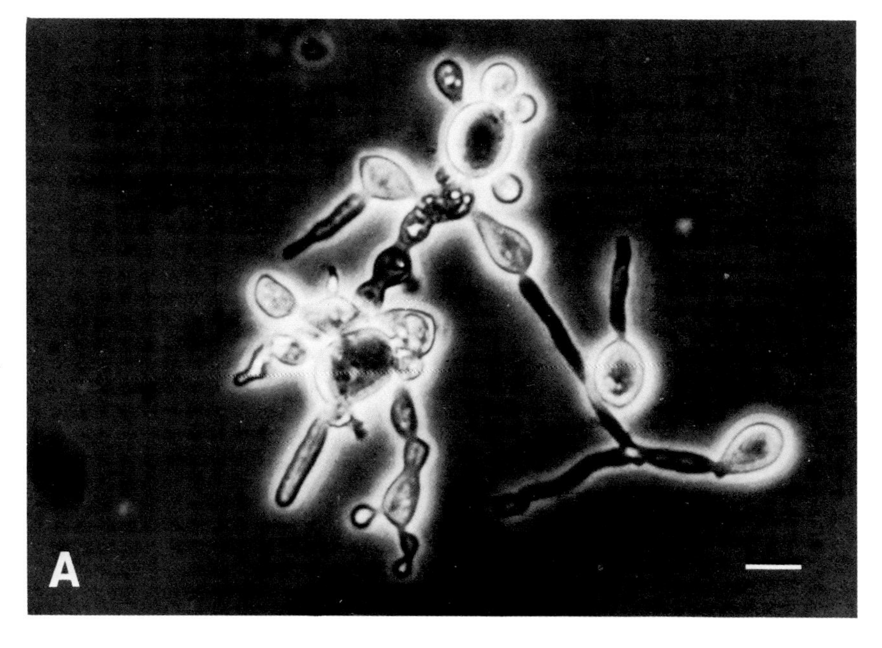

Figure 7. Effect of actinomycin D on the morphology of dimorphism of *P. brasiliensis*. Cultures of either M or Y form of *P. brasiliensis* in peptone–glucose broth containing 50 μg/ml of actinomycin D were set to transform at the permissive temperature. (A) Yeast cells transferred to 22°C; (B) hyphae transferred to 37°C. Photographs were taken 24 hr after the change of temperature. Similar morphological patterns are also produced in the presence of 10^{-5} M pactomycin or 0.5 μg/ml of anisomycin. Scale bars: 10 μm. (From Inlow, 1979.)

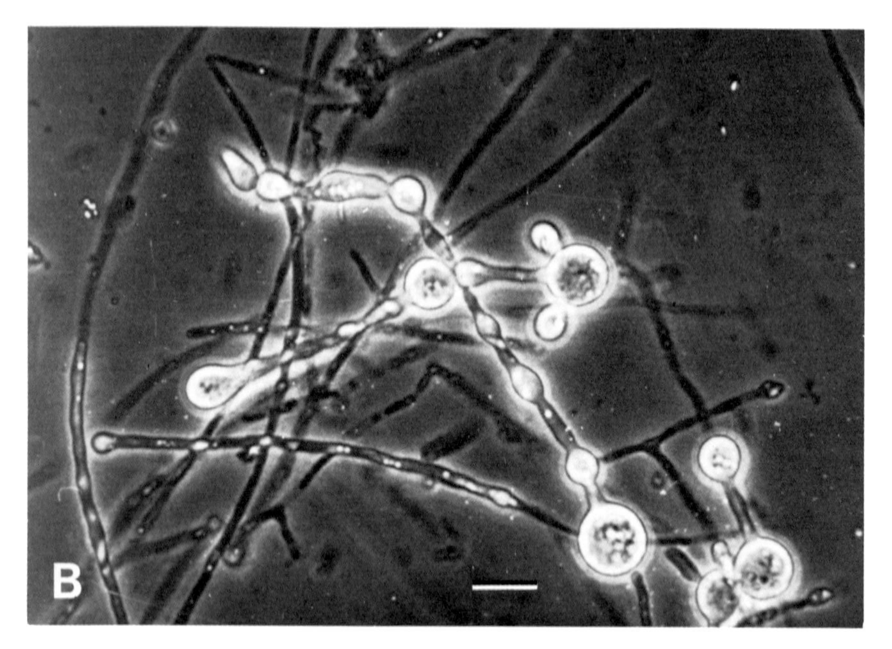

Figure 7. *(continued)*

4. CELL WALL AND DIMORPHISM

The role of the chemical composition of the fungal cell wall in the process of dimorphism has been stressed by several authors (Bartnicki-García, 1968; Cabib and Farkas, 1971). Kanetsuna *et al.* (1969, 1972) analyzed the chemical composition of *P. brasiliensis* cell walls and found that an α1-3-glucan was present in the Y form, whereas a β1-3-glucan replaced the former as the glucose polymer in the M form. These and other results led Kanetsuna *et al.* (1972) to propose a hypothesis to explain the morphological changes observed during transition from yeast to mycelium. This hypothesis was based on the assumption that a round shape is produced by a simultaneous synthesis of the whole cell wall and that a cylindrical shape is produced when the cell-wall synthesis is limited to the hyphal tip. Since the α1-3-glucan shapes the outer layer and chitin the inner layer in the yeast cell wall (Carbonell, 1969), these authors suggest that the low amounts of β-glucan may be localized in discrete islets in the yeast cell wall. Through an unknown mechanism that may involve the participation of β-glucanase and disulfide reductase, the yeast wall would soften around the β-glucan islets, allowing the formation of a bud.

At 37°C, the synthesis of a α-glucan and chitin is more active than that of β-glucan, and the high activity of disulfide reductase limits the frequency of disulfide links in the yeast-wall proteins. Both processes result in the formation of a daughter cell with the round shape characteristic of yeasts.

Conversely, at 22°C, the synthesis of α-glucan decreases and long β-glucan fibrils form in the budding places. In this way, the formation of a longitudinal shape is favored. Mycelial-wall proteins also have a higher degree of rigidity than yeast-wall proteins due to the higher amounts of disulfide bridges and low activity of disulfide reductase in the mycelial form. Therefore, a round shape is prevented. Mycelial proteins and chitin become interwoven with β-glucan fibrils, forming a single-layered cell wall that contrasts with the double-layered yeast wall in which α-glucan and chitin are distinctly separated (Kanetsuna *et al.,* 1972).

This hypothesis does not explain transition from hypha to yeast. Some evidence, though, suggested that yeasts of hyphal origin arise only in discrete parts of the hyphae (Kanetsuna *et al.,* 1972). Hence, during temperature increases from 22 to 37°C, the synthesis of β-glucan decreases while some cell-wall segments become softened by the combined action of β-glucanase and protein disulfide reductase. Simultaneously, the synthesis of α-glucan may start and a spherical yeast emerge.

Recently, Kanetsuna (1981) proposed a modification of his earlier hypothesis to explain phase transition. In it, the inhibition of α-glucan synthesis during temperature decreases results in the formation of a tunnel through which the M form extends. The linear fibrils of chitin, located in the inner layer of the yeast cell wall, are pressed between the tunnel and expanding cytoplasm and continue to grow in a linear fashion, allowing for the elongated shape characterisitic of hyphae. In this hypothesis, the role played by α-glucan is minimized in view of the evidence that α-glucan does not seem to be a permanent component of the yeast cell wall (G. San-Blas and F. San-Blas, 1977); therefore more permanent wall components such as chitin should play a more significant role in the process of dimorphism.

5. A MODEL OF DIMORPHISM

Although the hypotheses proposed by Kanetsuna (1972, 1981) hold true for the latest stages of dimorphism, i.e., the formation of typical hyphae or yeast cells, studies of dimorphic mutants suggest that qualitative changes in cell-wall composition do not seem to occur in the early stages of transition. For example, the mutant strain Pb229 is unable to complete the process of dimorphism or to grow at 37°C (Hallak *et al.*, 1982). When the M form of this strain is incubated at 37°C, some hyphal segments swell to produce both intercalary and terminal Y structures of variable sizes, some of which reach a diameter similar to that of mature Y wild-type cells (10–30 μm) (Figure 8). These Y structures, which resemble the transitional forms of the wild-type strain, are unable to separate and replicate autonomously. Further incubation results in total cellular deterioration (Figure 8C). The viability of the culture decreases to zero after 48 hr of incubation at 37°C. The process of dimorphism in this mutant is initated, as evidenced by the formation of Y structures, after the temperature is raised. Ultrastructurally, the cell wall of these Y structures formed at 37°C is indistinguishable from the cell wall of typical wild-type hyphae grown at 22°C. Chemical analysis reveals that the cell-wall glucan of these Y structures is polymerized as β1-3-glucan instead of the α1-3-glucan that is always reported as the main component in yeast walls of the wild-type strain of *P. brasiliensis.*

Observations with the electron microscope show that strain Pb229 induced to transform at 37°C is able to produce some morphologically typical Y cells by the same budding process as that described for the wild type (Figure 8D). However, since revertants to the wild- or a pseudowild-type strain were not recovered by continuous incubation of strain Pb229 at 37°C, it seems that the pseudorevertant Y cells observed with the electron microscope are unable to separate or multiply as single cells. The cell wall of the putative revertant Y cells is 150–200 nm thick and consists of an outer electron-thin layer and an inner electron-translucent layer. These aspects of size and structure are similar to those of the wild-type Y cells. Although chemical analysis of the cell wall of these revertents cannot be made by conventional methods, the ultrastructural morphology, the wall thickness, and the budding process that produced them suggest the presence of cell-wall α1-3-glucan.

The conclusions that may be derived from these observations in relation to dimorphism are twofold: (1) Contrary to an earlier report (Kanetsuna, 1972), α1-3-glucan does not seem to be responsible for the Y morphology of *P. brasiliensis.* (2) The early steps of M → Y transition, i.e., the swelling of hyphal segments to produce Y-like structures, does not require synthesis of α1-3-glucan, whereas this polysaccharide is essential for the late stage of M → Y transition, which involves the liberation and autonomous multiplication of the Y cells.

The mutation responsible for the phenotype shown by strain Pb229 must be associated with this late stage. Since this phenotype is expressed even in rich media where small molecules such as vitamins, amino acids, and bases are abundant, the mutation may result in a deficiency in the

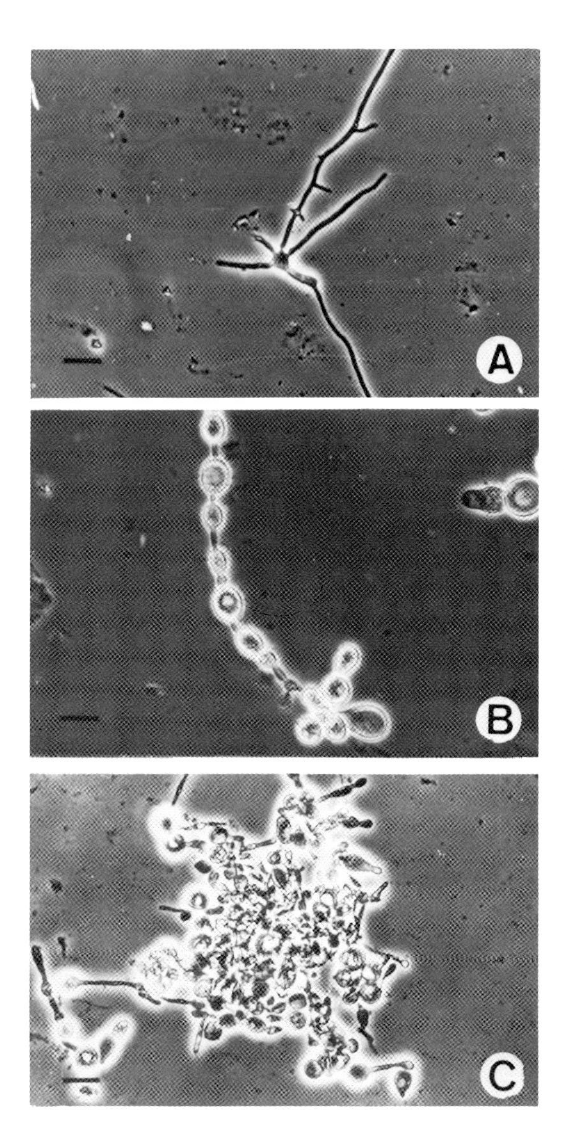

Figure 8. Light and electron micrographs of *P. brasiliensis* strain IVIC Pb229. (A) Mycelium grown at 23°C; (B) 24 hr at 37°C; (C) 72 hr at 37°C; (D) revertant Y cell originated by budding, still attached to the mother cell. Scale bars: (A–C) 10 μm; (D) 0.4 μm. (From F. San-Blas *et al.*, 1983.)

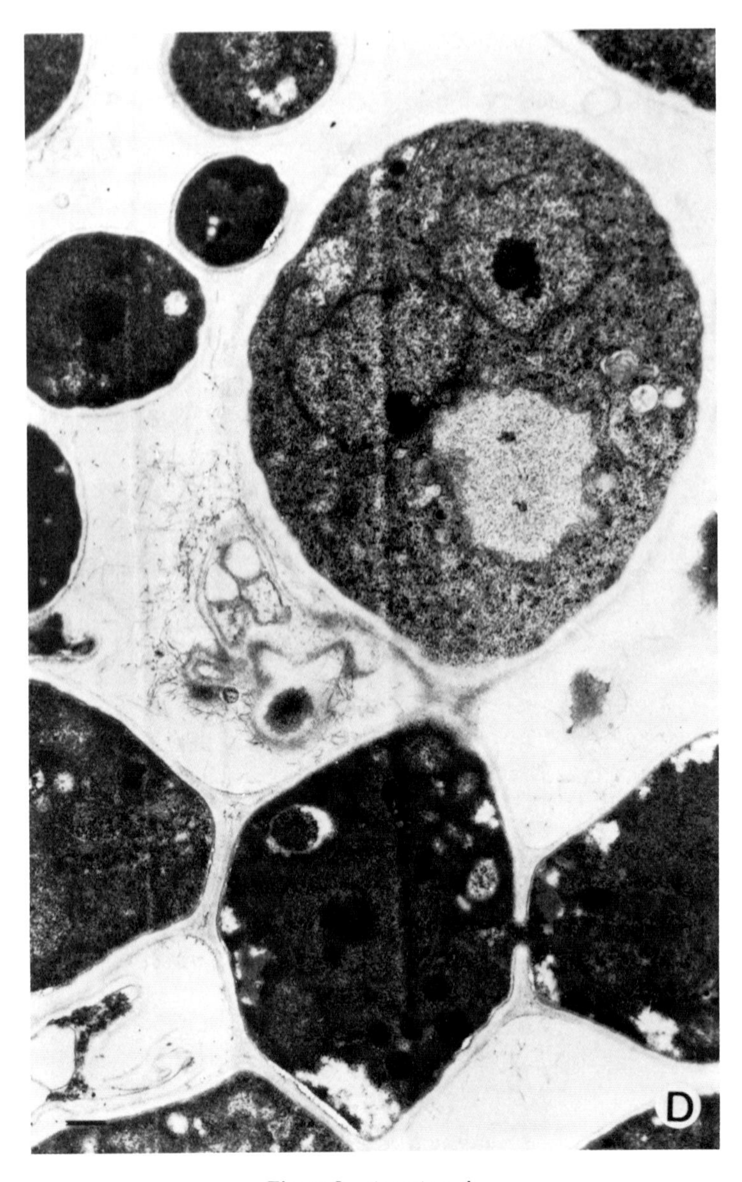

Figure 8. (*continued*)

synthesis of a macromolecule such as α1-3-glucan or in the uptake or incorporation of one or more of the small molecules. The inability of the mutant to grow at 37°C is not necessarily associated with its inability to synthesize this glucan. It is possible that the thermosensitive phenotype is a consequence of two or more different mutations.

Strain Pb267 of *P. brasiliensis* is another thermosensitive dimorphic mutant strain unable to grow at 37°C, while it grows at 22°C in a Y-like form (Figure 9A). Morphologically, the mutant Y-like cells are not as spherical as those observed in the wild-type strain grown at 37°C. Although some typical single ship's-wheel cells can be seen in the mutant strain at 22°C, most of the culture consists of oval isolated cells, many of which are able to produce short and wide pseudohyphae. Ultrastructurally, these pseudohyphae differ from wild-type hyphae not only in length and width, but also in the thickness of the cell wall (Figure 9B). Since chemical analyses of the mutant cell walls are not yet available, it is not known whether the thermosensitive phenotype shown by this mutant is related to some deficiency in the synthesis of a cell-wall component. The ability of this mutant to produce the pseudohyphae, even when unable to transform to the M form, supports the assumption that Y cells carry the enzymatic capabilities to elongage and initiate transition to the M form.

On the basis of the new accumulated data, we offer a modification of the models proposed by Kanetsuna *et al.* (1972) and Kanetsuna (1981) for the thermal dimorphism of *P. brasiliensis.* This new model (Figure 10) is also based on the assumption that a spherical form is produced by the simultaneous synthesis of the entire cell wall and that a cylindrical form is produced by synthesis in the apical region (Kanetsuna *et al.,* 1972). When Y cells are induced to form the mycelium, the synthesis of new RNA and proteins, as well as growth, stops for about 8 hr; the synthesis of α1-3-glucan decreases and mycelial buds are produced by the Y cells. At this early stage of transition, β1-3-glucan will not be synthesized unless the enzyme responsible for the synthesis of α1-3-glucan represents an allosteric enzymatic system that may change its quaternary structure as a result of a change in temperature. This gives the system the ability to synthesize β1-3-glucan. Alternatively, it may provide to activators or repressors the ability to modify the specificity of this glucan-synthesizing system.

The formation of the mycelial bud may occur as assumed by Kanetsuna *et al.* (1972). The β1-3-glucan present in the Y cell may exist as islets in the cell wall. Through the possible actions of the β-glucanase (a proposed constitutive enzyme in both the Y and the M form of *P. brasiliensis*) and protein disulfide reductase, a loss of rigidity at some of the islets

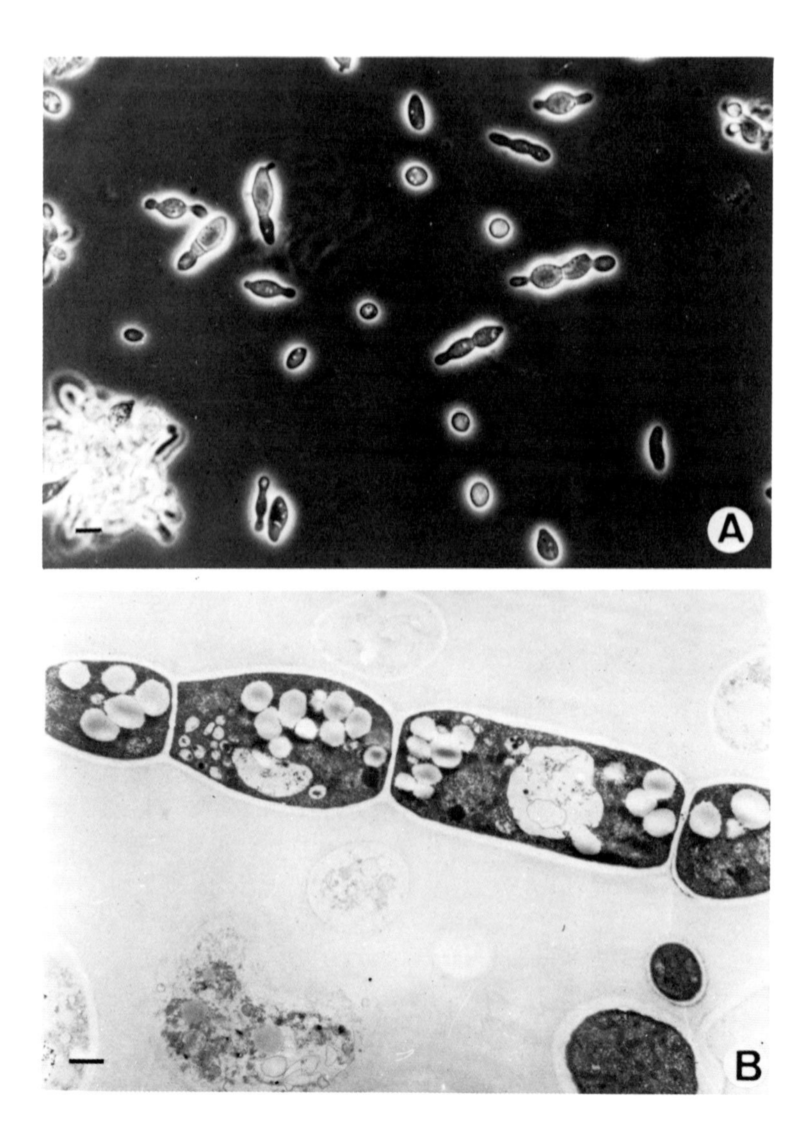

Figure 9. Light and electron micrographs of *P. brasiliensis* strain IVIC Pb267. (A) Culture grown at 23°C; (B) pseudohyphae. Scale bars: (A) 10 μm; (B) 1.25 μm.

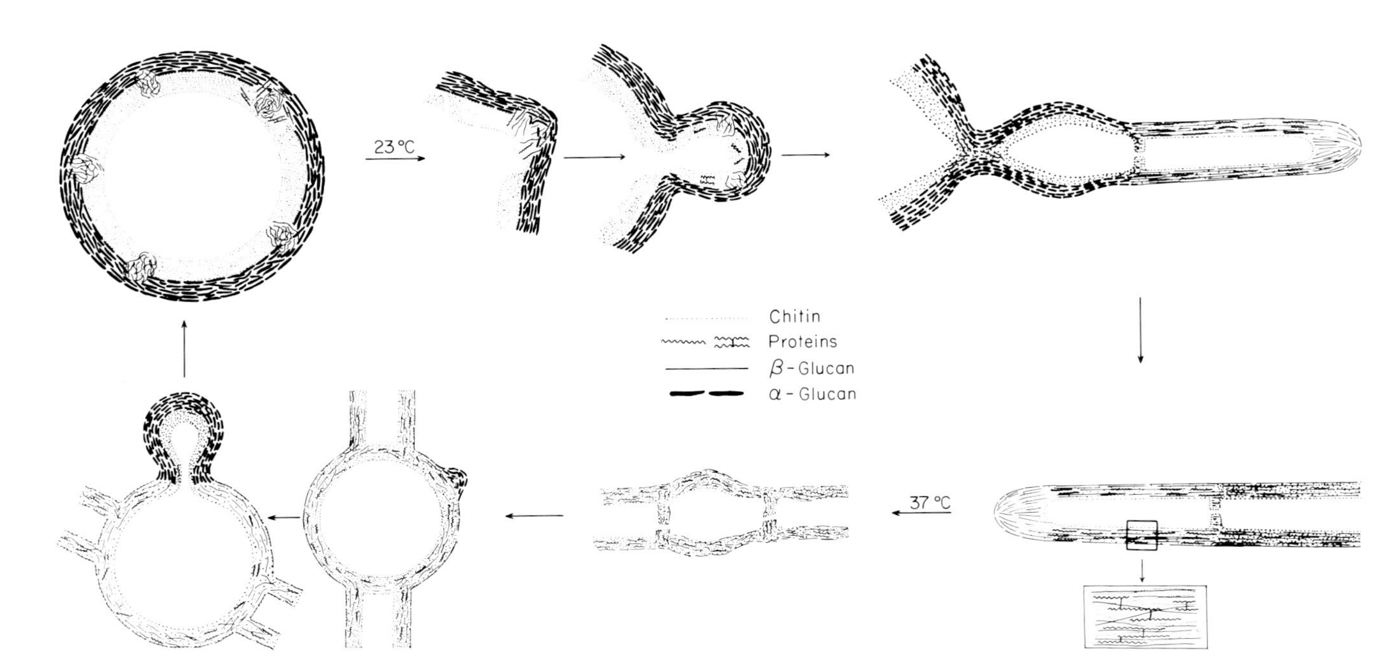

Figure 10. Hypothesis for the dimorphism of *P. brasiliensis*. (Modified from Kanetsuna *et al.*, 1972.)

in the wall may occur. The decrease in the rate of synthesis of α1-3-glucan and the internal pressure on the softened cell wall may then initiate the bud, the cell wall of which would at this initial stage of dimorphism still be made of α1-3-glucan and chitin (Figure 10). It is assumed that at this stage there would be no apical growth and that elongation of the mycelial bud would still be under the control of the Y cell. Later on, when synthesis of new proteins resumes, β1-3-glucan would be synthesized and apical growth resulting in the building of typical hyphae would proceed as suggested by Kanetsuna *et al.* (1972.)

The initiation of transition from the M form to the Y form also proceeds in the absence of RNA and protein synthesis. By an unknown mechanism induced by an increase in temperature, there is a decrease in the synthesis of β1-3-glucan (Kanetsuna *et al.*, 1972), which breaks the equilibrium between the synthesis of this polysaccharide and its degradation by β-glucanase. The cell wall softens and the internal pressure brings about a swelling of the interseptal space, initiating the formation of a yeast structure. The swelling of adjacent interseptal spaces in the hyphae creates chains of Y structures, forming transitional forms. At this stage of M $\rightarrow$ Y development, there is no synthesis of α1-3-glucan, which, as suggested by the behavior of the mutants described, seems to be required in the budding of these Y structures and, later on, in the formation and multiplication of typical yeast cells.

6. REGULATION OF GLUCAN SYNTHESIS IN *Paracoccidioides brasiliensis* CELL WALLS

To obtain more information on the mechanisms leading to the synthesis of polysaccharides prior to their localization in the cell wall, we have studied the *in vitro* synthesis of glucans of *P. brasiliensis* (G. San-Blas, 1979). Particulate preparations were obtained by centrifugation at 60,000*g* of wall-free-cytoplasmic extracts from strains Pb9 and Pb73. With both strains, yeast preparations were able to synthesize glucan from UDP-[^{3}H]glucose more efficiently at 37 than at 23°C (Figure 11). Other sugar nucleotides such as ADP-[^{14}C]glucose or GDP-[^{14}C]glucose were ineffective as precursors.

Particulate preparations obtained from stable mycelial cultures (i.e., either cultures older than 18 days after transition from the Y form or cultures maintained in the M form) were able to synthesize glucan from UDP-glucose more actively at 23 than at 37°C. The reverse was true for preparations obtained from yeast cultures undergoing transition to mycelia for less than 8 days (G. San-Blas, 1979). We may assume that the enzy-

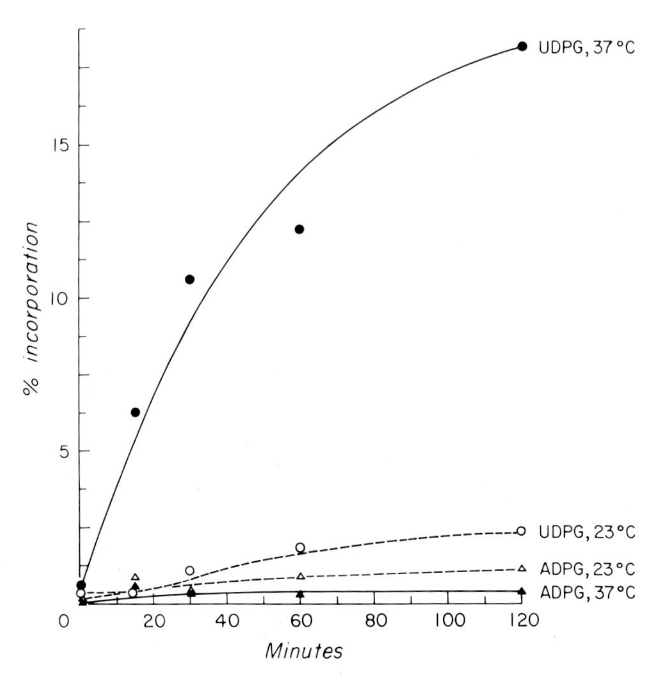

Figure 11. Incubation of particulate preparations from the Y form of *P. brasiliensis* with either UDP-[^{3}H]glucose or ADP-[^{14}C]glucose at different temperatures. (From G. San-Blas, 1979.)

matic system of the yeast glucan synthetase is still active after several days of initiation of transition and that its activity decreases progressively. Eventually, the activity is replaced by a glucan synthetase with a temperature optimum of 23°C, as expected for stable cultures of the M form. Though particulate preparations from both strains were as described above, preparations from strain Pb9 were 5–10 times less active in incorporating glucose into glucan than the corresponding preparations from strain Pb73 (F. San-Blas and G. San-Blas, unpublished results). This result could be interpreted as a consequence of either a less active enzyme or proportionally lower amounts of enzyme in the total protein content of the particulate preparation from strain Pb9.

Other differences between yeast and mycelial glucan synthetases concern the cationic requirements in both cases (G. San-Blas, 1979). The best stimulating cations for the yeast system (Table III) were $Ca^{2+} > Mg^{2+} > Fe^{2+} > Fe^{3+}$, at certain concentrations. Fe^{2+} and Fe^{3+}, at concentrations higher than 2 and 0.5 mM, respectively, and Zn^{2+} at any concentration, were inhibitory. With mycelial preparations, the stimulatory or inhibi-

Table III
Effect of Ions on Incorporation of Radioactivity into Glucan from UDP-[^{3}H]Glucose with Particulate Preparations of *P. brasiliensis*, Y form[a]

Concentration (mM)	Incorporation (%)					
	Mn^{2+}	Mg^{2+}	Fe^{2+}	Fe^{3+}	Ca^{2+}	Zn^{2+}
0.0	100.0	100.0	100.0	100.0	100.0	100.0
0.5	106.1	304.8	190.6	115.2	154.8	82.3
1.0	169.2	276.7	132.5	87.8	203.2	54.9
1.5	238.5	270.8	108.8	20.8	219.4	45.3
2.0	130.2	204.2	88.8	18.1	267.7	32.5
2.5	111.0	129.2	37.8	14.2	345.2	26.3

[a]From G. San-Blas (1979).

tory capacity of cations depended on the temperature at which the experiment was performed. At 23°C (Table IV), the stimulation followed the sequence $Fe^{3+} > Fe^{2+} > Mg^{2+}$. On the other hand, Zn^{2+} was inhibitory, although a slight stimulation was produced at 0.5 mM. The best stimulator of the reaction in yeasts was Ca^{2+}, which in turn did not influence the reaction in mycelial fractions at any temperature. However, Mn^{2+} was inhibitory in mycelia. At 37°C and at low concentrations (results not shown), the stimulation of incorporation in mycelial preparations was as follows: $Zn^{2+} > Fe^{3+} > Fe^{2+}$. However, at higher concentrations, these cations inhibited the process markedly. Also, Mg^{2+} and Mn^{2+} were weak inhibitors. EDTA was able to stimulate incorporation of glucose into glucan in yeast preparations (167–187% of controls) while inhibiting the

Table IV
Effect of Ions on Incorporation of Radioactivity into Glucan from UDP-[^{3}H]Glucose at 23°C with Particulate Prepations of *P. brasiliensis*, M Form[a]

Concentration (mM)	Incorporation (%)					
	Mn^{2+}	Mg^{3+}	Fe^{2+}	Fe^{3+}	Ca^{2+}	Zn^{2+}
0.0	100.0	100.0	100.0	100.0	100.0	100.0
0.5	97.9	107.1	151.2	162.1	98.6	119.3
1.0	89.7	110.7	152.2	210.9	95.1	95.5
1.5	85.2	114.3	140.1	187.5	93.5	63.3
2.0	74.8	121.5	130.6	147.2	91.3	59.3
2.5	72.7	134.0	22.9	22.7	96.6	4.9

[a]From G. San-Blas (1979).

same reaction in mycelia (75–84% of controls). This fact may be linked to a chelating effect on Fe^{2+} and Zn^{2+} ions, which inhibit the incorporation reaction in yeasts and stimulate it in mycelia.

A K_m of $1.25–2.00 \times 10^{-7}$ M for UDP-glucose was estimated for the glucan synthetase from yeastlike preparations. In mycelial fractions, this value ranged between 4.54 and 8.06×10^{-6} M. These low K_m's suggest a higher affinity for the substrate than other glycan synthetase systems as indicated by the K_m of 7.2×10^{-5} M for GDP-mannose in the synthesis of yeast mannan (Elorza *et al.*, 1977) and that for some chitin synthetases, i.e., 2.0×10^{-2} M for glucosamine in *Aspergillus flavus* (López-Romero and Ruiz-Herrera, 1976), $6–9 \times 10^{-3}$ M in *Saccharomyces carlbergensis* (Keller and Cabib, 1971), 1.58×10^{-3} M in *Aspergillus fumigatus* (Archer, 1977), and 5.0×10^{-4} M in *Mucor rouxii* (Ruiz-Herrera *et al.*, 1977).

The possibility that cytoplasmic factors may be operating as regulators in glucan synthesis is under study. Preliminary results suggest the possibility that the mycelial cytosol may contain factors that depress the activity of glucan synthetases at 23°C and that the yeast cytosol contains factors to depress the same activity at 37°C. This aspect of glucan regulation remains a matter for further studies.

Enzymatic degradation of synthesized glucans indicated that laminarinase (a β1-3-glucanase) digested between 83.2 and 95.0% of the yeast reaction product and between 77.4 and 84.4% of the mycelial product, whereas very little, if any, was hydrolyzed with either α1-3-glucanase or α-amylase (Figure 12). This result is somewhat unexpected, since it is known that the yeast cell wall of *P. brasiliensis* contains 95% of its glucan as α1-3-glucan (Kanetsuna and Carbonell, 1970) and also that synthesis of this polysaccharide occurs *in vivo* in this fungus (Kanetsuna *et al.*, 1972). Explanations for this apparent inability of yeast particulate preparations to synthesize α-glucan are not yet available. The possibility of sugar nucleotides other than UDP-glucose and the participation of dolichol intermediates in the reaction have been ruled out (G. San-Blas, 1979; F. San-Blas and G. San-Blas, unpublished results). Another possibility under study is that two glucan synthetases exist, one of them (α-glucan synthetase) being inactivated during the preparation procedure. The possibility that the cytoplasmic factors mentioned briefly above may be depressing β-glucan synthesis in favor of a α-glucan synthesis is also under consideration.

A tool to study biochemical processes is the use of antibiotics that block a given reaction. A few antibiotics have been reported that inhibit the synthesis of fungal cell-wall components. One is papulacandin B, an antibiotic produced by the deuteromycete *Papularia sphaerosperma.* It

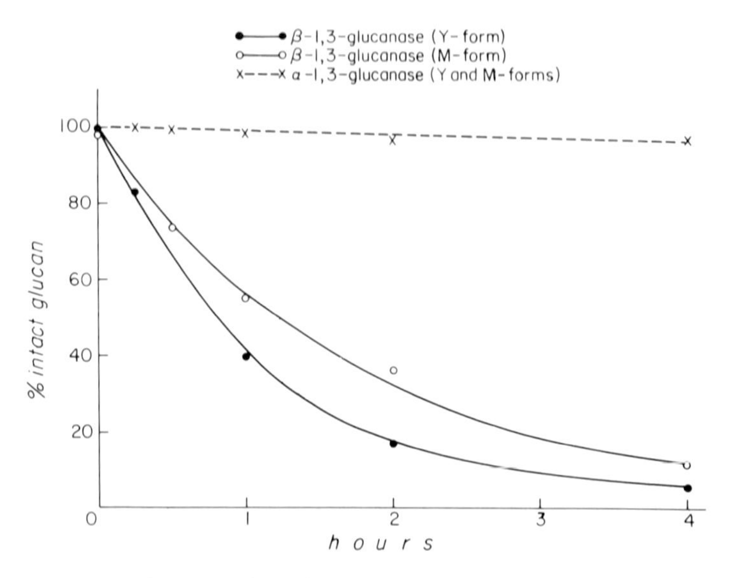

Figure 12. Enzymatic degradation of reaction products after incubation of particulate preparation with UDP-[^{3}H]glucose. (●——●) Yeast product digested with β1-3-glucanase; (○——○) mycelial product digested with β1-3-glucanase; (×----×) either yeast or mycelial product digested with α1-3-glucanase. (From G. San-Blas, 1979.)

has been reported as specific against yeasts, though inactive against filamentous fungi, bacteria, and protozoa (Traxler *et al.,* 1977). Its effect against *Saccharomyces cerevisiae* and *Candida albicans* is related to the selective inhibition of the synthesis of cell-wall glucan, which in turn provokes cell lysis by lack of a rigid support for the cytoplasmic material. *In vivo,* this antibiotic affects the M form of *P. brasiliensis* with the production of yeastlike structures at 23°C (Figure 13) (Dávila and San-Blas, unpublished results). At the same time, Y → M transition proceeds only to an incipient state (Figure 13), whereas M → Y transition is not affected. Although papulacandin B acts as an inhibitor of the glucan synthetase systems of *S. cerevisiae* (Baguley *et al.,* 1979) and *C. albicans* (Traxler *et al.,* 1977), this antibiotic is not able to block glucan synthesis *in vitro* in *P. brasiliensis* (Dávila and San-Blas, unpublished results). Whether this lack of inhibition is due to inhibition of β-glucan synthesis in favor of a α-glucan synthesis or to an actual failure to inhibit the glucan synthetase system in *P. brasiliensis* remains to be elucidated.

The main limitation of these studies resides in the fact that characterization of the enzyme was performed with crude membrane preparations. A better understanding of the biochemistry of these enzymes may

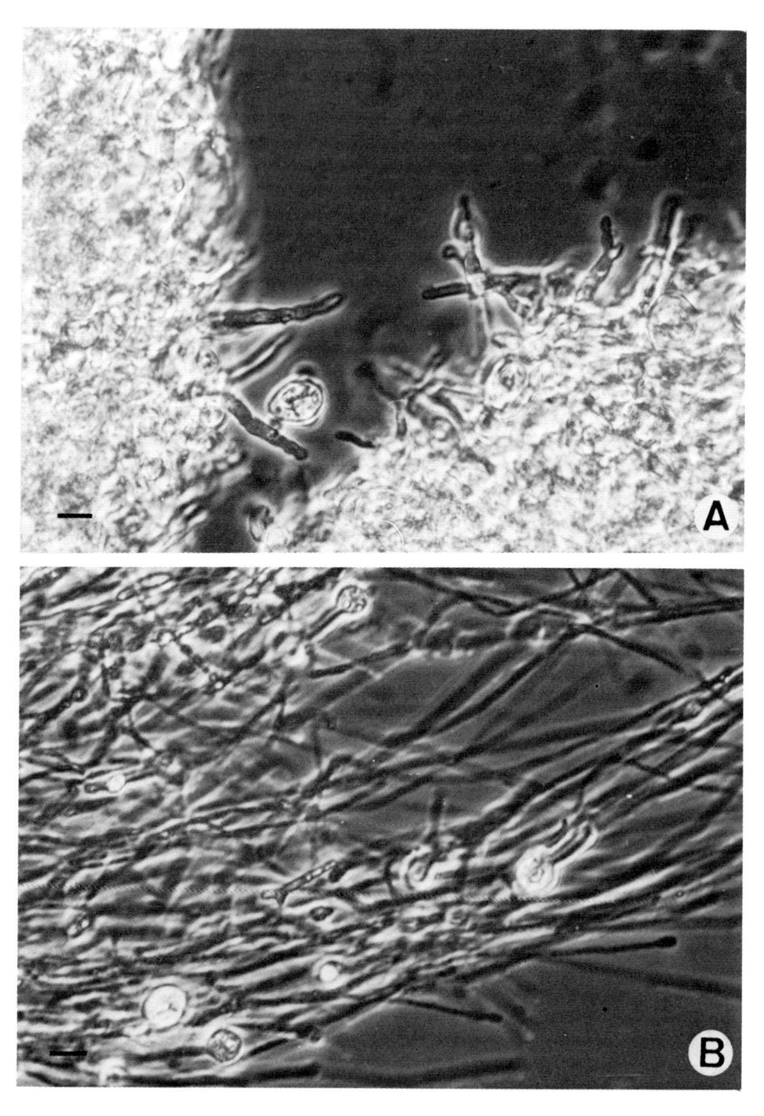

Figure 13. Effect of papulacandin B (5 μg/ml) on *P. brasiliensis*. (A) Y → M transition; (B) mycelia grown for 4 days. Scale bars: (A and B) 1 μm. (Dávila and San-Blas, unpublished results.)

be obtained if solubility is achieved. To this effect, separation of *P. brasiliensis* glucan synthetase from membrane fractions was attempted using detergents. These agents are frequently used to solubilize membrane-bound enzymes in an active form by disrupting the membranes where they reside. The results, particularly those with Triton X-100, indicated that yeast-membrane preparations treated with detergents for 1 hr at 4°C (Table V) increased the activity of glucan synthetase in the insoluble fraction without rendering the enzyme more soluble. When the detergents were used for more than 40 hr at −20°C (results not shown), the glucan synthetase was partially solubilized. This was particularly true when Brij 58 and Lubrol WX were used. Also, a higher enzymatic activity was observed in most of the insoluble fractions treated with detergents.

Conversely, none of the detergents tested (with the exception of Triton 770) released the glucan synthetase from mycelial preparations in a soluble form, although most of the detergents made the membrane preparations more active when compared to controls (Table V). These results indicate that glucan synthetases in *P. brasiliensis* have different characteristics in both forms of the fungus. Also, the different behaviors of the synthetases with the detergents may indicate that the lipid compositions of yeast and mycelial membranes of *P. brasiliensis* are different.

Table V
Extraction of Membrane Preparations from *P. brasiliensis* Strain Pb73

	Incorporation of [^{3}H]glucose into glucan (%)			
	Yeast phase		Mycelial phase	
Detergent (at 1% wt./vol.)	Insoluble fraction	Soluble fraction	Insoluble fraction	Soluble fraction
Brij 35	9.6	0.1	15.0	0.1
Brij 58	7.1	0.6	18.6	0.4
Lubrol WX	6.3	0.2	16.2	0.3
Nonidet P40	4.5	0.6	15.4	0.5
Tergitol 15-S-9	4.1	0.4	12.7	1.0
Tergitol NP10	4.3	0.3	12.5	1.3
Triton 770	19.3	0.2	19.8	2.3
Triton WR-1339	5.7	0.1	6.9	0.2
Triton X-100	5.8	0.1	13.0	0.4
Tween 20	5.6	0.8	10.4	0.8
Tween 40	6.6	0.4	9.9	0.2
Tween 60	10.6	0.3	11.0	0.2
Tween 80	7.0	0.2	11.0	0.2
Control	5.1	0.03	9.3	0.1

7. CONCLUSIONS

The pleomorphism characteristic of *P. brasiliensis,* the asynchrony of dimorphism, and, more important, the absence of a sexual phase in *P. brasiliensis* make it difficult to study the mechanism involved in the process of dimorphism. DNA determinations and other lines of research that would indicate whether *P. brasiliensis* is a haploid or polyploid organism have not been done. The multinucleate nature of *P. brasiliensis* may be responsible for the low rate of mutant induction and the instability of the mutant phenotypes obtained; to obtain stable mutants, all allelic genes for a given function must be simultaneously mutagenized. The absence of spores suitable for mutagenesis limits the application of this technique to the Y form, the multinucleate nature of which diminishes the efficiency of the technique. Despite these difficulties, it has been possible to isolate some apparently stable mutants affected in dimorphism. The understanding of the deficiencies affecting the mutants described herein, as well as others that are under study, will no doubt give more information on and a better understanding of the mechanisms involved in the process of dimorphism.

Enough evidence strongly supports a relationship between the process of biosynthesis and turnover of cell-wall constituents with dimorphism in *P. brasiliensis.* The isolation and study of the properties of cell-wall enzymatic systems, together with the study of mutants affected in these sytems, will help in understanding this process. The model proposed by Kanetsuna *et al.* (1972) to explain dimorphism in *P. brasiliensis,* although elegant, does not take into consideration the possible role played by α1-3-glucanase in the softening of cell walls of the yeast phase. The reason for this omission was the failure to detect this enzyme in cultures and in cell extracts of *P. brasiliensis.* Although its presence has been reported (Flores-Carreón *et al.,* 1979), reproducibility of these results has not been achieved. Since the survival of *P. brasiliensis* in tissue seems to depend on the presence of α1-3-glucan in the outermost layer of the yeast cell wall (G. San-Blas and F. San-Blas, 1977), the expression of α1-3-glucanase must be strictly controlled. However, we have recently isolated some mutant strains of *P. brasiliensis* that seem to express this enzyme in a derepressed state. On the other hand, it is possible to induce the expression of α-glucanase in the wild type of *P. brasiliensis* by using α1-3-glucan as the only source of carbon, although in this case the expression of the enzyme is lethal to the fungus. It is possible to assume that α1-3-glucanase plays a role in the dimorphism of *P. brasiliensis* and that an approach to the understanding of this process must include the study of the regulation and properties of this and other enzymes involved in the degradation and synthesis of cell-wall components.

REFERENCES

Archer, D. B., 1977, Chitin biosynthesis in protoplast fractions of *Aspergillus fumigatus*, *Biochem. J.* **164**:653–658.

Azuma, I., Kanetsuna, F., Tanaka, Y., Yammamura, Y., and Carbonell, L. M., 1974, Chemical and immunological properties of galactomannans obtained from *Histoplasma duboisii*, *Histoplasma capsulatum*, *Paracoccidiodes brasiliensis*, and *Blastomyces dermatitidis*, *Mycopathol. Mycol. Appl.* **54**:111–125.

Baguley, B., Rommele, G., Gruner, J., and Wehrli, W., 1979, Papulacandin B: An inhibitor of glucan synthesis in yeast spheroplasts, *Eur. J. Biochem.* **97**:345–351.

Bartnicki-García, S., 1968, Cell wall chemistry, morphogenesis, and taxonomy of fungi, *Annu. Rev. Microbiol.* **22**:87–108.

Cabib, E., and Farkas, V., 1971, The control of morphogenesis: An enzymatic mechanism for the initiation of septum formation in yeast, *Proc. Natl. Acad. Sci. U.S.A.* **68**:2052–2056.

Carbonell, L. M., 1969, Ultrastructure of dimorphic transformation in *Paracoccidioides brasiliensis*, *J. Bacteriol.* **100**:1076–1082.

Carbonell, L. M., 1972, Ultrastructure of *Paracoccidioides brasiliensis* in culture, in: *Paracoccidioidomycosis* (Pan American Health Organization, eds. Sci. Publ. No. 254), Proceedings of the First Pan American Symposium on Paracoccidioidomycosis, 1971, Medellín, Colombia, pp. 21–28.

Carbonell, L. M., and Pollak, L., 1968, Ultrastructura del *Paracoccidioides brasiliensis* en cultivos de la fase levaduriforme, *Mycopathol. Mycol. Appl.* **19**:184–204.

Carbonell, L. M., and Rodríguez, J., 1968, Mycelial phase of *Paracoccidioides brasiliensis* and *Blastomyces dermatitidis:* An electron microscope study, *J. Bacteriol.* **96**:533–543.

Ciferri, R., and Redaelli, P., 1936, *Paracoccidioidaceae*, n. fam. instuita per l'agente del granuloma paracoccidioide, *Biol. Ist. Sieroter. Milanese* **15**:97–102.

Elorza, M. V., Larriba, G., Villanueva, J. R., and Sentandreu, R., 1977, Biosynthesis of the yeast cell wall: Selective assays and regulation of some mannosyl transferase activities, *Antonie van Leeuwenhoek J. Microbiol. Serol.* **43**:129–142.

Emmons, C. W., 1959, Fungus nuclei in the diagnosis of mycoses, *Mycologia* **51**:227–236.

Flores-Carreón, A., Gomez-Villanueva, A., and San-Blas, G., 1979, β-1,3-Glucanase and dimorphism in *Paracoccidioides brasiliensis*, *Antonie van Leeuwenhoek J. Microbiol. Serol.* **45**:265–274.

Furtado, J. S., de Brito, T., and Freymuller, E., 1967, The structure and reproduction of *Paracoccidioides brasiliensis* in human tissue, *Sabouraudia* **5**:226–229.

Grivell, A., and Jackson, J., 1968, Thymidine kinase: Evidence for its absence from *Neurospora crassa* and some other micro-organisms, and the relevance of this to the specific labelling of deoxyribonucleic acid, *J. Gen. Microbiol.* **54**:307–317.

Hallak, J., San-Blas, F., and San-Blas, G., 1982, Isolation and wall analysis of dimorphic mutants of *Paracoccidioides brasiliensis*, *Sabouraudia* **20**:51–62.

Inlow, D., 1979, Estudios sobre el dimorfismo en *Paracoccidioides brasiliensis*, Thesis Ms.Sc., IVIC, Caracas, Venezuela.

Kanetsuna, F., 1972, Biochemical characteristics of *Paracoccidioides brasiliensis*, in: *Para-*

coccidioidomycosis, Proceedings of the First Pan American Symposium on Paracoccidioidomycosis, 1971, Medellín, Colombia, pp. 31–37.

Kanetsuna, F., 1981, Ultrastructural studies on the dimorphism of *Paracoccidioides brasiliensis, Blastomyces dermatitidies,* and *Histoplasma capsulatum, Sabouraudia* **19:**275–286.

Kanetsuna, F., and Carbonell, L. M., 1966, Enzymes in glycolysis and the citric acid cycle in the yeast and mycelial forms of Paracoccidioides brasiliensis, J. Bacteriol. **92:**1315–1320.

Kanetsuna, F., and Carbonell, L. M., 1970, Cell wall glucans of the yeast and mycelial forms of *Paracoccidioides brasiliensis, J. Bacteriol.* **101:**675–680.

Kanetsuna, F., Carbonell, L. M., Morena, R. E., and Rodréguez, J., 1969, Cell wall composition of the yeast and mycelial forms of *Paracoccidiodes brasiliensis, J. Bacteriol.* **97:**1036–1041.

Kanetsuna, F., Carbonell, L. M., Azuma, I., and Yamamura, Y., 1972, Biochemical studies on thermal dimorphism of *Paracoccidioides brasiliensis, J. Bacteriol.* **110:**208–218.

Keller, F. A., and Cabib, E., 1971, Chitin and yeast budding: Properties of chitin synthetase from *Saccharomyces cerevisiae, J. Biol. Chem.* **246:**160–166.

López-Romero, E., and Ruiz-Herrera, J., 1976, Synthesis of chitin by particulate preparations from *Aspergillus flavus, Antonie van Leeuwenhoek J. Microbiol. Serol.* **42:**261–276.

Lutz, A., 1908, Una mycose pseudo-coccidica localizada na boca e observada no Brasil: Contribuicao ao conhecimento das hyphoblastomycoses americanas, *Brasil Med.* **22:**121–124, 141–144.

Negroni, P., 1931, Estudio micológico sobre cincuenta casos de micosis observados en Buenos Aires, M.D. Thesis, Prensa Universitaria, Buenos Aires, Argentina.

Nickerson, W., and Edwards, G., 1949, Studies on the physiological basis of morphogenesis in fungi, *J. Gen. Physiol.* **33:**41–55.

Restrepo, A., 1970, A reappraisal of the microscopical appearance of the mycelial phase of *Paracoccidioides brasiliensis, Sabouraudia* **8:**141–144.

Ruiz-Herrera, J., López-Romero, E., and Bartnicki-García, S., 1977, Properties of chitin synthetase in isiolated chitosomes from yeast cells of *Mucor rouxii, J. Biol. Chem.* **252:**3338–3343.

San-Blas, F., and Centeno, S., 1977, Isolation and preliminary characterization of auxotrophic and morphological mutants of the yeastlike form of *Paracoccidioides brasilien sis, J. Bacteriol.* **129:**138–144.

San Blas, F., San-Blas, G., and Inlow D., 1980, Dimorphism in *Paracoccidioides brasiliensis,* in: *Medical Mycology* (Hans-Jurgen Preusser, ed.), Proceedings of Mycological Symposium XII International Congress of Microbiology, Munich, 1978, Gustav Fischer Verlag, Stuttgart, pp. 23–28.

San-Blas, F., San-Blas, G., Hallak, J., and Merino, E., 1983, Ultrastructure and cell wall chemistry of a thermosensitive mutant of *Paracoccidioides brasiliensis, Curr. Microbiol.* **8:**85–88.

San-Blas, G., 1979, Biosynthesis of glucans by subcellular fractions of *Paracoccidioides brasiliensis, Expt. Mycol.* **3:**249–258.

San-Blas, G., and San Blas, F., 1977, *Paracoccidioides brasiliensis:* Cell wall structure and virulence, a review, *Mycopathologia* **62:**77–86.

Traxler, P. Gruner, J., and Auden, J. A., 1977, Papulacandins, a new family of antibiotics with antifungal activity, *J. Antibiot.* **30:**289–296.

Chapter 6

Sporothrix schenckii

Luiz R. Travassos

1. INTRODUCTION

Sporothrix schenckii Hektoen and Perkins (1900) is a dimorphic fungus that occasionally infects humans to cause sporotrichosis, a chronic, usually benign disease involving cutaneous and subcutaneous tissues, often with associated lymphangitis and lymph-node enlargement. Cases of extracutaneous sporotrichosis have been reported with increasing frequency (Wilson *et al.*, 1967; Lynch *et al.*, 1970), involving mucous membranes and viscera, musculoskeletal tissues, the eye, and the central nervous system (Lurie, 1971). Disseminated infection may follow a state of decreased immunological responsiveness. In endemic areas, individuals may be resistant to sporotrichosis or develop a localized cutaneous form. Clinical types and the histopathology of sporotrichosis were reviewed by Lurie (1971).

Since the progression of sporotrichosis depends chiefly on the host immunological response, considerable attention has been given to the cell-surface components of *S. schenckii* and their capacity to react with antibodies, elicit immediate and delayed-type hypersensitivity reactions, or act as immunopotentiating agents. Chemical structures and some antigenic determinants have been characterized in both morphological phases of *S. schenckii* (Travassos and Lloyd, 1980).

Dimorphism in *S. schenckii,* besides being a suitable model for studies on the correlation of morphogenesis and growth conditions, also pro-

Luiz R. Travassos • Department of Mycology, Paulista School of Medicine, São Paulo, SP 04023, Brazil.

vides a system for investigation of the relationships between a host and a pathogenic fungus undergoing morphological and biochemical changes *in vivo. In vitro* requirements for phase transitions in *S. schenckii,* as well as the ultrastructure and surface reactivity of forms arising *in vivo* and *in vitro,* have been studied. Results obtained are reviewed in this chapter.

The geographic distribution and epidemiology of sporotrichosis were reviewed by Lurie (1971) and Mackinnon (1970). Studies on the natural habitats of *S. schenckii* led to the isolation of dimorphic, morphologically related fungi that were classified as *Ceratocystis* spp. Mixed cultures of *S. schenckii* and *Ceratocystis* have also been obtained (Mackinnon *et al.,* 1969). Since a particular species of *Ceratocystis* could be the ascigerous form of *S. schenckii* (Kendrick and Carmichael, 1973), several studies centered on the identification of convergent properties of *S. schenckii* and one or more species of the ascomycete. The taxonomic relationships of the *S. schenckii–Ceratocystis* spp. fungal complex were discussed by Mariat (1977). Analyses of polysaccharides and DNA-hybridization studies were used to compare phenotypic and genotypic characteristics of *S. schenckii* and its presumed ascigerous states. Nuclear magnetic resonance (^{13}C) spectroscopy of *S. schenckii* heteropolymers contributed to the establishment of new signal assignments and to the application of this method in the recognition of several other microbial polysaccharide structures (Gorin, 1981).

This chapter includes recent investigations on *S. schenckii* dimorphism, a description of recognized structures and properties of different cell types in comparison with those of *Ceratocystis* spp., and the possible correlation between surface components and fungal virulence.

2. MORPHOLOGICAL PHASE TRANSITION

The free-living form of *S. schenckii* consists of a mycelium. Elements of the mycelial phase are hyphae and conidia. Conidia can detach from hyphae, thus becoming independent cells potentially able to germinate into new hyphal elements. Sporotrichosis arises from the traumatic introduction of hyphae or conidia or both into the host tissue. These forms occur naturally in soil or plants or even on nonsporotrichotic human skin (Iwatsu, 1980). Parasitic yeastlike cells develop at the sites of infection. Yeasts usually originate from hyphae, but there is also evidence for their formation directly from conidia. The yeast phase is formed depending on environmental conditions such as temperature or availability of certain nutrients. In some culture media at 28–30°C, all three cell types—hyphae, conidia, and yeast forms—may occur simultaneously and are readily recognized.

Conversion of hyphal elements into the yeast phase is an important step in the identification of *S. schenckii*. Growth on glucose–cysteine blood agar at 37°C or inoculation into animals or tissue culture favors the phase transition. When mycelial fragments are inoculated into the testes of mice, the purulent exudate that accumulates after 2–3 weeks contains yeast cells. Mycelial particles can also convert into yeast cells at 37°C and high CO_2 tension in cultured guinea pig peritoneal macrophages (Hempel and Goodman, 1975). The yeast phase can be maintained in brain–heart infusion at 35–37°C. Morphological phase transition is reversible. By adding penicillin to the purulent exudate from a human lesion, Gonzalez-Ochoa and Soto-Pacheco (1950) observed that growth of *S. schenckii* was stimulated and that gram-stained round or oval cells gradually changed into fusiform and bacillary forms that gave rise to septate hyphae and conidia.

Colonies of the mycelial phase of *S. schenckii* formed at 25°C are flat, moist, initially dirty white and coarsely tufted, then turning brown or black with wrinkled surfaces. Colonies of the yeast phase at 37°C are moist and cream-colored. Slide cultures of the mycelial phase on malt extract agar at 22–25°C show the typical conidial morphology of *Sporothrix*. A description of cell morphology *in vitro* and *in vivo* is given in Section 2.1.

The form-genus *Sporothrix* and the type form-species *S. schenckii* do not resemble *Sporotrichum aureum* Link, the lectotype form-species of the form-genus *Sporotrichum* (Carmichael, 1962). The variety *S. schenckii* var. *luriei* (Ajello and Kaplan, 1969) differs from the type form-species of *Sporothrix* by the unusual cell types formed *in vivo:* Hyaline, thick-walled yeast forms (12–18 by 14–23 μm) were observed along with the usual much smaller yeast cells. *Sporothrix curviconia* and *S. inflata* are morphologically and antigenically related to *S. schenckii* (Ishizaki *et al.*, 1979a,b).

2.1. *Sporothrix schenckii* Cell Types: *In Vitro* and *in Vivo* Morphology

In vitro slide cultures of *S. schenckii* at room temperature consist of hyaline, septate hyphae (diameter 1–2 μm) and oval, pyriform, or elongated hyaline conidia (1.5–3 by 3–6 μm). Conidia emerge singly or in groups on small denticles along hyphae (radulaspores) or on apical sympodia (sympodulospores). Primary sympodulospores may germinate to form one or more sporogenous cells (sympodulae). These cells may bear secondary sympodulospores. Primary conidia may also produce secondary conidia directly on short sterigmata (Taylor, 1970a). Pathogenic strains of *S. schenckii* form spherical or conical (triangular) pigmented conidia (diameter 2.4–3.7 μm) that have thick walls and are inserted on larger pedicels (Nicot and Mariat, 1973). Triangular spores were first observed by Brown *et al.* (1947). Taxonomically, the pigmented macrospores of *S. schenckii* are characteristic of the species (Mackinnon *et al.*, 1969).

The yeast phase of *S. schenckii,* which is generally obtained at 35–37°C, consists of fusiform and ovoid cells (2.5–5 by 3.5–6.5 μm) that multiply by single or multiple budding. Yeast forms emerge from the sides and tips of hyphae. Conidia usually germinate into short hyphae that may give rise, under appropriate conditions, to yeast forms. The latter can also arise by fragmentation of chains of oidia that form inside hyphae (Garrison *et al.,* 1975). With the use of Muir's stain (Bailey and Scott, 1966), the presence of a distinct capsular-slime layer about the ovoid cells of *S. schenckii* yeast phase was observed. A halo effect was also a consistent observation when yeast forms were analyzed by electron microscopy of glutaraldehyde–osmium–fixed preparations in agar (Lane *et al.,* 1969).

A complex morphology of *S. schenckii* is observed *in vivo,* with predominance of round or oval yeast forms that may become cigar-shaped as lesions increase in size. Few yeasts are present in organs with invasive micronodular lesions. Cigar-shaped cells multiply actively around large suppurative lesions. Tissue forms of *S. schenckii* observed by Fukushiro *et al.* (1965) were round, spherical, and oval. Elongated, fusiform, and half-moon-shaped cells were also reported. Single or budding yeast forms inside giant cells were also round or spherical.

In many cases of sporotrichosis, the conventional microscopic inspection of purulent secretions and tissue sections is not successful in detecting fungal cells. Observation of yeast forms *in vivo* is possible by immunofluorescence staining (Section 4.4) and also by peroxidase-linked antibodies. The latter method was used to locate *S. schenckii* forms in tissue sections fixed in formaldehyde and embedded in paraffin without trypsinization (Russell *et al.,* 1979). To enrich for yeast elements in exudates, a preincubation at 37°C overnight before preparing smears was recommended (Lurie, 1963). Clusters of 100 or more fungal cells were observed. A colloidal iron capture method with safranin counterstaining was also used to demonstrate cigar-shaped forms in pathological tissues (Correa *et al.,* 1971). *In vivo,* yeast cells are gram-positive when viable and periodic-acid–Schiff–positive. Intracellular yeasts can be found in macrophages and giant cells. In biopsy material of spontaneous feline sporotrichosis, the intracellular budding yeast forms were surrounded by a halo with the inner electron-opaque layer consisting of microfibrillar material (Garrison *et al.,* 1979).

Hyphae are rarely seen in biological specimens. Their presence in tissue sections of human and murine sporotrichosis has occasionally been reported (Lii and Shigemi, 1973; Maberry *et al.*, 1966; Okudaira *et al.*, 1961). Filamentous forms arising from round forms present at the center of necrotic zones in infected mice were also observed (Lavalle *et al.*, 1963). Hyphae *in vivo* are short, occur in small numbers, and are not well resolved from cellular infiltrates, nuclear fragments, and stain particles (Lii and Shigemi, 1973). The host temperature and other factors seem to partially inhibit the apical growth process involved in the generation of the hyphal filament. Spherical cells are favored by isotropic wall deposition (Anderson, 1978). Okudaira *et al.* (1961) were able to induce the development of hyphae in tissues by administering amphotericin B or griseofulvin. The basis of these effects is unclear. Griseofulvin, which has no inhibitory activity against *S. schenckii in vitro,* may act as a vasodilator and possibly raise the local temperature (S. O. B. Roberts, 1980).

Spherical forms arising from cigar-shaped cells by gemulation can further differentiate by synthesizing a double membrane and depositing eosinophilic material from which radiating projections (1–12 μm) emerge, giving rise to asteroid bodies (Lavalle *et al.*, 1963). Such structures were frequently found in sporotrichotic primary and secondary lesions (Lurie, 1963; Moraes and Miranda, 1964) and were interpreted as being due to aggregation of antigen–antibody precipitates at the cell surface. Lurie (1971) suggested that when host resistance is high, cigar-shaped bodies change into chlamydospores. As antibodies react with the fungus, the asteroid eosinophilic material is deposited (Lurie and Still, 1969). Prevalence of asteroid-body formation can thus express host resistance to *S. schenckii.*

2.2. Growth Conditions and Cell Types

The yeast phase of *S. schenckii* develops in cultures containing as main nutrients casein hydrolysate or amino acids, glucose, thiamine, and biotin (Drouhet and Mariat, 1952b). Arginine and glycine can substitute for casein hydrolysate. Thiamine is an essential growth factor with its pyrimidine moiety being the effective requirement (Drouhet and Mariat, 1952a). The temperature of incubation is generally 37°C. An increased CO_2 tension is a very effective morphogenetic factor in *S. schenckii* (Romano, 1966). In a medium containing ammonium sulfate, asparagine, or arginine as N sources, yeast forms developed at 37°C provided the medium was sparged with a stream of air–CO_2 (95:5). Streams of N_2–air mixtures or air alone resulted in mycelial growth. Increased CO_2 tensions, obtained by incorporating carbonates into the medium and keeping the culture vessels tightly sealed, also effectively induce morphogenesis. In an appropriate chemically defined medium (Mendonça *et al.*,

1976) under these conditions, yeast cells formed in shaking cultures at both 25 and 37°C, indicating that temperature is not essential for phase transition. In this medium, the mycelial form can be obtained from conidia as a result of the combined effect of temperature (25°C) and low pH (4.0–5.0). Only hexoses are suitable C sources for the development of yeasts (Rodriguez-Del Valle *et al.*, 1983). The high glucose concentration is consistent with the observations by Nickerson and Mankowski (1953) that glucose is required for maintenance of the yeast shape, whereas its removal leads to filamentous growth in *Candida.* A nutritionally balanced medium for *S. schenckii* yeast phase was devised on the basis of other synthetic media developed for fastidious psychrophobic enteric yeasts (Travassos and Cury, 1971). A low oxidation–reduction potential favors the yeast phase of *S. schenckii* and *Histoplasma capsulatum* (Rippon, 1968, 1980). The Eh requirement can be satisfied by adding cysteine to the medium. With cells harvested at different incubation times, oxygen consumption was less in yeast forms of *S. schenckii* than in hyphae. Oxygen uptake decreased sharply with time (Mariat, 1968). This is in contrast to the activities of some other dimorphic fungi such as *Blastomyces dermatitidis* and *C. albicans,* which consume more oxygen in the yeast than in the mycelial phase (Nickerson and Edwards, 1949; Land *et al.*, 1975).

2.3. Morphologically Related *Ceratocystis*

Several species of *Ceratocystis* produce sympodulosporogenous anamorphs that are morphologically indistinguishable from that of *Sporothrix* (Taylor, 1970b). These are: *C. stenoceras, C. minor, C. multiannulata, C. narcissi, C. nigrocarpa, C. perparvispora, C. pilifera,* and possibly also *C. montia.* Cultures of five strains of *S. schenckii* and of seven *Ceratocystis* species were comparatively studied. All cultures at room temperature had septate hyphae with sympodulae from which ovate, elongate-ovate, or subcylindrical sympodulospores were produced acropetally. Glucose–blood agar cultures from viscera of inoculated animals consisted of budding, ovate to elongate-ovate yeastlike cells. On serial passages through mice, *S. schenckii* and the *Ceratocystis* species were macroscopically and microscopically identical on growing on Mycobiotic agar plates (Taylor, 1970b). Identification of *Ceratocystis* is made by observation of perithecium formation. Perithecia of *Ceratocystis* spp. failed to appear after animal passage.

In the absence of perithecium formation, the identification of *Ceratocystis* species as distinguished from *S. schenckii* is difficult. Conidia of all species agglutinate with an anti-*S. schenckii* serum, but this antigenic cross-reaction can be extended to morphologically unrelated fungi such as *C. ulmi.* The possibility that a particular species of *Ceratocystis* is the perfect form of *S. schenckii* is discussed in Section 3.1.

2.4. Ultrastructure of the Phase Transition

Ultrastructural comparison of the mycelial-to-yeast transition in *S. schenckii* with that of *Histoplasma farciminosum* and *Wangiella dermatitidis* (Oujezdsky *et al.*, 1973) showed that there is a direct budding process of yeast cells from hyphae by blastic action. Yeast-cell walls are 100–300 nm thick as compared with walls of hyphae (80–140 nm) and pigmented conidia (330 nm). Both yeast and conidial cell walls have two distinct layers. In conidia, the external 120-nm-thick layer may contain irregular granules that are pigmented particles (Mariat *et al.*, 1978). Hyphae of *S. schenckii* and morphologically related *Ceratocystis* show osmiophilic lipoprotein structures (Garrison *et al.*, 1977) that have possibly been mistaken for microendospores, endogenous spores, or ascospores. On cellular aging, they tend to degenerate with subsequent vacuolization. Micrographs by Findlay *et al.* (1979) also showed aspects of conidium formation that could erroneously be interpreted as the teleomorph of *S. schenckii.*

Characteristic of yeast cells of *S. schenckii* are the electron-dense microfibrils associated with the cell wall (Kitamura, 1965; Lurie and Still, 1969; Lane *et al.*, 1969). No microfibrils were observed at the surface of hyphae. Yeast cells emerging laterally or terminally from hyphae before or after septation show increased thickness of the microfibrillar material (Figures 1 and 2). When undergoing phase conversion, yeast cells of *S. schenckii, Paracoccidiodes brasiliensis, B. dermatitidis,* and *H. capsulatum* give rise to a transitional cell type that has a mixture of both yeastlike and hyphal characteristics. Intracytoplasmic membranes precede the formation of the transitional cells (Lane and Garrison, 1970; Garrison *et al.*, 1975). The observation that a yeast cell can also arise directly from conidia (Weise, 1931) has recently been confirmed by Garrison (see Chapter 2). Yeast cells arising by fragmentation of chains of oidia formed in hyphae (Howard, 1961) are also coated with dense microfibrillar material. Similar oidial cells were observed in *C. stenoceras* (Garrison *et al.*, 1976). Bud scars were shown in *S. schenckii* yeast forms (Garrison *et al.*, 1979), and multiple budding in these forms could reflect the abortive development of the mycelial phase (Salvin, 1947).

The ultrastructure of *S. schenckii* plasma membrane was studied by the freeze–fracture method (Maeda *et al.*, 1980). Two types of plasma membrane were observed in hyphae. The membrane either has a smooth appearance with randomly distributed particles about 8–12 nm in diam-

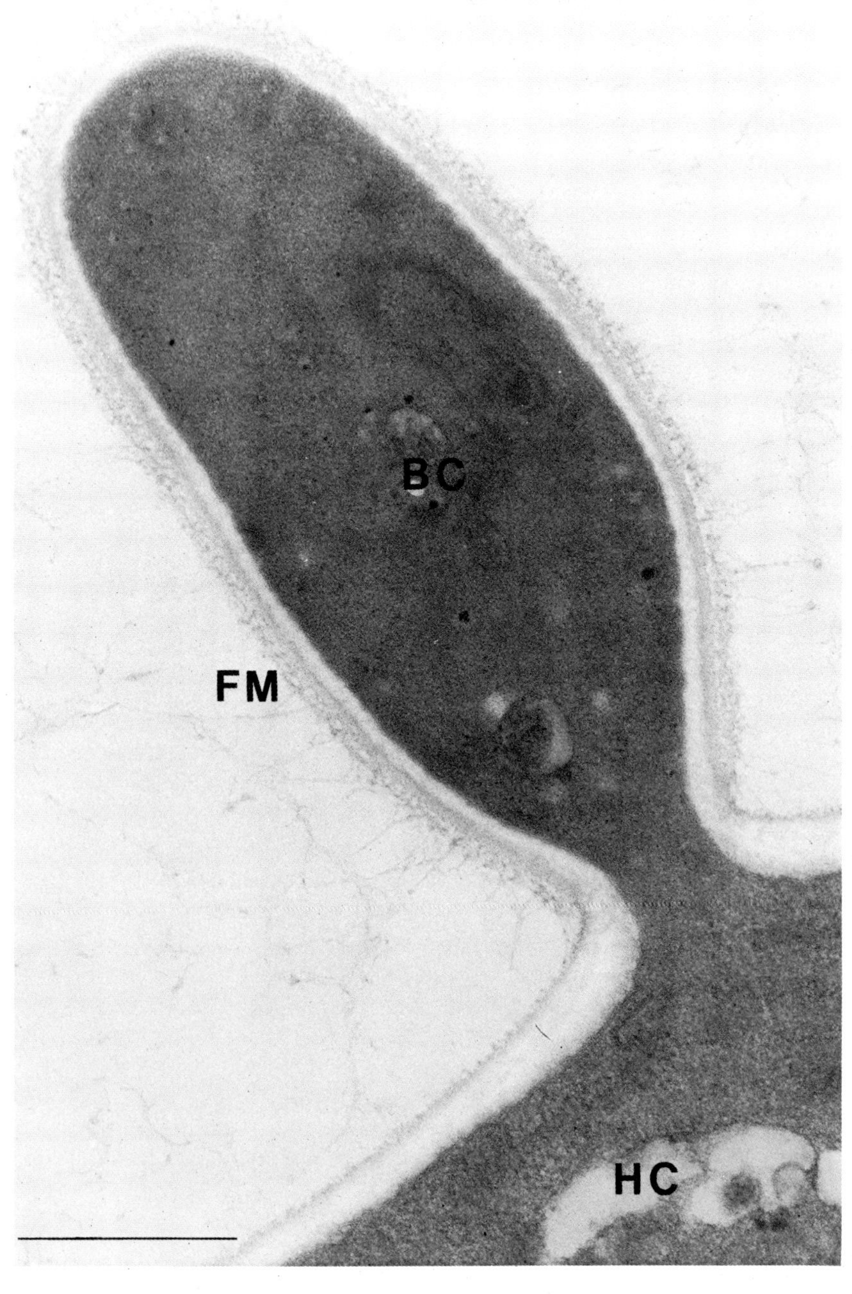

Figure 1. Thin section of a glutaraldehyde–OsO_4-fixed hypha bearing a young yeast bud clearly showing the wall-associated microfilbrillar material (FM). (HC) Hyphal cell; (BC) bud cell. Scale bar: 0.25 μm. (Courtesy of R. G. Garrison.)

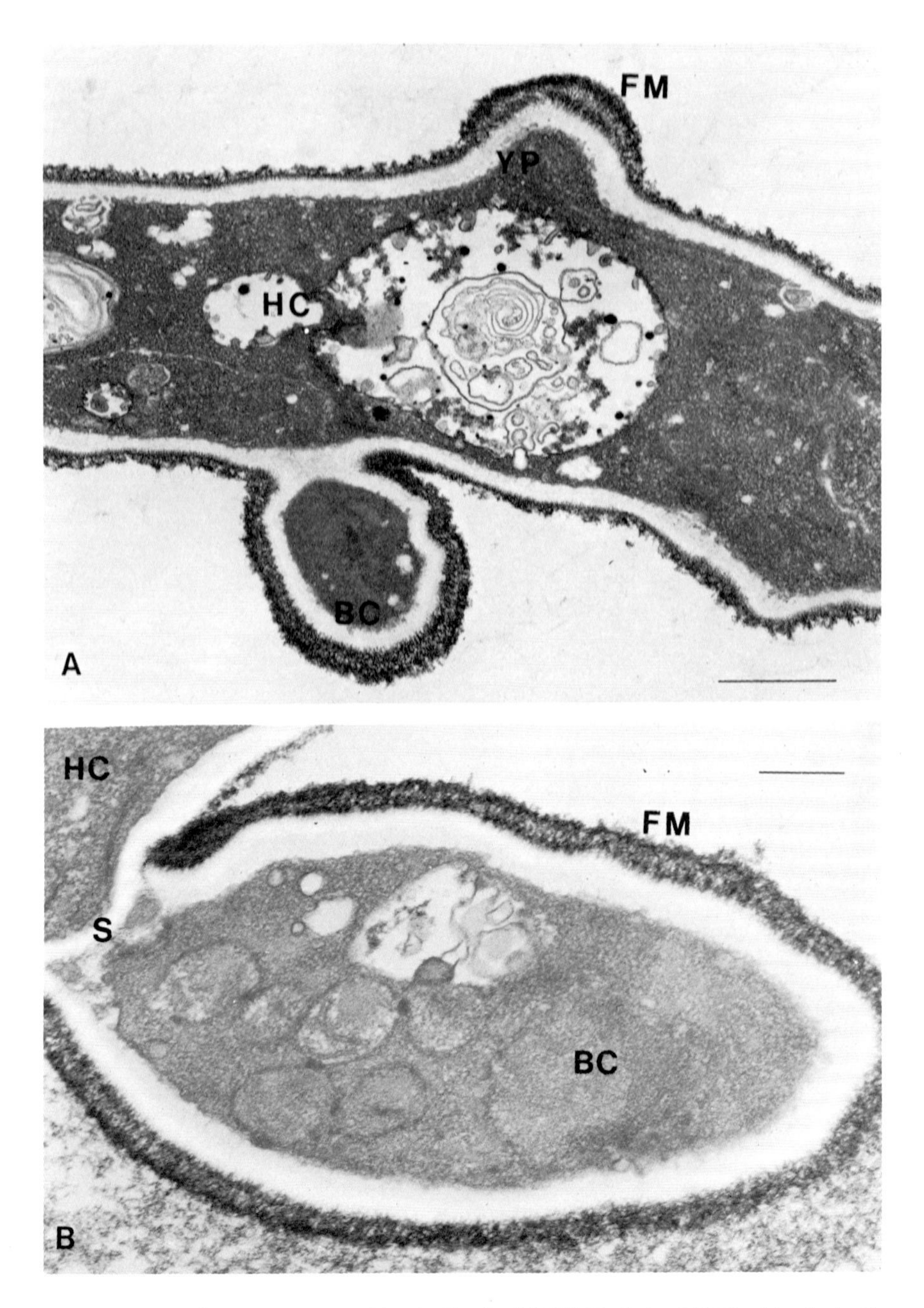

Figure 2. Mycelium-to-yeast transition in *S. schenkii.* (A) Hyphal cell (HC) with a bud cell (BC) and a yeast primordium (YP) both showing thick microfibrillar material (FM). Scale bar: 0.5 μm. (Courtesy of R. G. Garrison.) (B) HC and BC after septum (S) formation. Note the difference in thickness of the FM layer. Scale bar: 0.25 μm. Glutaraldehyde–dialyzed iron–osmium staining. (From Garrison *et al.,* 1975. Used with permission.)

eter as seen on the P-face (Figure 3) or shows irregularly shaped invaginations on both P- and E-faces. The E-face has fewer membrane particles than the P-face of hyphal plasma membrane. The cleavage faces of conidial membrane show rice-grain-like invaginations, whereas in yeast forms both faces show irregularly shaped invaginations or wrinkles (Figure 4). Young cells at the early logarithmic phase tend to have the smooth type of plasma membrane. Hyphae with invaginations in the membrane, which in turn increase the surface area, may be ready to divide or produce conidia.

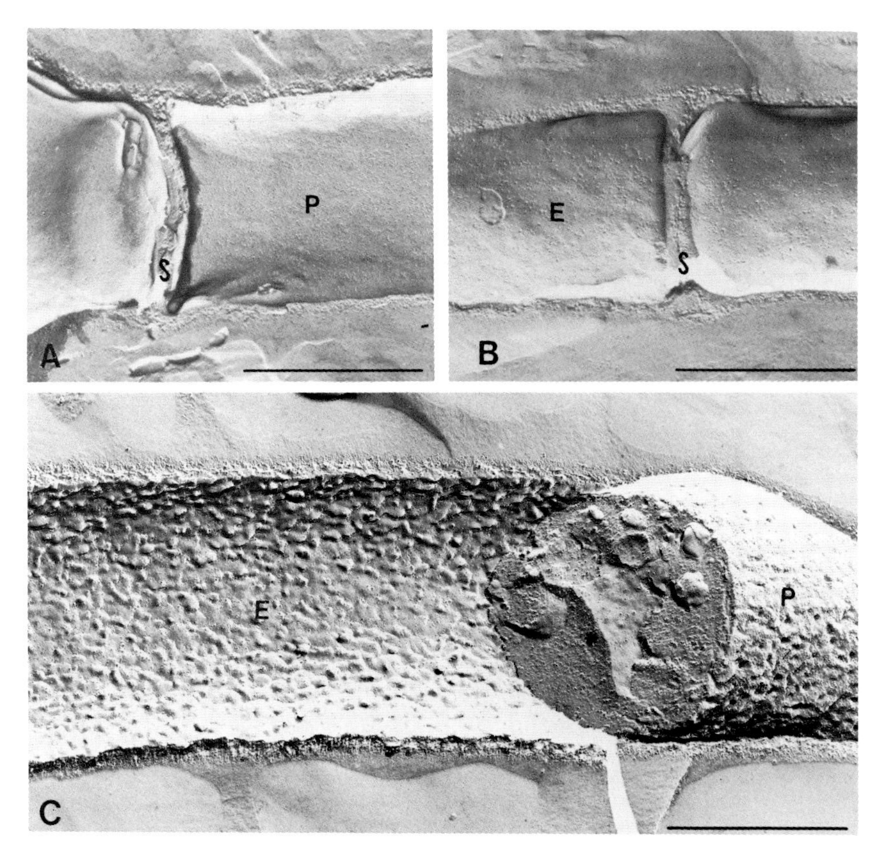

Figure 3. Freeze–fracture electron microscopy of the plasma membrane of hyphae. (A, B) P-face (P) of the smooth type of plasma membrane with globular particles; E-face (E) of the smooth type of membrane with a septum (S) perpendicular to the cell wall. (C) P- and E-face of the invaginated type of plasma membrane. (*) Cytoplasm. Scale bar: 1 μm. (Courtesy of M. Maeda.)

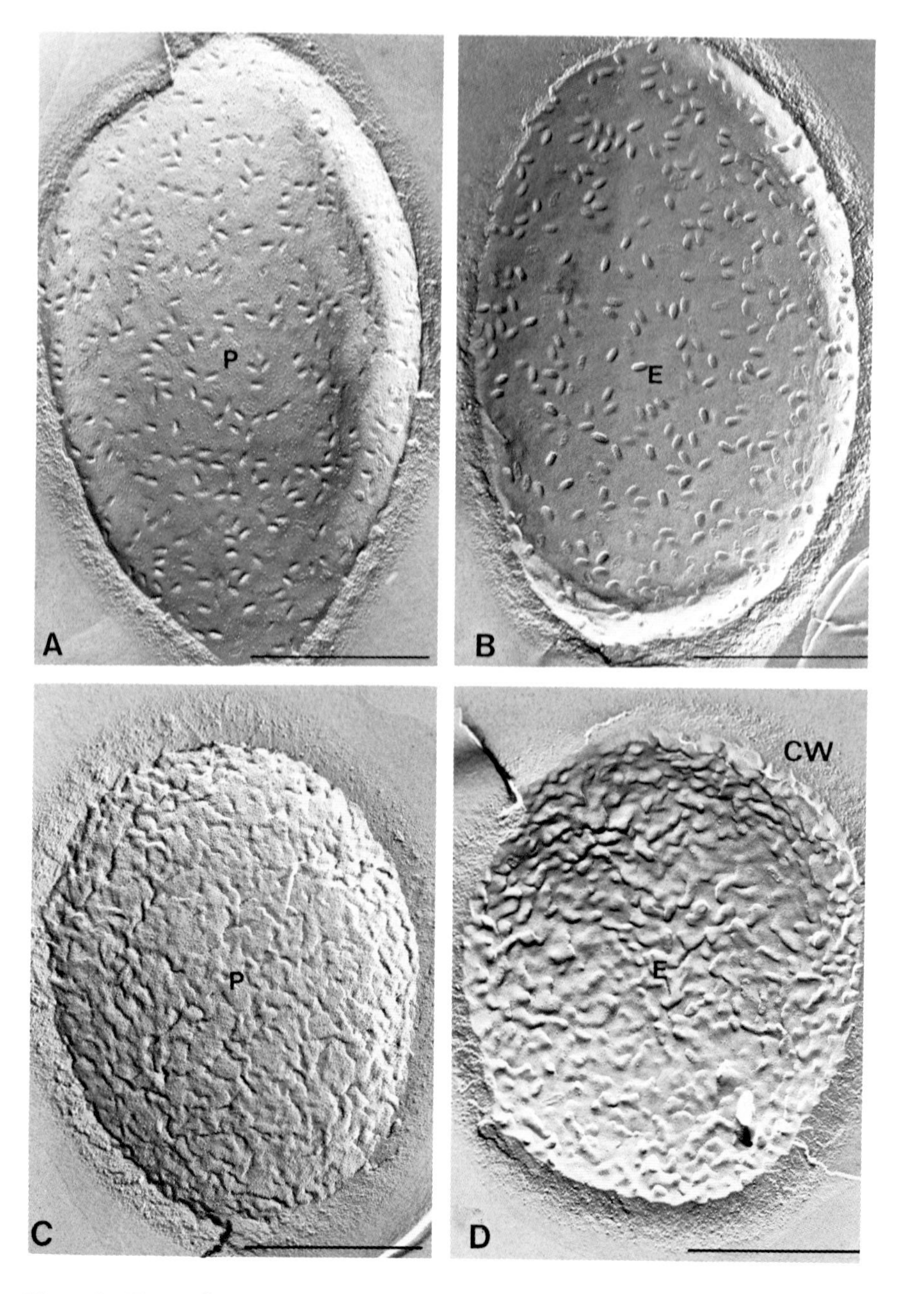

Figure 4. Freeze–fracture electron microscopy of the plasma membrane of a conidium (A, B) and a yeast form (C, D). (A) P-face with invaginations. (B) E-face with rice-grain-like protrusions. (C) P-face with irregular invaginations in a silkwormlike pattern. (D) E-face with protrusions and fewer particles. (CW) Cell wall. Scale bars: 1 μm. (Courtesy of M. Maeda.)

3. BIOCHEMICAL ACTIVITIES AND CELL CONSTITUENTS

Analysis by gel electrophoresis of *S. schenckii* yeast-cell extracts showed the presence of several enzymes including dehydrogenases, catalase, and peroxidases, as well as hydrolases such as acid and alkaline phosphatases, β-glucosidase, leucylaminopeptidase, aldolase, β-amylase, RNase, and DNase. Two esterases hydrolyzing butyrylthiocholine and β -naphthylacetate (Walbaum *et al.*, 1978), and neuraminidase, as well as lipolytic and fibrinolytic activities, were also detected in *S. schenckii* (Muller, 1975).

Yeast forms of *S. schenckii* were reported to assimilate urea, cysteine, glycine, cyanuric acid, and even a derivative of an s-triazine herbicide (Zeyer *et al.*, 1981a,b). Pathogenic strains assimilate guanidoacetic acid, creatine, and creatinine in the presence of thiamine (Staib *et al.*, 1974). Strains of *S. schenckii* growing at 37°C and assimilating creatine or creatinine caused visible muscle swelling and abcess formation when injected into mice (Staib *et al.*, 1972).

The phospholipids of *S. schenckii* and *C. stenoceras* were compared (Bièvre and Jourd'huy, 1974). Cardiolipin, phosphatidylethanolamine, -monomethylethanolamine, -serine, and -choline, lysophosphatidylethanolamine, and lysolecithin were identified. Phosphatidylinositol was found in *C. stenoceras,* but not in *S. schenckii.* Polar and neutral lipids were separated on silicic acid and fatty acids identified as their methyl esters (Bièvre and Mariat, 1975). Predominating are C16 and C18:2 acids. *Ceratocystis stenoceras* has C20:1 and C20 fatty acids that are absent in *S. schenckii* polar fractions. Long-chain fatty acids of 11 strains of *S. schenckii* grown on a defatted medium at 30°C were identified (Stretton and Dart, 1976). Predominating are C16, C18:1, and C18:2 fatty acids, but low proportions of C18 and C18:3 wcrc also found.

3.1. Teleomorph of *Sporothrix schenckii*

The question of the teleomorph of *S. schenckii* has been approached by comparing phenotypic as well as genotypic characteristics of *S. schenckii* and ascigerous species of *Ceratocystis.* As mentioned above, several species of *Ceratocystis* produced anamorphs indistinguishable from that of *S. schenckii.* Immunological properties as a criterion to single out the teleomorph of *S. schenckii* were not helpful because of the multiple cross-reactivity of antigens from *Ceratocystis* spp. (Ishizaki *et al.*, 1978). Purified rhamnomannans from *C. stenoceras, C. pilifera, C. minor,* and *C. ulmi* were equally precipitated by an antiserum raised against *S. schenckii* yeast forms (Lloyd and Travassos, 1975). One *Ceratocystis* species, *C.*

stenoceras, was thought to be a likely candidate for the teleomorph (Mariat, 1971) on the basis of morphological similarities, requirement for thiamine, growth at 37°C, and conversion to the yeast phase. *Ceratocystis stenoceras* could also be isolated from the same natural habitats as *S. schenckii* (Mariat, 1975). Genotypic studies described below, however, do not confirm that *C. stenoceras* is the teleomorph of *S. schenckii.*

By studying the properties of the DNAs from a number of strains of *S. schenckii,* it was observed that this form-species is rather homogeneous in accordance with earlier results on their purified rhamnomannans (Travassos *et al.,* 1974). The guanine plus cytosine (GC) contents of four *S. schenckii* DNAs were found to be very similar: average of 54.7 mole%. Two strains of *C. stenoceras* yielded DNAs with a GC proportion of 52.6 mole%. Other form-species of *Ceratocystis,* with the exception of *C. minor,* have DNAs with GC contents differing from those of *S. schenckii* DNAs (Mendonça-Hagler *et al.,* 1974). The GC contents of DNAs from six different strains of *S. schenckii* and two strains of *C. stenoceras* were independently determined in another laboratory with similar results (Bièvre and Mariat, 1981); averages of 54.3 and 52.4 mole% for *S. schenckii* and *C. stenoceras* DNAs, respectively, were obtained. The DNAs from four *S. schenckii* strains had a high degree of relative binding (range 70–100%) as determined by cross-hybridization experiments. The DNAs from *C. stenoceras* and *C. pilifera* have proportions of relative binding to *S. schenckii* DNA of only 30 and 35%, respectively (Mendonça-Hagler *et al.,* 1974). Data on the genotypic relationships of *C. minor* and *S. schenckii* are controversial. Determinations carried out with two different strains of *C. minor* showed GC proportions of 54.6 and 51.2 mole%. The DNA of the former strain bound to *S. schenckii* DNA with a homology of 75%. The analysis of the DNA properties of several other strains of *C. minor* should indicate whether this species is indeed more related to *S. schenckii* than other *Ceratocystis* species.

On the basis of the DNA base composition and hybridization experiments, Travassos and Lloyd (1980) suggested that different strains of *S. schenckii* are not the anamorphs of different *Ceratocystis* species, but rather that the species *S. schenckii* is the homogeneous imperfect form of one as yet unidentified *Ceratocystis* species.

4. CELL-SURFACE REACTIVITY AND COMPOSITION

Different surface components of *S. schenckii* were identified by direct and indirect methods. Differences in composition of cell walls from hyphae, conidia, and yeast cells were noted. The following sections review these results with the aim of presenting an integrated view of the surface structures of this fungus and their relevance to dimorphism and immunological reactivity.

4.1. Cell-Wall Composition in Different Cell Types

Cell-wall constituents are thought to determine the cell shape in fungi. In the case of dimorphic fungi, several attempts have been made to uncover differences in the composition of cell walls from different morphological phases. It should be pointed out that overall differences in cell-wall composition may not reflect specific alterations at sites where differentiation processes occur. Also, if cells are harvested at the stationary phase of growth, their cell walls may differ from those of exponentially growing cells (Gooday and Trinci, 1980). The composition of the medium and the growth conditions are also important in the expression of cell-surface polymers. Increases of temperature to induce the yeast phase may affect the synthesis of certain components not necessarily involved in determining the cell shape. Hence, interpretations of the morphogenetic significance of cell-wall alterations should be made with caution. In the case of *S. schenckii,* cell walls were obtained from actively growing cells cultured in different synthetic and semisynthetic media at 37 and 25°C (Previato *et al.,* 1979a). The media were selected to favor pure yeast–or mycelial-phase cultures. Cell walls were exhaustively washed, which makes it likely that the final preparations did not contain the loosely bound external layers characteristic of the yeast phase. Such layers, which contain among the chief constituents peptidorhamnomannans, galactomannans, sialoglycolipids, and amylose, are easily sloughed off into the medium. Their role in morphogenesis is unclear. Since the final yeast-cell-wall preparations contained substantial amounts of rhamnose and mannose, but only traces of galactose (Table I), it is probable that peptidorhamnomannans, along with soluble glucans but not galactomannans, are also firmly bound to the cell-wall matrix. According to Nickerson (1971), α-linked polymers such as rhamnomannans and soluble glucans that are bound to insoluble components may impart circularity to the wall. Filamentous hyphae would have a minimum of components imparting circularity. The relatively high amounts of rhamnomannans, as well as soluble glucans, in hyphae suggest a more complex correlation between surface polymers and cell shape.

The cell-wall composition of *S. schenckii* cell types (Table I) revealed that the conidial wall composition is closer to that of hyphae than of yeasts. Differences in amino acid composition of walls from both phases of *S. schenckii* were small and restricted to threonine, serine, lysine, argi-

Table I
Analyses of Cell Walls from Different *S. schenckii* Cell Types[a]

Analysis	Yeasts	Mycelium	Conidia
Neutral sugars	61 ± 1.3 (12)	44 ± 0.9 (12)	47 ± 1.0 (8)
Hexosamine	7.0 ± 0.4 (9)	7.0 ± 0.3 (9)	8.3 ± 0.6 (6)
Glucose as amylose	1.8 ± 0.0 (3)	1.6 ± 0.0 (3)	1.7 ± 0.0 (2)
Glucose[b]	48.1 ± 0.2 (3)	54.9 ± 0.9 (3)	57.9 ± 0.4 (2)
Mannose[b]	36.0 ± 0.8 (3)	28.8 ± 0.5 (3)	25.1 ± 0.5 (2)
Rhamnose[b]	15.7 ± 0.7 (3)	16.2 ± 0.9 (3)	17.0 ± 0.2 (2)
Galactose[b]	Trace	Trace	Trace
Lipids	18 ± 0.9 (9)	26 ± 1.3 (9)	19.6 ± 1.2 (6)
Phosphate	0.7 ± 0.0 (6)	1.2 ± 0.0 (6)	0.8 ± 0.0 (4)
Total N	2.9 ± 0.1 (6)	3.9 ± 0.1 (6)	4.5 ± 0.1 (4)
N of chitin	0.5	0.5	0.6
N as protein[c]	14.3	21.2	24.3
Protein[d]	14.4 ± 0.7 (3)	21.7 ± 1.0 (3)	24.2 ± 0.5 (2)
Total recovery[e]	101.1	99.9	99.9

[a]From Previato *et al.* (1979a); used with permission. Values (± S.D.), unless otherwise indicated, are percentages of cell-wall weight and averages of several determinations (in parentheses) on two (conidia) or three (yeast or mycelium) different cell-wall preparations.
[b]Values are percentages of total carbohydrate.
[c](Total N − N of chitin) × 6.25.
[d]Determined by amino acid analysis.
[e]Total for neutral sugars, hexosamine, lipids, phosphate, and protein analyses.

nine, and glutamic acid (Previato *et al.*, 1979a). Cysteine was not detected. Yeast walls have higher carbohydrate and lower lipid contents than hyphal walls. Lipid fractions from mycelial and conidial walls have remarkably similar composition of fatty acids. Different proportions of saturated and unsaturated fatty acids were obtained for the yeast walls with the identification of C18:3 (linolenic) acid as a unique component of the yeast phase. A direct correlation between linolenic acid and cyclic AMP (cAMP) has been established in *Neurospora crassa* (Scott *et al.*, 1973). Dimorphism induced by temperature variation may depend on membrane lipid alterations (e.g., linolenic acid) that may affect enzymes such as adenylate cyclase or phosphodiesterase (Stewart and Rogers, 1978).

Although several differences in the composition of cell walls from yeasts and hyphae of *S. schenckii* have been noted, no model for a sequence of events leading to the phase transition can be advanced at present. It seems clear that no single polymer alone is responsible for the alterations in the physicochemical properties of *S. schenckii* cell walls. Soluble and insoluble glucans that may have a role in the transformation of other dimorphic fungi have very similar chemical structures in *S.*

schenckii yeast or mycelial walls (Previato *et al.*, 1979b). The similarity in composition of the conidial and hyphal walls observed in *S. schenckii* is in accordance with a morphogenetic process by which conidia are formed by a blowing out of the fertile hyphal wall (Cole, 1976).

4.2. Reactivity with Lectins

Of 17 lectins tested, only concanavalin A (Con A) and a lectin from *Limulus polyphemus* (limulin) were able to agglutinate *S. schenckii* yeast cells (Alviano *et al.*, 1982). Reactions with Con A and limulin were inhibited by methyl-α-D-mannoside and *N*-acetylneuraminic acid, respectively, confirming the specificities of lectin binding. Reactivity with limulin was due partly to the presence at the cell surface of sialoglycolipids (Section 4.3). Reaction with Con A is still not completely understood. That the residues recognized by this lectin are mannose units is inferred from the fact that bacterial fimbriae of type 1 also agglutinate *S. schenckii* yeast cells. Purified rhamnomannans from *S. schenckii* that did not contain terminal nonreducing units of α-D-mannopyranose (Travassos *et al.*, 1977) did not precipitate Con A on a double-diffusion test. The corresponding peptidopolysaccharides, crude or fractionated with Cetavlon, precipitated Con A at 5 mg/ml. Fungal peptidopolysaccharides may contain, in addition to long-chain polymers, short mannose-containing oligosaccharide chains usually O-linked to serine or threonine residues in the peptide (Lloyd, 1970; Ballou, 1976). Presumably, similar short chains in *S. schenckii* peptidopolysaccharides are responsible for the Con A reaction, but this has not been further investigated. Cell-wall components reacting with Con A in yeast forms and yeast primordia on hyphae were located by use of fluorescent Con A staining and a cytochemical method using Con A–horseradish peroxidase–diaminobenzidine (Travassos *et al.*, 1977). Hyphal walls were weakly reactive. The surface material reactive with Con A in yeast forms and conidia (Figures 5 and 6) was eventually shed into the suspension medium. In addition to the peptidorhamnomannans, neutral galactomannans also occur at the cell surface of yeast forms, and they may have variable proportions of 2-O-substituted and nonreducing end units of α-D-mannopyranose that react with Con A.

4.3. Anionic Groups

The microfibrillar material that is present along the outermost surface of yeast cell walls stains heavily with acidified dialyzed iron (Garrison *et al.*, 1975). Labeling with cationized ferritin (CF) was also stronger

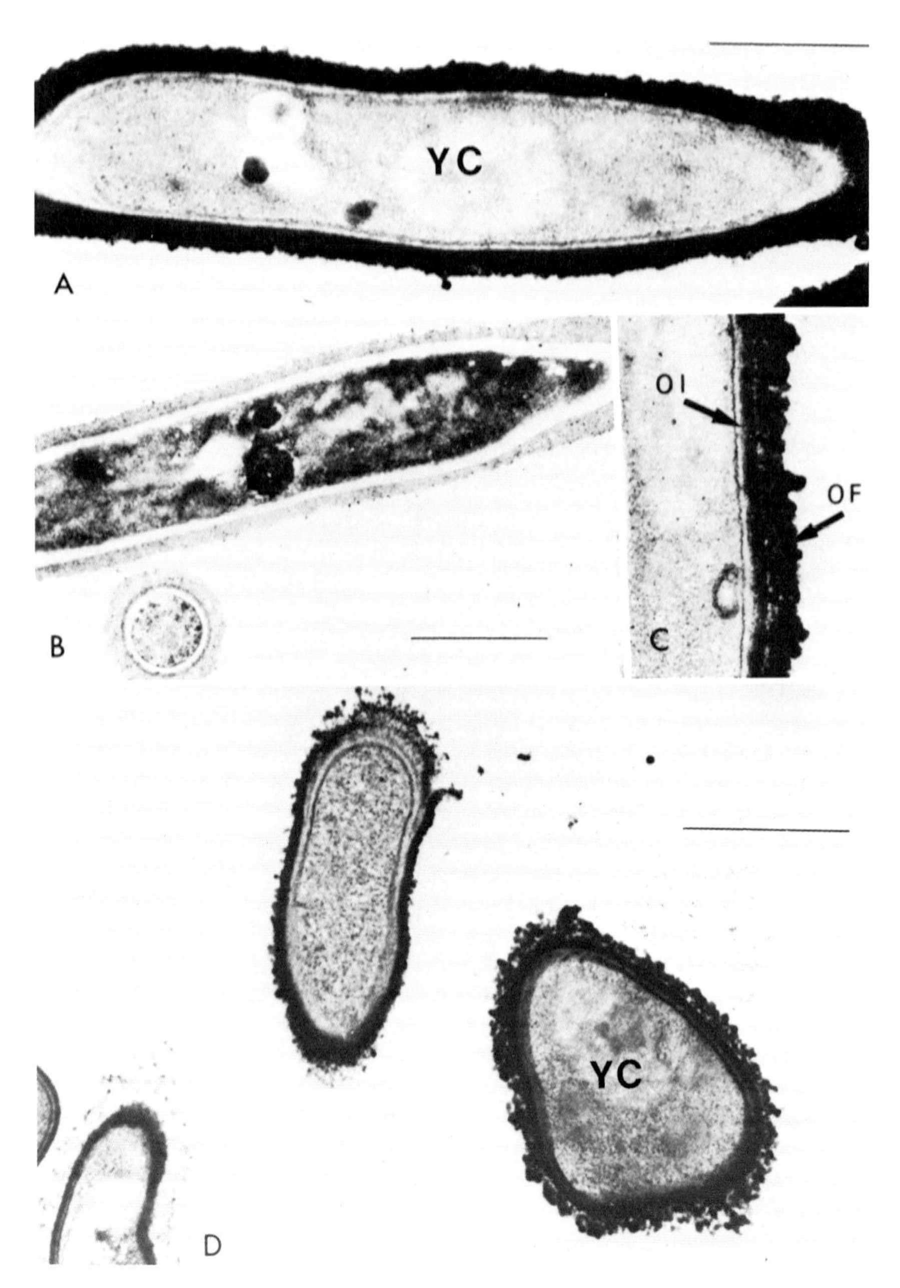

Figure 5. Reactivity of yeast cells (YC) of *S. schenckii* with concanavalin A. Two layers of reactive material, inner sublayer (OI) and fibrillar sublayer (OF), were observed (C). The strong reactivity in (A) is inhibited by adding methyl-α-D-mannoside (B). The reaction of different cells with Con A, regarding the outer layers of the cell wall, is heterogeneous. Scale bars: (A, B, D) 1 μm; (C) 0.5 μm. (From Travassos *et al.*, 1977. Used with permission.)

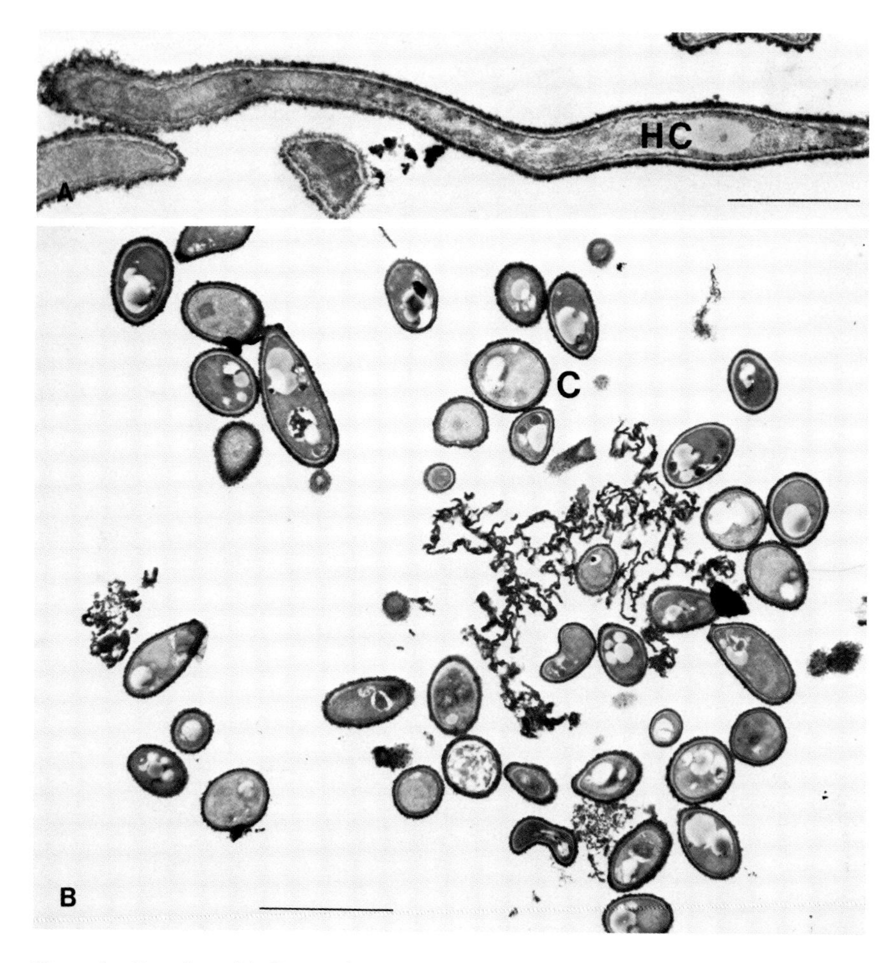

Figure 6. Reaction with Con A of hyphal (HC) and conidial (C) cells. (A) The reactive cell-wall layer is thinner than that in the yeast forms. Scale bar: 1 μm. (B) Homogeneous reaction of conidia with Con A. Ribbons of reactive material are released into the medium. Scale bar: 5 μm. (From Travassos *et al.*, 1977. Used with permission.)

on the outer sublayer of the external layer of the cell wall. After binding CF, the outer sublayer was shown in several cells to detach from the cell wall as long ribbons of electron-dense material. In some instances, a single CF-reactive layer would detach from the cell, leaving behind the remaining cell-wall structure, which had virtually no CF-reactive anionic groups (Figure 7). Visualization of both the outer and inner sublayers was best with the colloidal iron hydroxide method at low pH (Benchimol *et al.*, 1979).

Anionic groups in *S. schenckii* seem to be associated with a complex material that is weakly bonded to the inner portion of the cell wall and apparently is not essential for cell viability. Apart from the acidic amino acids present in the peptidorhamnomannans that can react with CF, sialic acid residues responsible for the reactivity with colloidal iron hydroxide (CIH) at pH 1.8 were also detected in *S. schenckii.* Neuraminidase-treated cells became unreactive with CIH (Alviano *et al.*, 1982). Sialic acid residues either are located on the peptidopolysaccharide com-

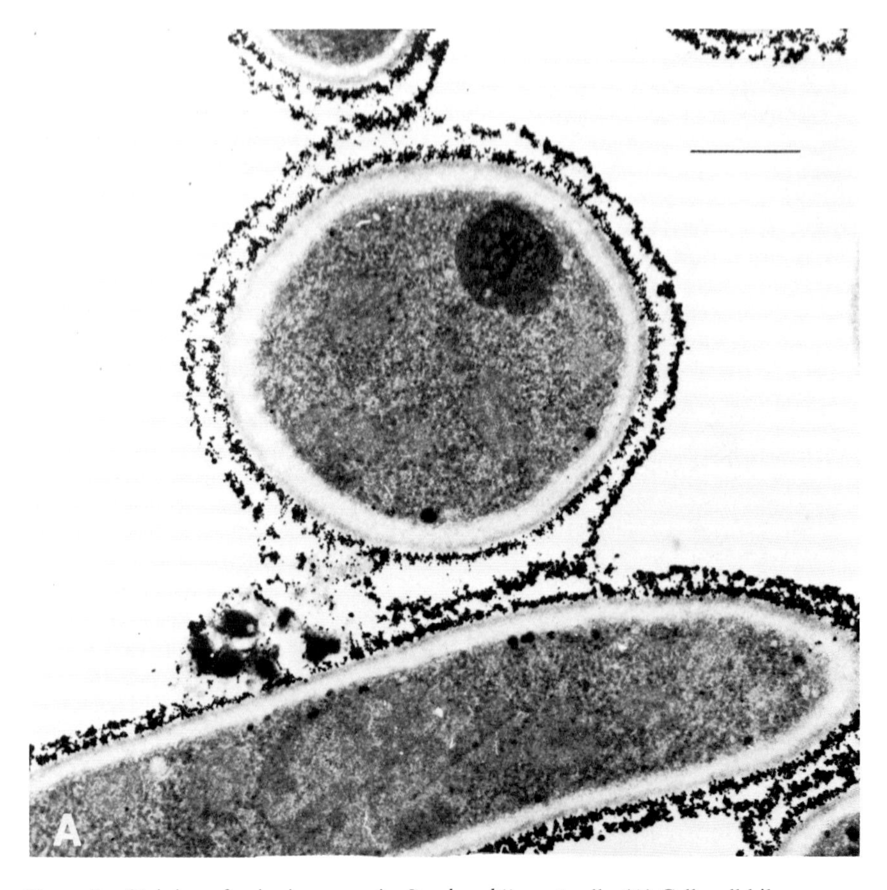

Figure 7. Staining of anionic groups in *S. schenckii* yeast cells. (A) Cell-wall bilayer reactivity with colloidal iron hydroxide. Scale bar: 0.5 μm. (B) Detachment of the outer layer of surface components reacting with ferritin. (↑) Sites of detachment. Scale bar: 0.5 μm. (From Benchimol *et al.*, 1979. Used with permission.)

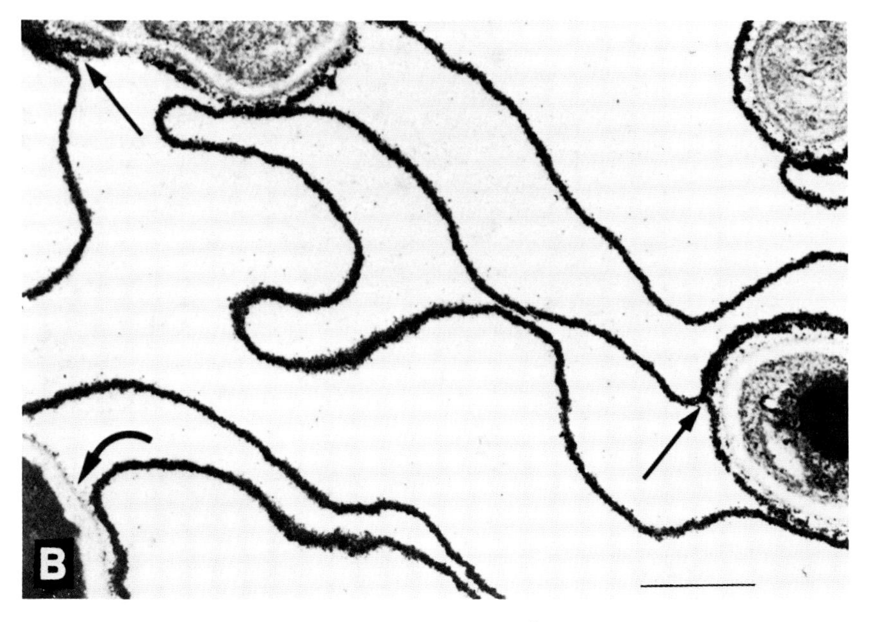

Figure 7. *(continued)*

plexes or are constituents of polar glycolipids. A hydrolysate of a polar glycolipid fraction from *S. schenckii* yeast forms had *N*-glycolylneuraminic acid units identified by thin-layer chromatography. Sialoglycolipids may be bound to the peptidopolysaccharide complexes: The loosely bound outer layer of *S. schenckii* cell wall reacts with CIH and with Con A (Travassos and Alviano, 1981).

4.4. Immunofluorescence Reactions

Fluorescent anti-*S. schenckii* rabbit globulins stain both yeast and mycelial forms in culture or in clinical specimens (Kaplan and Ivens, 1960). The reaction was negative with 47 strains of 21 heterologous species of fungi (Kaplan, 1970). In several patients with sporotrichosis as diagnosed by positive cultures for *S. schenckii,* fluorescent antibodies detected cigar-shaped, oval, elliptical, bacilliform, and globose cells in smears of lesion exudates. Culturally negative cases were also negative by fluorescent antibody staining. Since very few cells are present in lesion exudates, several microscopic fields had to be inspected.

Rabbit sera were raised against acetone-dried cells of *S. schenckii* previously grown in a supplemented yeast–nitrogen–base medium at both 37 and 25°C. Sera were cross-absorbed with the heterologous morphological phase to yield reagents reactive mainly with hyphal (AH) or yeast (AY) antigens. By using the indirect immunofluorescence technique, it was shown that the AY antiserum was strongly reactive with yeast forms either free or emerging from hyphae, whereas hyphae were poorly reactive or negative with this serum (Lloyd *et al.*, 1978). The AY serum also stained conidia, attached to hyphae or free, suggesting a similarity between yeast and conidial surface antigens. Conversely, the AH antiserum reacted strongly with hyphal cell walls and was negative or very weakly reactive with yeast forms or conidia (Figure 8).

Antisera against yeast cells of *S. schenckii* gave positive indirect immunofluorescence reactions with conidia and mycelia of *C. stenoceras* and *C. ulmi*. Perithecia and ascospores were unreactive (Harada *et al.*, 1976).

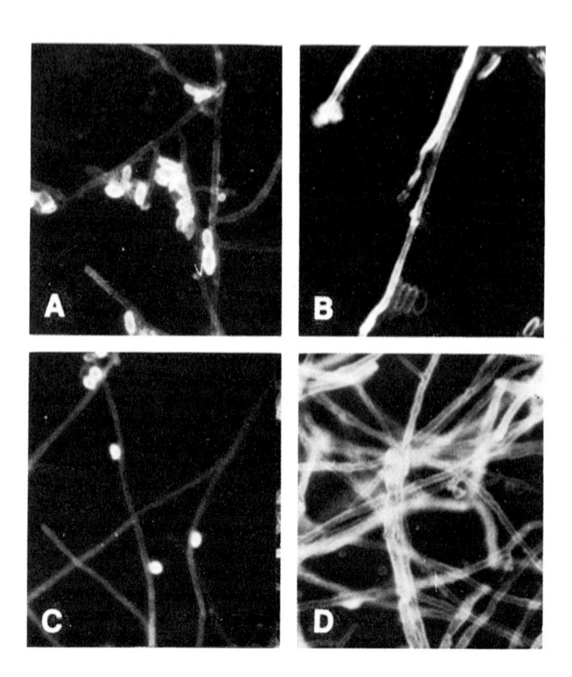

Figure 8. Immunofluorescent staining of *S. schenckii* cell types. (A, C) The absorbed serum reacting with yeast antigens gives a strong reaction with budding cells and conidia on hyphae while reacting very poorly with hyphae. (B, D) Strong reaction of hyphae and almost negative reaction of yeast cells with the absorbed serum recognizing mycelial antigens. (From Lloyd *et al.*, 1978. Used with permission.)

4.5. Surface Components and Yeast Phagocytosis

The ingestion of *S. schenckii* yeasts by thioglycollate-elicited mouse peritoneal macrophages was studied by Oda *et al.* (1983). Opsonization of yeasts with Con A at subagglutinating concentrations greatly increased the phagocytosis. With unopsonized yeasts, the phagocytosis apparently depended on the reactivity of fungal cell-surface components with appropriate receptors on the macrophage membrane. Neuraminidase treatment of yeasts increased the ingestion of unopsonized cells 7.7-fold. Sugars known to be present on the cell surface of *S. schenckii,* such as rhamnose, mannose, and galactose, partially inhibited phagocytosis (40–50% reduction of phagocytic indexes of control systems). Isolated *S. schenckii* rhamnomannan and galactomannan were also inhibitors.

The best inhibitor of phagocytosis was *N*-acetylglucosamine (GlcNAc), which, however, is not a prominent component of *S. schenckii* cell wall (Previato *et al.,* 1979a). GlcNAc inhibited binding of yeasts to macrophages at 4°C as well as the ingestion of yeasts by macrophages pretreated with this sugar. The phagocytosis of sensitized erythrocytes or latex particles was unaffected by GlcNAc under the same conditions. The inhibitory effect of GlcNAc is probably related to the specificity of certain receptors on the membrane of mouse peritoneal macrophages. A (mannose/glucosamine)-reacting receptor that also binds *Candida krusei* has been identified in alveolar macrophages (Warr, 1980).

While the role of sialic acid residues in protecting *S. schenckii* from phagocytosis *in vivo* seems clear, before an efficient antibody response is effective, the protection against phagocytosis by exocellularly released peptidorhamnomannan–galactomannan complexes (Benchimol *et al.,* 1979) will depend on the expression of specific receptors on macrophages at the site of infection.

5. *Sporothrix schenckii* POLYSACCHARIDES

In recent years, several polysaccharides of *S. schenckii* have been studied and their fine structures determined by conventional chemical analysis, including methylation–fragmentation techniques, and by spectroscopic methods. The soluble polysaccharides characterized were rhamnomannans, galactomannans, and glucans. Rhamnomannans are present in all strains of *S. schenckii,* but are also found in a variety of nonpathogenic fungi mainly of the genus *Ceratocystis.* Differences in the fine structures of rhamnomannans as related to dimorphism were demonstrated and correlated well with the reactivity of different cell types with specific antisera that recognized different rhamnose-containing antigenic determinants. Less specific antigens of *S. schenckii* are the galactomannans with galactofuranose side chains as the main antigenic determinants. Soluble and insoluble glucans were characterized in cell walls from different *S. schenckii* cell types, but their relationship to dimorphism is unclear.

5.1. Rhamnomannans at Different Growth Temperatures

Peptidorhamnomannans accumulate in the culture medium of *S. schenckii* and can be directly isolated along with soluble glucans and galactomannans. The sugar constituents in these polymers were initially identified by Aoki *et al.* (1967) and Ishizaki (1970). Partial purification of rhamnomannans was achieved either by Cetavlon precipitation of the borate complexes at pH 8.5 and chromatography on diethylaminoethyl (DEAE)–Sephadex (Lloyd and Bitoon, 1971) or by precipitation with Fehling's reagent (Travassos *et al.*, 1973, 1974).

The rhamnomannans of *S. schenckii* are α-linked structures having very few or no α-D-mannopyranosyl nonreducing end units. Rhamnose side chains can be removed by mild acid hydrolysis (pH 1.1 at 100°C), which yields an $\alpha(1 \rightarrow 6)$-mannopyranan as determined by methylation analysis. Single-unit rhamnosyl or dirhamnosyl side chains were detected in *S. schenckii* rhamnomannan (Figure 9, structures I and II). Monorhamnosyl side chains are characteristic of rhamnomannans isolated at 37°C or from the yeast phase. Dirhamnosyl side chains are formed mostly by *S. schenckii* cultures grown at 25°C or in the mycelial phase. The question of whether these side chains respond to temperature variation or are phenotypes linked to the morphological phase was answered as follows: Yeast cells of *S. schenckii* were grown with shaking at both 25 and 37°C in the synthetic medium of Mendonça *et al.* (1976) with ammonium carbonate. Cultures at both temperatures contained 100% of yeast forms. The rhamnomannans extracted from these cells had only monorhamnosyl side chains, as indicated by methylation analysis and ^{13}C nuclear magnetic resonance (^{13}C NMR) spectroscopy. Rhamnomannans with structure I (Figure 9) seem, then, to be characteristic of yeast forms irrespective of the incubation temperature (Mendonça *et al.*, 1976). Temperature effect was reflected in the presence of 4-O- and 2,4-di-O-substituted α-D-mannopyranose units in the rhamnomannan. At 37°C, such units were absent in the rhamnomannan of one *S. schenckii* strain. By shifting the growth temperature to 25°C, these units were synthesized and incorporated into rhamnomannans of both yeast forms and mycelium. The probable structure containing 4-O- and 2,4-di-O-substituted man-

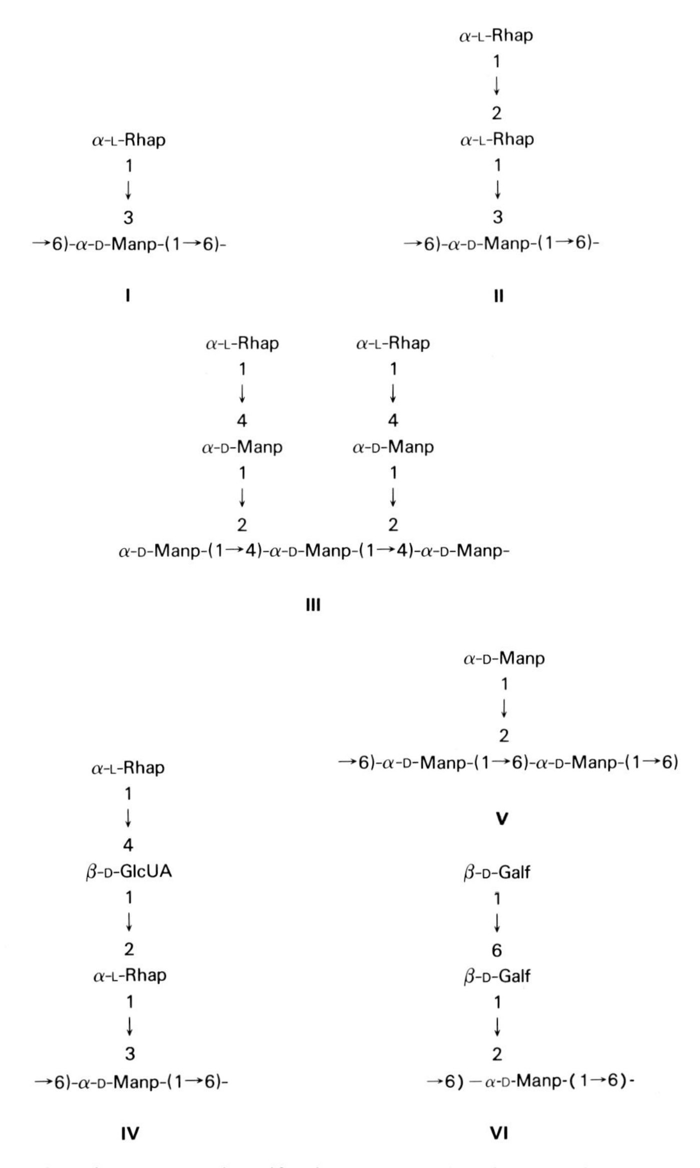

Figure 9. Fine structures identified in polysaccharides from *S. schenckii* and *C. stenoceras*.

nopyranose units is depicted in Figure 9 (structure III). One strain of *S. schenckii* when growing at 25°C in a semisynthetic medium formed a conidialess mycelial culture after short incubation. Rhamnomannans from hyphae contained high proportions of dirhamnosylrhamnomannans. In another medium favoring sporulation at 25°C, a mycelial culture of the same *S. schenckii* strain was filtered through gauze to separate free conidia. The rhamnomannan isolated from such conidia had less than 10% of side chains containing (1 → 2)-linked dirhamnosyl residues (Travassos and Mendonça-Previato, 1978). It seems, therefore, that conidia have predominantly monorhamnosylrhamnomannans with some 4-O- and 2,4-di-O-substituted α-D-mannopyranose units, much like the rhamnomannans formed by yeast cells growing at 25°C. Results on the distribution of monorhamnosylrhamnomannans in yeast forms and conidia and of dirhamnosylrhamnomannans in hyphae are in accordance with the immunofluorescence staining of cell walls with specific sera (Lloyd *et al.*, 1978).

5.2. Rhamnomannans of *Ceratocystis*

Several species of *Ceratocystis* form rhamnomannans (Spencer and Gorin, 1971) having structures similar to those characterized in *S. schenckii* polysaccharides. Exocellular polysaccharides from *C. stenoceras* were precipitated with Fehling's solution and fractionated by DEAE–cellulose chromatography. Elution with dilute acid gave a rhamnomannan having a (1 → 6)-linked α-D-mannopyranan as the main chain substituted at positions O-3 by α-L-rhamnopyranosyl units and an acidic rhamnomannan containing 4-O-substituted glucuronic acid units (Gorin *et al.*, 1977). The probable side chains of *C. stenoceras* rhamnomannan are depicted in Figure 9 (structures I and IV). Since the ^{13}C NMR spectrum of *C. stenoceras* rhamnomannan does not contain signals at δ_c 103.7 and 96.6, which arise from C-1's of *O*-α-L-rhamnopyranosyl-(1 → 2)-α-L-rhamnopyranosyl side chains, this polysaccharide differs from *S. schenckii* rhamnomannan obtained at 25°C. Dirhamnosyl side chains seem, then, to be characteristic of *S. schenckii* mycelial rhamnomannans. β-Glucuronic acid units may also be present in some *S. schenckii* rhamnomannans as inferred from the minor peaks at δ_c 105.3–105.5 observed in their ^{13}C NMR spectra (Travassos *et al.*, 1974). Since signals at δ_c 97.3 and 81.6 were absent in these spectra, it is likely that the side chains of *S. schenckii* rhamnomannans differ from those of *C. stenoceras* acidic rhamnomannan. However, in one *S. schenckii* strain, initially regarded as a pathogenic mutant of *C. stenoceras,* a neutral monorhamnosylrhamnomannan was isolated with high proportions of 4-O- and 2,4-di-O-substituted α-D-mannopyranosyl residues along with an acidic rhamnomannan similar to that of *C. stenoceras,* except for the concomitant presence of dirhamnosyl side chains. Such structures were identified by ^{13}C NMR spectroscopy (Travassos *et al.,* 1978).

The rhamnomannan from *C. ulmi* is similar to *S. schenckii* rhamnomannan formed at 37°C (Figure 9, structure I). No 2,4-di-O-substituted α-D-mannopyranose units were detected. Longer side chains with (1 → 2)-linked α-L-rhamnopyranose units were also suggested, but a dirhamnosyl structure as found in *S. schenckii* is unlikely because the 2-O-linked rhamnose units were stable to partial acid hydrolysis (Strobel *et al.,* 1978). Peptidopolysaccharides from *C. ulmi* are also shed into the medium, bind Con A, and have most of the carbohydrate chains O-linked to the peptide.

5.3. Nuclear Magnetic Resonance Spectroscopy and Polysaccharide Structure

NMR spectroscopy (^{13}C) has been used to fingerprint *S. schenckii* and *C. stenoceras* rhamnomannans (Travassos *et al.,* 1974). Acidic rhamnomannans of *C. stenoceras* gave spectra clearly differing from those of *S. schenckii* rhamnomannans as shown by the absence of signals at δ_c 103.5, 99.7, and 96.5 in the C-1 region and the presence of signals at δ_c 105.4, 97.0, 81.4, and 75.0, which correspond to different side-chain structures in the *C. stenoceras* polysaccharide (Table II). Rhamnomannans of *S. schenckii* obtained at 37°C gave spectra differing from those of rhamnomannans from both *S. schenckii* and *C. stenoceras* obtained at 25°C (Figure 10). The lack of longer side chains was inferred from the absence of signals at δ_c 105.4, 103.5, 96.6, and 80.2 (Table III). Depending on the strain, rhamnomannans from yeast forms of *S. schenckii* obtained at 37°C as well as the mycelial rhamnomannans gave spectra with C-1 peaks at δ_c 102.3 and 100.1 corresponding to 4-O- and 2,4-di-O-substituted α-D-mannopyranose units. Assignments of ^{13}C signals in the NMR spectra were made by comparing spectra of purified oligosaccharides and polysaccharides of known structure and of methylglycosides. In the case of methylglycosides used as standards, assignments of signals from *S. schenckii* NMR spectra were made by prediction of the effects of O-substitution on chemical shifts (Gorin and Mazurek, 1975). Signals arising from carbons of the α-D-(1 → 6)-linked D-mannopyranan main chain were assigned in spectra of polysaccharides isolated after Smith degradation or after mild acid hydrolysis of the neutral rhamnomannan. In the case of the yeast rhamnomannan, several signals were assigned in comparison with the chemical shifts of carbons from methyl-α-L-rhamnopyr-

Table II
Structures of *S. schenckii* and *C. stenoceras* Rhamnomannans and Galactomannans: Assignments of ^{13}C NMR Signals of Side Chains of Polysaccharides Obtained at 25°C[a]

Polysaccharide	Signal δ_c (ppm)[b]	C	Structure[c]
Rhamnomannan (*S. schenckii*)	103.7	C-1	α-L-Rhap nonreducing end unit of α-L-Rhap-(1 → 2)-α-L-Rhap
	102.3	C-1	4-O-substituted α-D-Manp of α-L-Rhap-(1 → 4)-α-D-Manp-(1 → 2)-α-D-Manp
	98.2	C-1	α-L-Rhap nonreducing end unit of α-L-Rhap-(1 → 3)-α-D-Manp
	96.8	C-1	2-O-substituted α-L-Rhap of α-L-Rhap-(1 → 2)-α-L-Rhap-(1 → 3)-α-D-Manp
	80.3	C-2	2-O-substituted α-L-Rhap
Rhamnomannan (*C. stenoceras*)	105.6	C-1	4-O-substituted β-D-GlcUA
	102.4	C-1	α-L-Rhap nonreducing end unit of α-L-Rhap-(1 → 4)-β-D-GlcUA
	98.3	C-1	α-L-Rhap nonreducing end unit of α-L-Rhap-(1 → 3)-α-D-Manp
	97.3	C-1	2-O-substituted α-L-Rhap of α-L-Rhap-(1 → 4)-β-D-GlcUA-(1 → 2)-α-L-Rhap
	81.6	C-2	2-O-substituted α-L-Rhap of α-L-Rhap-(1 → 4)-β-D-GlcUA-(1 → 2)-α-L-Rhap
	80.3	C-4	4-O-substituted β-D-GlcUA
Galactomannan (*S. schenckii* or *C. stenoceras*)	109.5	C-1	β-D-Galf nonreducing end unit of β-D-Galf-(1 → 6)-β-D-Galf and β-D-Galf-(1 → 6)-α-D-Manp
	107.2-107.6	C-1	β-D-Galf of β-D-Galf-(1 → 2)-α-D-Manp
	70.7	C-6	β-D-Galf O-6-substituted of β-D-Galf-(1 → 6)-β-D-Galf
	71.3	C-5	β-D-Galf O-6 substituted of β-D-Galf-(1 → 6)-β-D-Galf
	64.5	C-6	O-6 Unsubstituted β-D-Galf
	78.5	C-3	β-D-Galf units
	82.6-83.1	C-2	β-D-Galf units
	84.8-85.0	C-4	β-D-Galf units

[a] Structures are shown in Figure 9.
[b] Signals represent chemical shifts at 70°C.
[c] (Rhap) Rhamnopyranose; (Manp) mannopyranose; (GlcUA) glucopyranosyluronic acid; (Galf) galactofuranose.

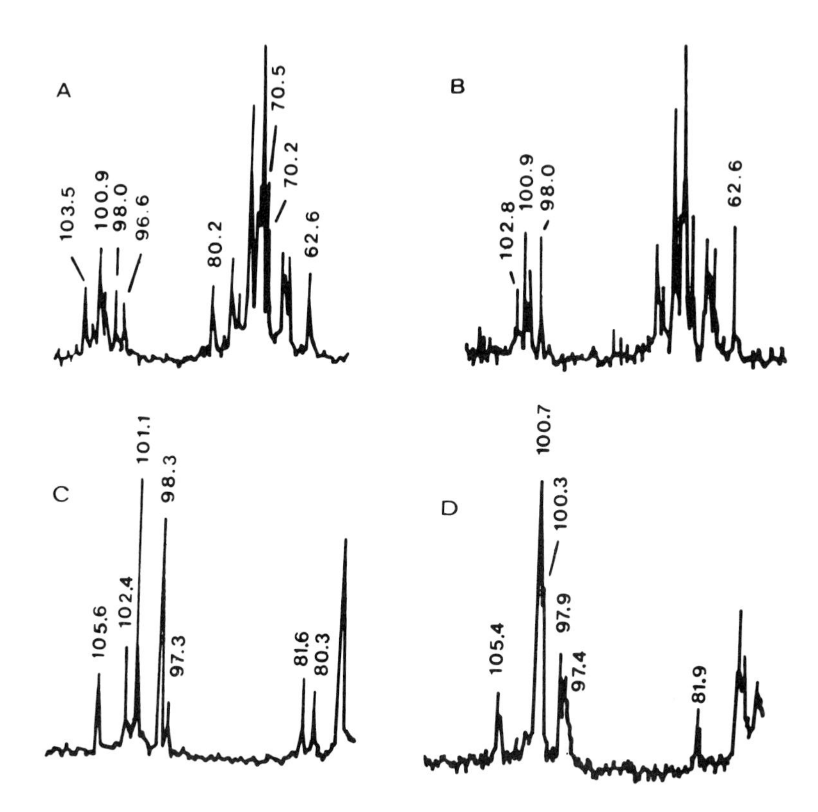

Figure 10. Partial ^{13}C NMR spectra of *S. schenckii* and *C. stenoceras* rhamnomannans. (A) *Sporothrix schenckii* rhamnomannan of the mycelial phase; (B) *S. schenckii* rhamnomannan of the yeast phase with 4-O- and 2,4-di-O-α-D-mannopyranose units; (C) *C. stenoceras* acidic rhamnomannan; (D) acid-degraded polysaccharide of *C. stenoceras.*

Table III
Assignments of Signals in the ^{13}C NMR Spectrum of an *S. schenckii* Rhamnomannan Obtained at 37°C

	Signals, δ_c (70°C)[a] (ppm)						
Structure	C-1	C-2	C-3	C-4	C-5	C-6[b]	CH_3
α-L-Rhamnopyranose nonreducing end units	98.3	(72.0-71.9)		73.6	70.4	—	18.4
3,6-di-O-substituted α-D-mannopyranose units	101.1	67.6	76.6	66.3	72.4	67.3	—

[a]Signals in the δ_c 66.3–76.6 region have values corrected for 70°C (+0.6 ppm), since they were originally obtained at 33°C (Gorin *et al.*, 1977).
[b]Trace amounts of 4-O-substituted α-D-mannopyranose units were detected in this rhamnomannan; a trace of a signal at δ_c. 62.8 (O-6—unsubstituted α-D-Manp units) was present in this spectrum.

anoside and methyl-α-D-mannopyranoside and with spectra of polysaccharides obtained by growing *S. schenckii* with D-[6-$^2H_2$]glucose or D-glucose containing twice the natural abundance of ^{13}C in the C-2 position (Gorin *et al.*, 1977). In the case of *C. stenoceras* glucuronorhamnomannans, some assignments were made by comparison with spectra of the acid-degraded polysaccharide, which lacked signals at δ_c 102.4 and 80.3, indicating the removal of a terminal unit of α-L-rhamnose (1 → 4)-linked to a β-D-glucuronic acid unit (Figure 10).

^{13}C NMR spectroscopy was also helpful in determining the structure of *S. schenckii* and *C. stenoceras* galactomannans. β-Galactofuranose units were identified by comparison with the chemical shifts of ^{13}C signals of methyl-β-D-galactofuranoside and the nonreducing end unit of 5-O-β-linked galactotetraose from *Penicillium charlesii* (Gorin and Mazurek, 1975; Mendonça *et al.*, 1976). Correct assignments of the C-1 signals from *S. schenckii* galactomannans were made after a series of model disaccharides were studied showing that the shifts of the C-1 from β-D-galactofuranose depended on the position of substitution on the mannosyl residue or adjacent galactofuranose unit (Gorin *et al.*, 1981). Thus, a value of δ_c 109.7 was observed for a (1 → 6) linkage, δ_c 107.7 for a (1 → 2) linkage and δ_c 106.5 for a (1 → 3) linkage. *Sporothrix schenckii* and *C. stenoceras* galactomannans gave spectra (Figure 11) with signals at δ_c 109.5, 107.6, and 107.1, suggesting (1 → 6) and (1 → 2) linkages (Mendonça-Previato *et al.*, 1980). Signal assignments in spectra of *S. schenckii* and *C. stenoceras* galactomannans are in Table II.

Structures of *S. schenckii* soluble glucans were confirmed by ^{13}C NMR spectra in comparison with spectra of gentiobiose, β-laminaribiose,

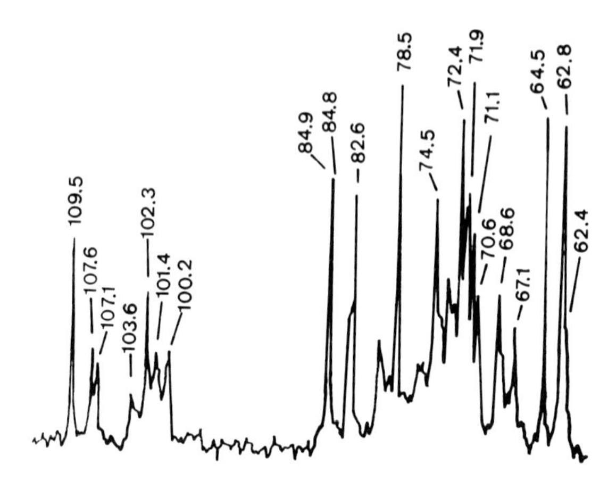

Figure 11. ^{13}C NMR spectrum of *S. schenckii* galactomannan. (From Mendonça-Previato *et al.*, 1980. Used with permission.)

β-cellobiose, laminarin, and a (1 → 6)-linked β-glucan (Previato *et al.*, 1979b).

5.4. Galactomannans

A Fehling's-reagent-precipitable galactomannan was isolated from a conidialess mycelium culture of one *S. schenckii* strain (Mendonça *et al.*, 1976). It contained α-D-mannopyranose and β-D-galactofuranose nonreducing end units and mainly 6-O- and 2,6-di-O-substituted α-D-mannopyranose units. An α(1 → 6)-linked mannopyranan main chain was determined by removal of the α-D-mannopyranose units of the side chains by exo-D-mannosidase. The linkage of the galactofuranose units to the mannan core was not determined. The main structure of this polysaccharide is shown in Figure 9 (structure V). Other galactomannans have been isolated from *S. schenckii* and *C. stenoceras*. In contrast to the one described above, they were not precipitated by Fehling's reagent. These galactomannans accumulated in the medium of mycelial cultures at 25°C along with amylose. A possible structure in these galactomannans is shown in Figure 9 (structure VI). β-D-Galactofuranose units are in side chains of a mannan core, which contains α(1 → 6)- and α(1 → 2)-linked mannopyranose units. They are (1 → 6)-linked to each other (^{13}C NMR C-1 signal at δ_c 109.5) and are in turn at least partly (1 → 2)-linked to the mannan core (C-1 signals at δ_c 107.6 and 107.2).

Several other form-species of *Sporothrix* grown in liquid media were found to accumulate galactose- and mannose-containing polysaccharides (Ishizaki *et al.*, 1979b). Only those form-species closely related to *S. schenckii*—*S. curviconia, S. inflata,* and *S. schenckii* var. *luriei*—contained polysaccharides with rhamnose in addition to galactose and mannose. Galactomannans of *S. schenckii* and *C. stenoceras* differ from those of several species of *Aspergillus* (Barreto-Bergter *et al.*, 1980, 1981) in that they do not contain side chains of (1 → 5)-linked β-galactofuranose units (^{13}C NMR signals at δ_c 108.3–108.5).

5.5. Glucans in Different Cell Types

Alkali-soluble and -insoluble glucans were isolated from *S. schenckii* cell walls of both yeast and mycelial phases (Previato *et al.*, 1979b). The proportions of β(1 → 3), β(1 → 4), and β(1 → 6) linkages in these glucans were determined by methylation–fragmentation analysis and quantitative periodate oxidation (Table IV). Both mycelial and yeast glucans have β(1 → 3)-linked block-type structures and consecutive (1 → 6)- and (1 → 4)- linked oxidizable units. The β-configuration and linkages of *S. schen-*

Table IV
Proportions (%) of Linkages in Soluble and Insoluble Glucans from Different *S. schenckii* Cell Types[a]

Linkages	Yeasts	Conidia	Hyphae
Insoluble glucans			
$\beta(1 \rightarrow 3)$	66	65	65
$\beta(1 \rightarrow 4)$	5	10	9
$\beta(1 \rightarrow 6)$	29	25	26
Soluble glucans			
$\beta(1 \rightarrow 3)$	44	45	45
$\beta(1 \rightarrow 4)$	28	31	29
$\beta(1 \rightarrow 6)$	28	24	26

[a]From Previato *et al.* (1979b). Used with permission.

ckii glucans were confirmed by ^{13}C NMR (C-1 signals at δ_c 103.8 and 104.0) and hydrolysis with exo- and endo-$\beta(1 \rightarrow 3)$-glucanase of *Arthrobacter luteus* and a mixture of $\beta(1 \rightarrow 3)$- and $\beta(1 \rightarrow 6)$-endoglucanases of *Bacillus circulans.* Linear polymers containing mixed $\beta(1 \rightarrow 4)$-, $\beta(1 \rightarrow 6)$-, and $\beta(1 \rightarrow 3)$-linked D-glucopyranose units as in *S. schenckii* are rather uncommon structures in fungi.

The insoluble linear glucan of *S. schenckii* at 10 mg/kg per day and following a standard therapy schedule (Tarnowski, 1975) caused regression of Sarcoma 180 implanted in mice. This activity parallels antitumor properties of other fungal glucans (Whistler *et al.*, 1976).

6. IMMUNOCHEMISTRY OF *Sporothrix schenckii* ANTIGENS

Efforts have been made to locate *S. schenckii* antigens in different cell types as well as to identify antigenic determinants reacting with antibodies or eliciting delayed-type reactions. Well-characterized antigenic determinants are the rhamnose-containing side chains of yeast and mycelial rhamnomannans, but it is obvious that several other structures are important in determining the overall immunological reactivity of *S. schenckii* in infected tissues.

6.1. Antigenic Determinants and Cross-Reactions

Well-characterized *S. schenckii* antigens that were used in immunodiffusion and immunoelectrophoresis tests were obtained by Ishizaki (1970) and by Lloyd and Bitoon (1971). Preparations consisted of peptidorhamnomannans with a contamination of 1–5% of galactose. The antigen from the yeast phase precipitated antibodies from sera of patients with sporotrichosis, but not from sera of normal individuals or patients with other fungal diseases. Since the antigenic determinants in the *S. schenckii* antigen contain rhamnose end units, cross-reactions would be expected with microbial antigens that also contain rhamnose. Reciprocal cross-reactions between *S. schenckii* and several types of *Streptococcus pneumoniae* were reported. Cross-agglutination reactions of both pneumococcal and *S. schenckii* antisera were inhibited by purified pneumococcal S substances (Neill *et al.*, 1955). Cross-reactions were also observed with certain strains of *Leuconostoc mesenteroides*, group B *Streptococcus* (Nakamura *et al.*, 1977), *Klebsiella pneumoniae* K47 (Ishizaki *et al.*, 1979a), rhamnose-containing polysaccharides of 60 species of *Ceratocystis, Europhium,* and *Graphium* that produce exoconidia (Ishizaki *et al.*, 1978), and other species of *Sporothrix* that also synthesize rhamnomannans (Ishizaki *et al.*, 1979b).

Polysaccharides with different rhamnose-containing determinants are expressed on hyphal or on yeast and conidial cell walls of *S. schenckii.* This was shown by chemical analysis of isolated polymers and by immunofluorescent staining of the different cell types (Travassos and Lloyd, 1980). Rabbit sera were raised against an *S. schenckii* strain synthesizing a rhamnomannan at 25°C with a high proportion (~85%) of (1 → 2)-linked dirhamnosyl side chains (Travassos *et al.*, 1973, 1978). At 37°C, rhamnomannans contained mostly monorhamnosyl side chains. The serum raised against cells grown at 25°C precipitated the homologous rhamnomannan and the rhamnomannan from another strain of *S. schenckii* grown at 25°C, but reacted very poorly with the corresponding rhamnomannans isolated from cultures grown at 37°C (Lloyd and Travassos, 1975). The serum raised against cells grown at 27°C precipitated equally well the rhamnomannans obtained at 25 and 37°C. This serum also precipitated rhamnomannans from four species of *Ceratocystis.* The serum raised against cells grown at 25°C reacted poorly with *Ceratocystis* polysaccharides. These results were interpreted as follows: (1) *Sporothrix schenckii* mycelial cultures grown at 25°C form a specific determinant that is probably the α(1 → 2)-linked dirhamnosyl side chain, absent in *Ceratocystis* rhamnomannans or in *S. schenckii* rhamnomannans obtained at 37°C. (2) The reactivities of the rhamnomannans from *Ceratocystis* and *S. schenckii* obtained at 25 and 37°C with the serum raised against *S. schenckii* cells grown at 37°C or in the yeast phase were due to the presence in all polymers of variable proportions of monorhamnosyl side chains. Inhibition experiments with *O*-α-L-rhamnopyranosyl-(1 → 2)-*O*-α-L-rhamnopyranosyl-(1 → 3)-D-mannopyranose and *O*-α-L-rhamnopyranosyl-(1 → 3)-D-mannopyranose confirmed those assumptions (Lloyd and Travassos, 1975). Antibodies raised against the monorhamnosyl side chains were much less specific than those recognizing the dirhamnosyl determinant, and this presumably explains the wide range of cross-reactivity between *S. schenckii* yeast antigens and the rhamnose-containing antigens from *Ceratocystis, Graphium,* and some bacteria.

In addition to the rhamnomannans, *S. schenckii* yeasts also contain antigenic galactomannans. Determinants involved in the cross-reactions of fungal galactomannans contain one or more units of D-galactofuranose units. An anti-*Hormodendrum* serum that reacted with *S. schenckii* yeast forms (Travassos and Lloyd, 1980) had a specificity for β-D-galactofuranose units and thus also reacted with galactomannans from *Aspergillus fumigatus, Exophiala werneckii,* and *Trichophyton rubrum* (Suzuki and Takeda, 1977). By using a rabbit antiserum against the yeast form of *S. schenckii,* additional cross-reactions with pathogenic fungi were detected (Ishizaki *et al.,* 1981). Such reactions were inhibited by absorbing the serum with cells of *E. werneckii* or by adding galactose. Addition of mannose or absorption with *S. cerevisiae* did not abolish serum reactivity. Cross-reactive galactomannans of *S. schenckii* are minor antigens and, depending on the preparations employed for serological tests, may be absent. They tend to be released into the culture medium and are easily removed from the cell wall by washing. Specific reactions for *S. schenckii* using agglutination and precipitin tests have been reported (Karlin and Nielsen, 1970; G.D. Roberts and Larsh, 1971; Seeliger, 1968). Rhamnomannans precipitated by Fehling's reagent may contain only traces of galactose and should be the choice antigen for specific reactions for *S. schenckii.*

6.2. Delayed Hypersensitivity and Other Cell-Mediated Reactions

Skin tests with soluble and cellular antigens of *S. schenckii* yeast forms have long been used in the diagnosis of sporotrichosis or to detect previous immunosensitizing contact with this fungus (Gonzalez-Ochoa and Figueroa, 1947). By using several antigenic preparations including soluble cytoplasmic components and defatted and detergent-extracted cell walls that were further treated with pronase and ribonuclease, Nielsen (1968) observed that only those preparations containing treated or untreated cell walls gave results comparable to those with the whole-yeast antigen. Sensitivity to sporotrichin is greater with the yeast-phase than with the mycelial-phase antigen. Delayed hypersensitivity was tested in 14 patients with cutaneous sporotrichosis by using ethanol-precipitated culture filtrates of the yeast forms of *S. schenckii, C. stenoceras, C. ulmi,*

C. ips, and *C. minor* (Ishizaki *et al.,* 1976). Extensive cross-reactions were obtained, with the reactivity of the *C. stenoceras* antigen showing the best correlation with that of sporotrichin.

An immunologically active *S. schenckii* peptidopolysaccharide able to induce both immediate and delayed hypersensitivity reactions was isolated by extraction with phenol (Noguchi, 1972). After treatment with 16 mM periodate, the oxidized antigen still elicited delayed-type reactions, but was no longer active in the passive cutaneous anaphylaxis test. Treatment with papain gave a glycopeptide fraction that reacted with an anti-*S. schenckii* rabbit serum, but had a decreased capacity to elicit delayed-type reactions (Shimonaka *et al.,* 1975). Results indicate that the determinants for delayed hypersensitivity responses are present in the peptide moieties of the peptidopolysaccharide complexes. Other human pathogenic species do not produce antigens inducing a delayed-type reaction in animals sensitized to *S. schenckii* (Nielsen, 1968).

Cell-mediated immunity in sporotrichosis was also evaluated by the lymphocyte transformation method (Plouffe *et al.,* 1979). Six patients with systemic sporotrichosis had deficient cell-mediated immunity as determined by decreased lymphocyte transformation in response to phytohemagglutinin as compared to normal individuals. Most patients with sporotrichosis showed positive *in vitro* lymphocyte transformation tests in response to yeast forms of *S. schenckii.* Lymphocyte transformation induced by a mycelial antigen was also obtained in a patient with sporotrichotic arthritis (Steele *et al.,* 1976). Transfer factor was successfully used to control the disease in two patients with protracted illnesses and abnormalities of cell-mediated immunity.

In cats infected with the nematode *Brugia malayi,* which produces lymphatic dysfunction, inoculation of *S. schenckii* resulted in more severe lesions and rapid spread to other sites in the body as compared to cats infected only with *S. schenckii* (Barbee *et al.,* 1977). Macdonald *et al.* (1980) observed that subcutaneous and skin lesions that developed in cats inoculated with *S. schenckii* regressed within 31–88 days to complete resolution. To assess whether spontaneous healing of lesions also corresponded to complete elimination of the fungus, animals were inoculated with methyl-prednisolone sodium succinate to suppress immune responses. Lesions reappeared at the same site or at sites close to that of the initial infection 4–9 weeks after treatment with the suppressor. Results suggest that viable fungal elements can be sequestered in tissues for up to 6 months and that healed lesions may be reactivated after immunosuppression.

Experimental sporotrichosis induced in congenitally athymic (nude) mice *(nu/nu)* showed a great susceptibility of these animals to intravenous inoculation of *S. schenckii*. However, elimination of the fungus began on day 8, whereas delayed hypersensitivity to a soluble *S. schenckii* antigen was detected in *nu/+* mice only on day 17 after inoculation, indicating that host resistance does not depend solely on cellular immunity (Shiraishi *et al.*, 1979). Hachisuka and Sasai (1981) inoculated *S. schenckii* intracutaneously in cyclophosphamide-treated mice. Cyclophosphamide severely affects the humoral immune system of chicks and mice without having much effect on the cellular immune compartment. The lesion that developed in cyclophosphamide-treated mice inoculated with *S. schenckii* enlarged strikingly up to the 8th day. After 12 days, the size of the lesion was similar to that of untreated mice, suggesting that a nonhumoral immune mechanism became effective in checking growth of the lesions in both treated and control mice. Several observations in humans and experimental animals suggest that humoral immunity is important as a defense mechanism in early infection. Mixed granulomas of human sporotrichosis contain plasma cells (Lurie, 1971). The dermal infiltrate of guinea pigs inoculated with *S. schenckii* had decreased T-cell and increased B-cell numbers (Hachisuka and Sasai, 1980). A self-limited lymphatic disease was obtained in Syrian hamsters by cutaneous footpad inoculation. Primary infection increased the resistance to reinfection, and sera from infected animals had persistent agglutinin titers against the yeast phase (Charoenvit and Taylor, 1979). Resistance to disseminated infection, as induced by increasing the inoculum, was enhanced by subcutaneous inoculation of crude ribosomal preparations or trypsinized cell walls from *S. schenckii* yeast forms.

Results presented in this section seem to indicate that both humoral and cellular immune responses are effective against growth of lesions and spread of sporotrichosis.

7. PERSPECTIVES

In the last 30 years, studies on *S. schenckii* have evolved from observations on the mycology, clinical forms, and serology of sporotrichosis in infected animals and humans (Norden, 1951). More recent contributions have focused on the chemical nature of antigens and other surface components of *S. schenckii*, the ultrastructure, and the phenotypic and genotypic comparison of this hyphomycete and related species of *Ceratocystis* (Travassos and Lloyd, 1980). Ecological and epidemiological studies, as well as observations to define the role of humoral and cellular immunity in sporotrichosis, have also been reported.

The possibility of obtaining purified components from *S. schenckii* permits determination of their effects on the development of the infection and their capacity to elicit specific immune responses. The relevance of antigen shedding can thus be evaluated in relation to the effectiveness of the immune defense mechanisms.

Purified galactose-free rhamnomannans are now available for the specific serological diagnosis of sporotrichosis. Further studies are necessary to understand their biosynthesis and the induction of enzymes characteristic of each morphological phase. A better knowledge of the organization of the various cell-wall components is also required. Methods involving selective extraction procedures, digestion by specific enzymes, and electron microscopy should be helpful.

Dimorphism in *S. schenckii* has not been clearly correlated with the overall chemical composition of the cell wall. New methods should be introduced to detect localized or discrete alterations in cells already committed to morphogenesis. Other differential markers such as cAMP levels and fatty acid synthesis should be sought to explain dimorphism. Differences in the lipid contents of yeast forms (e.g., linolenic acid) in comparison with the mycelium, as already noted, suggest promising lines of research in *S. schenckii.*

The teleomorph of *S. schenckii* is still unknown. Results obtained so far point to one definite species of *Ceratocystis* being the ascigerous form. On the basis of GC analyses and DNA–DNA hybridization studies, several morphologically related species, including *C. stenoceras,* do not seem to be the perfect form of *S. schenckii.* The phylogenetic relationships of *C. minor* and *S. schenckii* are not clear. A greater number of strains of this species should be investigated in this respect. The search for an as yet unrecognized *Ceratocystis* species that represents the teleomorph of *S. schenckii* should stimulate additional ecological studies.

REFERENCES

Ajello, L., and Kaplan, W., 1969, A new variant of *Sporothrix schenckii, Mykosen* **12:**633–644.

Alviano, C. S., Pereira, M. E. A., Souza, W., Oda, L. M., and Travassos, L. R., 1982, Sialic acids are surface components of *Sporothrix schenckii* yeast forms, *FEMS Microbiol. Lett.* **15:**223–227.

Anderson, J. G., 1978, Temperature-induced fungal development, in: *The Filamentous Fungi,* Vol. 3, *Developmental Mycology* (J. E. Smith and D. R. Barry, eds.), Edward Arnold, London, pp. 358–375.

Aoki, Y., Nakayoshi, H., Asaga, S., and Ono, M., 1967, Studies on the immunologically active substances in fungi, *Jpn. J. Med. Mycol.* **8:**284–291.

Bailey, W. R., and Scott, E. G., 1966, *Diagnostic Microbiology,* 2nd ed., C. V. Mosby, St. Louis.

Ballou, C., 1976, Structure and biosynthesis of the mannan component of the yeast cell envelope, *Adv. Microb. Physiol.* **14**:93–158.

Barbee, W. C., Ewert, A., and Folse, D., 1977, The combined effect of a cutaneo-lymphatic fungus, *Sporothrix schenckii*, and a lymphatic-dwelling nematode, *Brugia malayi*, *Trop,. Geogr. Med.* **29**:65–73.

Barreto-Bergter, E., Travassos, L. R., and Gorin, P. A. J., 1980, Chemical structure of the D-galacto-D-mannan component from hyphae of *Aspergillus niger* and other *Aspergillus* spp., *Carbohydr. Res.* **86**:273–285.

Barreto-Bergter, E., Gorin, P. A. J., and Travassos, L. R., 1981, Cell constituents of mycelia and conidia of *Aspergillus fumigatus*, *Carbohydr. Res.* **95**:205–218.

Benchimol, M., Souza, W., and Travassos, L. R., 1979, Distribution of anionic groups at the cell surface of different *Sporothrix schenckii* cell types, *Infect. Immun.* **24**:912–919.

Bièvre, C., and Jourd'huy, C., 1974, Etude comparative des phospholipides de plusieurs souches de *Ceratocystis stenoceras* et *Sporothrix schenckii*, *C.R. Acad. Sci. Paris* **278**:53–55.

Bièvre, C., and Mariat, F., 1975, Composition en acides gras des lipides polaries et neutres de *Sporothrix schenckii* et de *Ceratocystis stenoceras*, *Sabouraudia* **13**:226–230.

Bièvre, C., and Mariat, F., 1981, Etude de la composition en bases de l'acide desoxyribonucleique de souches de *Sporothrix schenckii* et de *Ceratocystis*, *Ann. Microbiol. Paris* **132B**:281–284.

Brown, R., Weintraub, D., and Simpson, M. W., 1947, Timber as a source of sporotrichosis infection, *Proc. Mine Med. Off. Assoc.* **27**:5–33.

Carmichael, J. W., 1962, *Chrysosporium* and some other aleurosporic hyphomycetes, *Can. J. Bot.* **40**:1137–1173.

Charoenvit, Y., and Taylor, R. L., 1979, Experimental sporotrichosis in Syrian hamsters, *Infect. Immun.* **23**:366–362.

Cole, G. T., 1976, Conidiogenesis in pathogenic hyphomycetes. I. *Sporothrix, Exophiala, Geotrichum*, and *Microsporum*, *Sabouraudia* **14**:81–98.

Correa, C. N. M., Gottschalk, A. F., and Correa, W. M., 1971, Esporotricose: Coloração histológica das navetas por método de captura do ferro coloidal, *Arq. Inst. Biol. Sao Paulo* **38**:163–165.

Drouhet, E., and Mariat, F., 1952a, Action de qualques composes pyrimidiques sur la croissance de *Sporotrichum schenckii*, *Ann. Inst. Pasteur* **82**:114–118.

Drouhet, E., and Mariat, F., 1952b, Etude des facteurs déterminant le développement de la phase levure de *Sporotrichum schenckii*, *Ann. Inst. Pasteur* **83**:506–514.

Findlay, G. H., Vismer, H. F., and Liebenberg, N. W., 1979, Spore ultrastructure in *Sporothrix schenckii*, *Mycopathologia* **69**:167–170.

Fukushiro, R., Kagawa, S., Nishiyama, S., Takahashi, H., and Ishikawa, H., 1965, Die Pilzelemente im Gewebe der Hautsporotrichose des Menschen, *Hautarzt* **16**:18–25.

Garrison, R. G., Boyd, K. S., and Mariat, F., 1975, Ultrastructural studies of the mycelium-to-yeast transformation of *Sporothrix schenckii*, *J. Bacteriol.* **124**:959–968.

Garrison, R. G., Boyd, K. S., and Mariat, F., 1976, Etude sur l'ultrastructure de la transformation mycelium-levure du *Sporothrix schenckii* et du *Ceratocystis stenoceras*, *Bull. Soc. Mycol. Med.* **5**:69–74.

Garrison, R. G., Mariat, F., Boyd, K. S., and Fromentin, H., 1977, Ultrastructural observations of an unusual osmiophilic body in the hyphae of *Sporothrix schenckii* and *Ceratocystis stenoceras*, *Ann. Microbiol. Paris* **128B**:319–337.

Garrison, R. G., Boyd, K. S., Kier, A. B., and Wagner, J. E., 1979, Spontaneous feline sporotrichosis: A fine structural study, *Mycopathologia* **69**:57–62.

Gonzalez-Ochoa, A., and Figueroa, E. S., 1947, Polisacáridos del *Sporotrichum schenckii*, datos inmunollógicos: Intra-dermoreacción en el diagnóstico de la esporotricosis, *Rev. Inst. Salubr. Enferm. Trop. Mexico City* **8**:143–153.

Gonzalez-Ochoa, A., and Soto-Pacheco, R., 1950, Desarollo del *Sporotrichum schenckii* en el pus obtenido de gomas esporotricosicas: Algunos datos sobre su ciclo evolutivo, *Rev. Inst. Salubr. Enferm. Trop. Mexico City* **11**:3–19.

Gooday, G. W., and Trinci, A. P. J., 1980, Wall structure and biosynthesis in fungi, in: *The Eukaryotic Microbial Cell* (G. W. Gooday, D. Lloyd, and A. P. J. Trinci, eds.), Cambridge University Press, London, pp. 207–251.

Gorin, P. A. J., 1981, Carbon-13 nuclear magnetic resonance spectroscopy of polysaccharides, *Adv. Carbohydr. Chem. Biochem.* **38**:13–104.

Gorin, P. A. J., and Mazurek, M., 1975, Further studies on the assignments of signals in ^{13}C magnetic resonance spectra of aldoses and derived methylglycosides, *Can. J. Chem.* **53**:1212–1223.

Gorin, P. A. J., Haskins, R. H., Travassos, L. R., and Mendonça-Previato, L., 1977, Further studies on the rhamnomannans and acidic rhamnomannans of *Sporothrix schenckii* and *Ceratocystis stenoceras, Carbohydr. Res.* **55**:21–33.

Gorin, P. A. J., Barreto-Bergter, E., and Cruz, F. S., 1981, The chemical structure of the D-galacto-D-mannan component of *Trypanosoma cruzi:* ^{13}C N.M.R. shift dependence on structure of D-galactose to D-mannose linkage, *Carbohydr. Res.* **88**:177–188.

Hachisuka, H., and Sasai, Y., 1980, Subpopulations of lymphocytes in the infiltrate of experimental sporotrichosis, *Mycopathologia* **71**:167–169.

Hachisuka, H., and Sasai, Y., 1981, Development of experimental sporotrichosis in normal and modified animals, *Mycopathologia* **76**:79–82.

Harada, T., Nishikawa, T., and Hatano, H., 1976, Antigenic similarity between *Ceratocystis* species and *Sporothrix schenckii* as observed by immunofluorescence, *Sabouraudia* **14**:211–215.

Hektoen, L., and Perkins, C. F., 1900, Refractory subcutaneous abcesses caused by *Sporothrix schenckii,* a new pathogenic fungus, *J. Exp. Med.* **5**:77–89.

Hempel, H., and Goodman, N. L., 1975, Rapid conversion of *Histoplasma capsulatum, Blastomyces dermatitidis,* and *Sporothrix schenckii* in tissue culture, *J. Clin. Microbiol.* **1**:420–424.

Howard, D. H., 1961, Dimorphism of *Sporotrichum schenckii, J. Bacteriol.* **81**:464–469.

Ishizaki, H., 1970, Some antigenic substances from culture filtrate of *Sporotrichum schenckii, Jpn. J. Dermatol. Ser. B* **80**:16–23.

Ishizaki, H., Nakamura, Y., Kariya, H., Iwatsu, T., and Wheat, R. W., 1976, Delayed hypersensitivity cross-reactions between *Sporothrix schenckii* and *Ceratocystis* species in sporotrichotic patients, *J. Clin. Microbiol.* **3**:545–547.

Ishizaki, H., Wheat, R. W., Kiel, D. P., and Conant, N. F., 1978, Serological cross-reactivity among *Sporothrix schenckii, Ceratocystis, Europhium* and *Graphium* species, *Infect. Immun.* **21**:585–593.

Ishizaki, H., Kurata, Y., Nakamura, Y., and Wheat, R. W., 1979a, Serological cross-reactivity between *Klebsiella pneumoniae* K47 and *Sporothrix* species, *Curr. Microbiol.* **2**:355–356.

Ishizaki, H., Nakamura, Y., and Wheat, R. W., 1979b, Comparative immunochemical studies on *Sporothrix* species, *J. Dermatol.* **6**:317–320.

Ishizaki, H., Nakamura, Y., and Wheat, R. W., 1981, Serological cross-reactivity between *Sporothrix schenckii* and various unrelated fungi, *Mycopathologia* **73**:65–68.

Iwatsu, T., 1980, A strain of *Sporothrix schenckii* isolated from nonsporotrichotic human skin scrapings, *Mycopathologia* **71**:37–38.

Kaplan, W., 1970, The fluorescent antibody technique in the diagnosis of mycotic diseases, in: *Proceedings of the International Symposium on Mycoses*, Pan American Health Organization, Washington, D.C., pp. 86–95.

Kaplan, W., and Ivens, M. S., 1970, Fluorescent antibody staining of *Sporotrichum schenckii* in cultures and clinical materials, *J. Invest. Dermatol.* **35**:151–159.

Karlin, J. V., and Nielsen, H. S., Jr., 1970, Serological aspects of sporotrichosis, *J. Infect. Dis.* **121**:316–327.

Kendrick, W. B., and Carmichael, J. W., 1973, Hyphomycetes, in: *The Fungi*, Vol. IVA (G. C. Ainsworth, F. K. Sparrow, and A. S. Sussman, eds.), Academic Press, New York, pp. 323–509.

Kitamura, K., 1965, *Sporotrichum schenckii:* An electron microscopic study, *Jpn. J. Dermatol.* **75**:285–304.

Land, G. A., McDonald, W. C., Stejernholm, R. L., and Friedman, L., 1975, Factors affecting filamentation in *Candida albicans:* Changes in respiratory activity of *Candida albicans* during filamentation, *Infect. Immun.* **12**:119–127.

Lane, J. W., and Garrison, R. G., 1970, Electron microscopy of the yeast to mycelial phase conversion of *Sporotrichum schenckii*, *Can. J. Microbiol.* **16**:747–749.

Lane, J. W., Garrison, R. G., and Field, M. F., 1969, Ultrastructural studies on the yeastlike and mycelial phases of *Sporotrichum schenckii*, *J. Bacteriol.* **100**:1010–1019.

Lavalle, P., Novales, J., and Mariat, F., 1963, Esporotricosis, in: *Congreso Mexicano de Dermatologia, Memorias*, Sociedad Mexicana de Dermatologia, Mexico City, pp. 276–287.

Lii, S.-L., and Shigemi, F., 1973, Demonstration of hyphae in human tissue of sporotrichosis, with statistics of cases reported from Tokushima, *Tokushima J. Exp. Med.* **20**:69–92.

Lloyd, K. O., 1970, Isolation, characterization, and partial structure of peptido-galactomannans from the yeast form of *Cladosporium werneckii*, *Biochemistry* **9**:3446–3453.

Lloyd, K. O., and Bitoon, M. A., 1971, Isolation and purification of a peptido-rhamnomannan from the yeast form of *Sporothrix schenckii:* Structural and immunochemical studies, *J. Immunol.* **107**:663–671.

Lloyd, K. O., and Travassos, L. R., 1975, Immunochemical studies on L-rhamno-D-mannans of *Sporothrix schenckii* and related fungi by use of rabbit and human antisera, *Carbohydr. Res.* **40**:89–97.

Lloyd, K. O., Mendonça-Previato, L., and Travassos, L. R., 1978, Distribution of antigenic polysaccharides in different cell types of *Sporothrix schenckii* as studied by immunofluorescent staining with rabbit antisera, *Exp. Mycol.* **2**:130–137.

Lurie, H. I., 1963, Histopathology of sporotrichosis: Notes on the nature of the asteroid body, *Arch. Pathol.* **75**:421–437.

Lurie, H. I., 1971, Sporotrichosis, in: *The Pathologic Anatomy of Mycoses: Human Infection with Fungi, Actinomyces and Algae* (E. Uehlinger, ed.), Springer-Verlag, New York, pp. 614–675.

Lurie, H. I., and Still, W. J. S., 1969, The "capsule" of *Sporotrichum schenckii* and the evolution of the asteroid body: A light and electron microscopic study, *Sabouraudia* **7**:64–70.

Lynch, P. J., Voorhees, J. J., and Harrell, E. R., 1970, Systemic sporotrichosis, *Ann. Intern. Med.* **73**:23–30.

Macdonald, E., Ewert, A., and Rietmeyer, J. C., 1980, Reappearance of *Sporothrix schenckii* lesions after administration of Solu-Medrol® to infected cats, *Sabouraudia* **18**:295–300.

Mackinnon, J. E., 1970, Ecology and epidemiology of sporotrichosis, in: *Proceedings of the International Symposium on Mycoses,* Pan American Health Organization, Washington, D.C., pp. 169–181.

Mackinnon, J. E., Conti-Diaz, I. A., Gezuelle, E., Civila, E., and Luz, S., 1969, Isolation of *Sporothrix schenckii* from nature and considerations on its pathogenicity and ecology, *Sabouraudia* **7**:38–45.

Maeda, M., Kitajima, Y., and Mori, S., 1980, Ultrastructure of plasma membrane in *Sporothrix schenckii* as revealed by the freeze-fracture method, *J. Electron Microsc.* **29**:236–241.

Mariat, F., 1968, Respiration des phases levure et filamenteuse de *Sporotrichum schenckii,* champignon dimorphique pathogène de l'homme, *C. R. Acad. Sci.* **266**:2064–2066.

Mariat, F., 1971, Adaption de *Ceratocystis* a la vie parasitaire chez l'animal: Etude de l'aquisition d'un pouvoir pathogène comparable a celui de *Sporothrix schenckii, Sabouraudia* **9**:191–205.

Mariat, F., 1975, Observations sur l'écologie de *Sporothrix schenckii* et de *Ceratocystis stenoceras* en Corse et en Alsace, provinces françaises indemnes de sporotrichose, *Sabouraudia* **13**:217–225.

Mariat, F., 1977, Taxonomic problems related to the fungal complex *Sporothrix schenckii/ Ceratocystis* spp., in: *Recent Advances in Medical and Veterinary Mycology* (K. Iwata, ed.), University of Tokyo Press, pp. 265–270.

Mariat, F., Garrison, R. G., Boyd, K. S., Rouffaud, M. A., and Fromentim, H., 1978, Premières observations sur les macrospores pigmentées de *Sporothrix schenckii, C.R. Acad. Sci.* **286**:1429–1432.

Mayberry, J. D., Mullins, J. F., and Stone, O. J., 1966, Sporotrichosis with demonstration of hyphae in human tissue, *Arch. Dermatol.* **93**:65–67.

Mendonça, L., Gorin, P. A. J., Lloyd, K. O., and Travassos, L. R., 1976, Polymorphism of *Sporothrix schenckii* surface polysaccharides as a function of morphological differentiation, *Biochemistry* **15**:2423–2431.

Mendonça-Hagler, L. C., Travassos, L. R., Lloyd, K. O., and Phaff, H. J., 1974, Deoxyribonucleic acid base composition and hybridization studies on the human pathogen *Sporothrix schenckii* and *Ceratocystis* species, *Infect. Immun.* **9**:934–938.

Mendonça-Previato, L., Gorin, P. A. J., and Travassos, L. R., 1980, Galactose-containing polysaccharides from the human pathogens *Sporothrix schenckii* and *Ceratocystis stenoceras, Infect. Immun.* **29**:934–939.

Moraes, M. A. P., and Miranda, E. V., 1964, Sobre a presença de formações radiadas (asteróides) na esporotricose, *Rev. Inst. Med. Trop. Sao Paulo* **6**:5–11.

Muller, H. E., 1975, Uber das Vorkommen von Neuraminidase bei *Sporothrix schenckii* und *Ceratocystis stenoceras* und ihre Bedeutung fur die Ökologie und den Pathomechanismus dieser Pilze, *Zentralbl. Bakteriol. Parasitenkd. Infektionskr. Hyg. Abt. 1 Orig.* **232**:365–372.

Nakamura, Y., Ishizaki, H., and Wheat, R. W., 1977, Serological cross-reactivity between group B *Streptococcus* and *Sporothrix schenckii, Ceratocystis* species and *Graphium* species, *Infect. Immun.* **16**:547–549.

Neill, J. M., Castillo, C. G., and Pinks, A. H., 1955, Serological relationships between fungi and bacteria. I. Cross reactions of *Sporotrichum schenckii* with pneumococci, *J. Immunol.* **74**:120–125.

Nickerson, W. J., 1971, Biochemical bases of cellular shape, in: *Recent Progress in Microbiology* (A. Perez-Miravete and D. Pelaez, eds), Assoc. Mexicana Microbiologia, Mexico City, pp. 123–129.

Nickerson, W. J., and Edwards, G. A., 1949, Studies on the physiological bases of morphogenesis in fungi. I. The respiratory metabolism of dimorphic pathogenic fungi, *J. Gen. Physiol.* **33**:41–55.

Nickerson, W. J., and Mankowski, Z., 1953, Role of nutrition in the yeast-shape in *Candida, Am. J. Bot.* **40**:584–592.

Nicot, J., and Mariat, F., 1973, Caractères morphologiques et position systématique de *Sporothrix schenckii,* agent de la sporotrichose humaine, *Mycopathol. Mycol. Appl.* **49**:53–65.

Nielsen, H. S., Jr., 1968, Biological properties of skin test antigens of yeast form *Sporotrichum schenckii, J. Infect. Dis.* **118**:173–180.

Noguchi, T., 1972, Immunochemical studies on *Sporotrichum schenckii,* I. Extraction and chemical composition of the immunologically active substances, *Acta Sch. Med. Univ. Gifu* **20**:335–343.

Norden, A., 1951, Sporotrichosis: Clinical and laboratory features and a serologic study in experimental animals and humans, *Acta. Pathol. Microbiol. Scand. Suppl.* **89**:1–119.

Oda, L. M., Kubelka, C. F., Alviano, C. S., and Travassos, L. R., 1983, Ingestion of yeast forms of *Sporothrix schenckii* by mouse peritoneal macrophages, *Infect. Immun.* **39**:497–504.

Okudaira, M., Tsubura, E., and Schwartz, J., 1961, A histopathological study of experimental murine sporotrichosis, *Mycopathologia* **14**:284–296.

Oujezdsky, K. B., Grove, S. N., and Szaniszlo, P. J., 1973, Morphological and structural changes during the yeast-to-mold conversion of *Phialophora dermatitidis, J. Bacteriol.* **113**:468–477.

Plouffe, J. F., Jr., Silva, J., Jr., Fekety, R., Reinhalter, E., and Browne, R., 1979, Cell-mediated immune responses in sporotrichosis, *J. Infect. Dis.* **139**:152–157.

Previato, J. O., Gorin, P. A. J., and Travassos, L. R., 1979a, Cell wall composition in different cell types of the dimorphic species *Sporothrix schenckii, Exp. Mycol.* **3**:83–91.

Previato, J. O., Gorin, P. A. J., Haskins, R. H., and Travassos, L. R., 1979b, Soluble and insoluble glucans from different cell types of the human pathogen *Sporothrix schenckii, Exp. Mycol.* **3**:92–105.

Rippon, J. W., 1968, Monitored environmental system to control cell growth, morphology and metabolic rate in fungi by oxidation–reduction potentials, *Appl. Microbiol.* **16**:114–121.

Rippon, J. W., 1980, Dimorphism in pathogenic fungi, *CRC Crit. Rev. Microbiol* **8**:49–97.

Roberts, G. D., and Larsh, H. W., 1971, The serologic diagnosis of extracutaneous sporotrichosis, *Am. J. Clin. Pathol. 56:597–600.*

Roberts, S. O. B., 1980, Treatment of superficial and subcutaneous mycoses, in: *Antifungal Chemotherapy* (D. C. E. Speller, ed.), J. Wiley, New York, pp. 225–283.

Rodriguez-Del Valle, N., Rosario, M., and Torres-Blasini, G., 1983, Effects of pH, temperature, aeration and carbon source on the development of the mycelial or yeast forms of *Sporothrix schenckii* from conidia, *Mycopathologia* **82**:83–88.

Romano, A. H., 1966, Dimorphism, in: *The Fungi,* Vol. II (G. C. Ainsworth and A. S. Sussman, eds.), Academic Press, New York and London, pp. 181–209.

Russell, B., Beckett, J. H., and Jacobs, P. H., 1979, Immunoperoxidase localization of *Sporothrix schenckii* and *Cryptococcus neoformans, Arch. Dermatol.* **115**:433–435.

Salvin, S. B., 1947, Multiple budding in *Sporotrichum schenckii, J. Bacteriol.* **81**:464–469.

Scott, W. A., Mishra, N. C., and Tatum, E. L., 1973, Biochemical genetics of morphogenesis in *Neurospora, Brookhaven Symp. Biol.* **25**:1–18.

Seeliger, H. P. R., 1968, Serology as an aid to taxonomy, in: *The Fungi,* Vol. III (G. C. Ainsworth and A. S. Sussman, eds.), Academic Press, New York and London, pp. 597–624.

Shimonaka, H., Noguchi, T., Kawai, K., Hasegawa, I., Nasawa, I., and Ito, Y., 1975, Immunochemical studies of chemical and enzymatic modification of the antigenic compounds upon immediate and delayed reactions. *Infect. Immun.* **11**:1187–1194.

Shiraishi, A., Nakagaki, K., and Arai, T., 1979, Experimental sporotrichosis in congenitally athymic (nude) mice, *RES J. Reticuloendothel. Soc.* **26**:333–336.

Spencer, J. F. T., and Gorin, P. A. J., 1971, Systematics of the genera *Ceratocystis* and *Graphium:* Proton magnetic resonance spectra of the mannose-containing polysaccharides as an aid in classification, *Mycologia* **63**:387–402.

Staib, F., Randhawa, H. S., and Blisse, A., 1972, Observations on experimental sporotrichosis of the muscle, *Zentralbl. Bakteriol. Parasitenkd. Infektionskr. Hyg. Abt. 1 Orig.* **221**:250–256.

Staib, F., Sethi, K. K., and Blisse, A., 1974, Assimilation von Kreatinin, Kreatin und Guanidoessigsäure durch *Ceratocystis stenoceras* Stamm IP-1013-70 von F. Mariat, *Zentralbl. Bakteriol. Parasitenkd. Infektionskr. Hyg. Abt. 1 Orig.* **226**:402–405.

Steele, R. W., Cannady, P. B., Jr., Moore, W. L., Jr., and Gentry, L. O., 1976, Skin test and blastogenic responses to *Sporotrichum schenckii, J. Clin. Invest.* **57**:156–160.

Stewart, P. R., and Rogers, P. J., 1978, Fungal dimorphism: A particular expression of cell wall morphogenesis, in: *The Filamentous Fungi,* Vol. 3, *Developmental Mycology* (J. E. Smith and D. R. Berry, eds.), Edward Arnold, London, pp. 164–196.

Stretton, R. J., and Dart, R. K., 1976, Long-chain fatty acids of *Sporothrix (Sporotrichum) schenckii, J. Gen. Microbiol.* **3**:635–636.

Strobel, G., Alfen, N., Hapner, K. D., McNeil, M., and Albersheim, P., 1978, Some phytotoxic glycopeptides from *Ceratocystis ulmi,* the Dutch elm disease pathogen, *Biochim. Biophys. Acta* **538**:60–75.

Suzuki, S., and Takeda, N., 1977, Immunochemical studies on the galactomannans isolated from mycelia and culture broths of three *Hormodendrum* strains, *Infect. Immun.* **17**:483–490.

Tarnowski, G. S., 1975, Approaches to the immunotherapy of experimental tumours, in: *Host Defense against Cancer and Its Potentiation* (D. Mizuna, ed.), University Park Press, Baltimore, pp. 389–396.

Taylor, J. J., 1970a, The nature of the secondary conidia of *Sporothrix schenckii, Mycopathol. Mycol. Appl.* **41**:379–382.

Taylor, J. J., 1970b, A comparison of some *Ceratocystis* species with *Sporothrix schenckii, Mycopathol. Mycol. Appl.* **42**:233–240.

Travassos, L. R., and Alviano, C. S., 1981, Cell surface structures of *Sporothrix schenckii* in relation to pathogenicity, *An. Acad. Bras. Cienc.* **53**:847.

Travassos, L. R., and Cury, A., 1971, Thermophilic enteric yeasts, *Annu. Rev. Microbiol.* **25**:49–74.

Travassos, L. R., and Lloyd, K. O., 1980, *Sporothrix schenckii* and related species of *Ceratocystis, Microbiol. Rev.* **44**:683–721.

Travassos, L. R., and Mendonça-Previato, L., 1978, Synthesis of monorhamnosyl L-rhamno-D-mannans by conidia of *Sporothrix schenckii, Infect. Immun.* **19**:1–4.

Travassos, L. R., Gorin, P. A. J., and Lloyd, K. O., 1973, Comparison of the rhamnomannans from the human pathogen *Sporothrix schenckii* with those from the *Ceratocystis* species, *Infect. Immun.* **8**:685–693.

Travassos, L. R., Gorin, P. A. J., and Lloyd, K. O., 1974, Discrimination between *Sporothrix schenckii* and *Ceratocystic stenoceras* rhamnomannans by proton and carbon-13 magnetic resonance spectroscopy, *Infect. Immun.* **9**:674–680.

Travassos, L. R., Souza, W., Mendonça-Previato, L., and Lloyd, K. O., 1977, Location and biochemical nature of surface components reacting with concanavalin A in different cell types of *Sporothrix schenckii, Exp. Mycol.* **1**:293–305.

Travassos, L. R., Mendonça-Previato, L., and Gorin, P. A. J., 1978, Heterogeneity of the rhamnomannans from one strain of the human pathogen *Sporothrix schenckii* determined by ^{13}C nuclear magnetic resonance spectroscopy, *Infect. Immun.* **19:**1107–1109.

Walbaum, S., Duriez, T., Dujardin, L., and Biguet, J., 1978, Etude d'un extrait de *Sporothrix schenckii* (forme levure): Analyse electrophorétique et immunoelectrophorétique; charactérisation des activités enzymatiques, *Mycopathologia* **63:**105–111.

Warr, G. A., 1980, A macrophage receptor for (mannose/glucosamine) glycoproteins of potential importance in phagocytic activity, *Biochem. Biophys. Res. Commun.* **93:**737–745.

Weise, F. C., 1931, Sporotrichosis in Connecticut, *N. Engl. J. Med.* **205:**951–955.

Whistler, R. L., Bushway, A. A., Singh, P. P., Nakahara, W., and Tokuzen, R., 1976, Noncytotoxic antitumor polysaccharides, *Adv. Carbohydr. Chem.* **32:**235–275.

Wilson, D. E., Mann, J. J., Bennett, J. E., and Utz, J. P. 1967, Clinical features of extracutaneous sporotrichosis, *Medicine* (Baltimore) **46:**265–279.

Zeyer, J., Bodmer, J., and Hutter, R., 1981a, Rapid degradation of cyanuric acid by *Sporothrix schenckii, Zentralbl. Bakteriol. Parasitenkd. Infektionskr. Hyg. Abt. 1 Orig. Reihe C* **2:**99–110.

Zeyer, J., Bodmer, J., and Hutter, R., 1981b, Microbial degradation of ammeline, *Zentralbl. Bakteriol. Parasitenkd. Infektionskr. Hyg. Abt. 1 Orig. Reihe C* **2:**289–298.

Part III

Fungi with Yeast and Hyphal Tissue Morphologies

Chapter 7

Candida albicans

David R. Soll

1. GENERAL INTRODUCTION

The dimorphic yeast *Candida albicans* is capable of growing in culture as an ellipsoidal bud or as an elongate hypha. The growth phenotype depends on environmental conditions and the growth history of the cells (Evans *et al.*, 1974, 1975; Chaffin and Sogin, 1976; Shepherd and Sullivan, 1976; Soll and Bedell, 1978; Mitchell and Soll, 1979a; Odds, 1979; Bell and Chaffin, 1980; Buffo *et al.*, 1984; Soll and Herman, 1983). Although most noted for genital infections, *C. albicans* can invade a variety of tissues and is one of the most pervasive fungal pathogens in man (Odds, 1979). It is a commensal inhabitant of the human body, increasing in concentration and invading tissue usually in response to changes in the physiology of the host. Although both growth forms are found in infected tissue (Mackenzie, 1964; Odds, 1979), it seems likely that the elongating hypha penetrates tissue, leaving in its path lateral colonies of budding cells that in turn give rise to new penetrating hyphae.

In the past few years, excellent reviews have been written on the pathogenicity of *Candida* (Odds, 1979), anti-*Candida* chemotherapy (Speller, 1980), the immunological response to *Candida* (Rogers and Balish, 1980), the role of zinc in *Candida* growth and dimorphism (Soll, 1985), and the *Candida* cell cycle (Soll, 1984). Because of space limitations, this chapter will focus on selected information on the molecular basis of phenotypic conversion between the two growth forms and in no way represents an extensive review of all the information so far gathered

David R. Soll • Department of Biology, University of Iowa, Iowa City, Iowa 52242.

on this organism. It is hoped that an understanding of the molecular basis of dimorphism in *C. albicans* will assist in the development of new strategies of therapy.

2. PHENOTYPIC REPERTOIRE OF *Candida albicans*

The budding growth form of *C. albicans* is similar to that of the intensively studied budding yeast *Saccharomyces cerevisiae* (Matile *et al.*, 1969). Cells are round to ellipsoidal and are encased in a cell wall. A fully mature cell exhibits an average diameter of approximately 4 μm (Bedell *et al.*, 1980; Herman and Soll, 1984). During normal cell replication, an evagination forms as an outpocketing of plasma membrane and wall and increases to a volume close to, but not equal to, that of the mother cell (Figure 1). During growth, a septum contiguous with the cell wall grows centripetally at the junction of mother cell and bud, pinching the plasma membrane on either side of the septum. Cell separation occurs at this point. As in *Saccharomyces,* bud and birth scars can be visualized on the

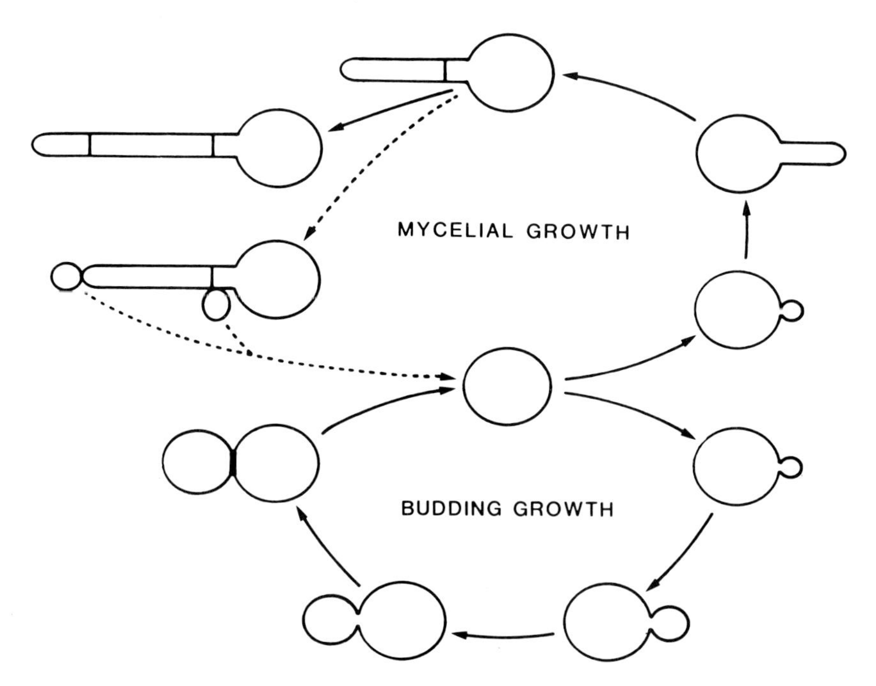

Figure 1. Major growth forms of *Candida albicans.* (----) Conversion of the hyphal form to the budding form.

surfaces of mother and daughter cells, respectively (Shannon and Rothman, 1971; Scherwitz *et al.*, 1978). The budding cell contains a normal repertoire of eukaryotic organelles, including a single nucleus, mitochondria, endoplasmic reticulum, ribosomes, lipid granules, and vacuole (Shannon and Rothman, 1971; Miller *et al.*, 1974; Yamaguchi *et al.*, 1974; Persi and Burnham, 1981). Nuclear division in *C. albicans* appears to be similar to that in *Saccharomyces* (Byers, 1981). The nuclear membrane does not break down during nuclear division, and the mitotic apparatus consists of microtubules attached to disks of dense material lying along the nuclear envelope (Figure 2) that have been referred to in *Saccharomyces* as spindle pole bodies (Byers, 1981).

A thick-walled ellipsoidal cell, which has been observed both in infected tissues (Heinemann *et al.*, 1961) and under prolonged culture conditions (Miller *et al.*, 1974), has been referred to as a chlamydospore.

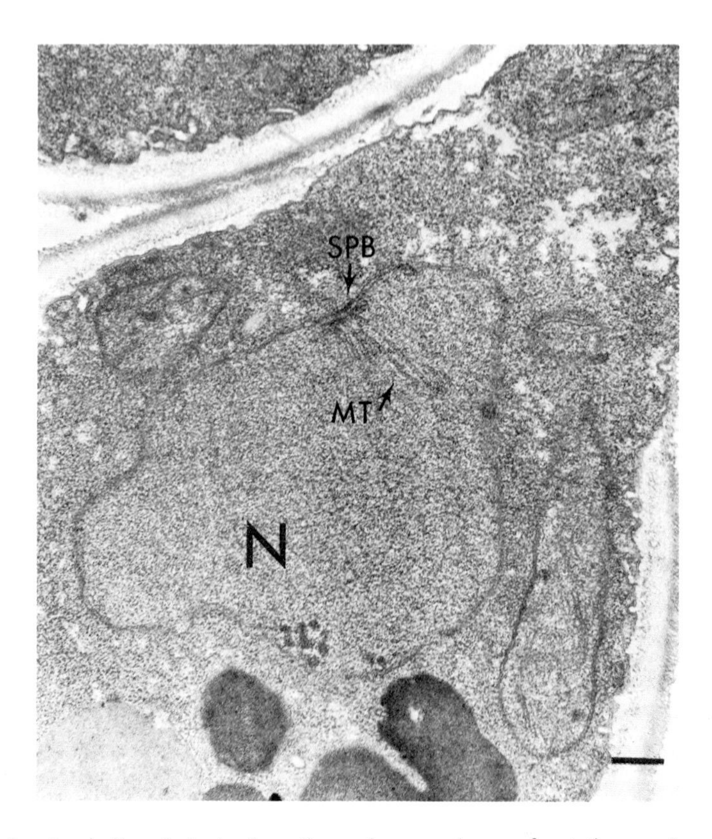

Figure 2. A spindle pole body along the nuclear membrane of a stationary-phase singlet undergoing hypha formation. (SPB) Spindle pole body; (MT) mictrotubule; (N) nucleus. Scale bar: 0.2 μm.

This cell type may represent a stationary-phase phenotype or even a terminal phenotype of the budding form (Nickerson and Mankowski, 1953; Miller and Finnerty, 1979; Shannon, 1981).

In the hyphal form, *C. albicans* grows apically (Braun and Calderone, 1978) as a compartmentalized tube or filament (see Figure 1), each compartment containing a single nucleus and separated by a distinct septum with a central pore (Scherwitz *et al.*, 1978; Gow *et al.*, 1980). Hyphal compartments contain the same organelles as budding cells (Yamaguchi *et al.*, 1974), and the diameter of a hypha is usually about one third the diameter of a comparable budding cell (Herman and Soll, 1984). A hypha can form as an appendage of an ellipsoidal cell or, on occasion, as a lateral extension from a preexisting hypha. During hyphal growth, daughter cells do not separate from mother cells, even after nuclear division is complete (Soll *et al.*, 1978) and a septum is formed. Therefore, one or more steps involved in the process of cell separation or septal maturation during the budding form of growth do not occur during hyphal growth. Scanning electron micrographs of the budding and hyphal forms of *C. albicans* are presented in Figure 3.

Candida can also grow as a pseudohypha, a form intermediate between the ellipsoidal yeast and elongate hypha. In pseudohyphae, cells are longer than normal buds, but more ellipsoidal than hyphal tubes. Cells form apically, do not normally separate, and taper at cell–cell junctions. Conditions that are intermediate to those conducive to bud or hypha formation may result in the pseudohyphal form (Buffo *et al.*, 1984).

3. MINIMUM REQUIREMENTS FOR GROWTH IN CULTURE

In any systematic analysis of the regulation of phenotype in a dimorphic organism, it is necessary to develop sets of environmental conditions that promote and support the alternative growth phenotypes exclusively. The alternative sets of conditions should be as similar as possible in order to present a minimum number of environmental determinants of phenotype. Unfortunately, many of the comparisons of the alternative growth forms of *C. albicans* have employed diverse environmental conditions, including media of different and sometimes undefined composition and temperatures varying as much as 13°C. Such varying environmental conditions may result in different growth rates and in differences in cell physiology that are the direct result of the differing environments and not necessarily basic to the alternative phenotypes, a point that must be kept in mind when assessing biochemical comparisons of the alternative growth forms.

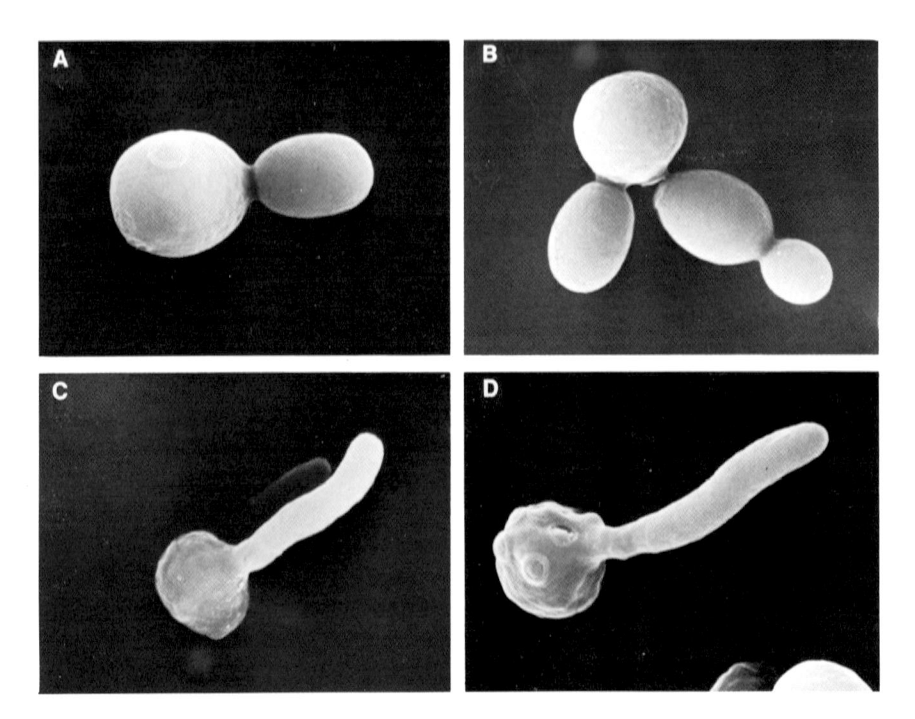

Figure 3. Scanning electron micrographs of budding and hypha-forming cells. (A) A stationary-phase singlet that has formed a daughter bud; (B) a budded cell undergoing secondary bud formation; (C) a stationary-phase singlet that has formed a daughter hypha; (D) a singlet with a longer hypha comparable in growth time to the budded cell in (B).

Although a number of undefined media have been repeatedly employed for *in vitro* studies of growth and dimorphism (e.g., malt extract, rice cream, serum, hay infusion, proteose peptone, yeast extract), *C. albicans* will grow with generation times of less than 2 hr in simple defined media and produce either growth form when suspended in simple buffered medium containing glucose, biotin, inorganic salts, and amino acids (as examples, see Mardon *et al.*, 1971; Saltarelli, 1973; Land *et al.*, 1975; Lee *et al.*, 1975; Manning and Mitchell, 1980a). Growth of *C. albicans* has also been demonstrated to be dependent on specific trace metals (Vaughn and Weinberg, 1978; Soll *et al.*, 1981a). *Candida* is capable of growing under both aerobic and anaerobic conditions (Szawathowski and Hamilton-Miller, 1975) and contains an alternative oxidative pathway that crosses the standard pathway at cytochrome B (Kott *et al.*, 1976; Shepherd *et al.*, 1978).

A number of specific molecules have been demonstrated to affect the growth form of *C. albicans* under select conditions, including *N*-acetylglucosamine (GlcNAc) (Simonetti *et al.*, 1974; Sullivan and Shepherd, 1982), methionine (Mardon *et al.*, 1969), proline and ammonium (Land *et al.*, 1975; Dabrowa *et al.*, 1976), carbon dioxide (Mardon *et al.*, 1969), sulfhydryl compounds (Nickerson and Van Rij, 1949), zinc (Yamaguchi, 1975; Bedell and Soll, 1979; Soll *et al.*, 1981a; Soll, 1985), and serum or serum peptides (Taschdjian *et al.*, 1960; Barlow and Aldersley, 1974; Chattaway and O'Reilly, 1976). However, certain defined media will support both growth forms, the determining factor being either temperature or pH (Evans *et al.*, 1974; Lee *et al.*, 1975; Auger and Joly, 1977; Soll *et al.*, 1981b; Buffo *et al.*, 1984). In general, the budding phenotype is prevalent at low temperature or low pH and the hyphal phenotype is prevalent at high temperature plus high pH. However, some strains appear capable of forming hyphae at low temperature and low pH (Bedell and Soll, 1979; Hrmová and Drobnica, 1981; Soll, 1985).

During growth, *C. albicans* releases into the culture medium metabolites that can affect pH, the rate of growth, and the growth form (Saltarelli, 1973; Soll and Bedell, 1978; Hazen and Cutler, 1979). Although Lingappa *et al.* (1969) originally claimed that phenethyl alcohol and tryptophol were produced by *C. albicans* and functioned as autoinhibitors of growth, more recent studies indicate that these molecules do not function in this role (Hazen and Cutler, 1979; Soll *et al.*, 1981a). However, Hazen and Cutler (1979) have presented evidence that a low-molecular-weight molecule, designated "MARS," is released from budding cells and selectively inhibits hypha formation without affecting pH. Since cells will form either buds or mycelia in perfusion chambers in which the turnover of supporting medium precludes MARS accumulation (Soll and Herman, 1983), this molecule is not an essential component of the cell's soluble environment for the expression of the budding phenotype, although it may still play a role intracellularly.

4. A SIMPLE METHOD FOR REGULATING DIMORPHISM EMPLOYING pH AS THE SOLE DETERMINING FACTOR

In recent years, simple methods have been developed for obtaining synchronous bud or mycelium formation in entire populations of cells, the sole determining environmental factor being either temperature or pH (Buffo *et al.*, 1984). Cells in defined medium at 25°C grow exclusively in the budding form (Lee *et al.*, 1975; Chaffin and Sogin, 1976; Soll and Bedell, 1978) and may enter stationary phase on depletion of zinc or another essential ingredient of the medium, e.g., glucose (Soll *et al.*, 1981a). In the former case, cells accumulate as singlets in G_1 of the cell cycle, in a fashion similar to zinc-starved *Saccharomyces* (Johnston and

Singer, 1978); in the latter case, cells still accumulate as singlets, but cell volume is far more heterogeneous (Bedell and Soll, 1979; Soll *et al.*, 1981a; Anderson and Soll, 1984; Soll 1985). In either case, when stationary-phase cells are released into fresh medium at 37°C and pH 4.5, they synchronously and exclusively form buds and continue to grow in the budding form (Soll *et al.*, 1981b). However, when stationary-phase cells are released into the same medium at 37°C, but at pH 6.7, they synchronously and exclusively form hyphae and then continue to grow in the hyphal form as long as the pH remains above 6.0. At pHs between 5.5 and 6.5, released stationary-phase cultures initially form elongate daughter cells that revert to the budding mode of growth and intermediate phenotypes (Buffo *et al.*, 1984).

Dimorphism can also be regulated by releasing stationary-phase cells into the same medium at high pH, but at temperatures below 34°C for hyphal induction (Buffo *et al.*, 1984). The exact temperature and pH transition points may vary slightly according to the growth history of the cells, the composition of the initial growth medium and release medium, or the strain.

The use of temperature or pH or both to regulate the phenotype of outgrowing populations may be superior to the use of different nutrient media, since it seems more likely that the latter method may be prone to physiological differences not necessarily basic to the alternative phenotypes. For instance, GlcNAc, which has been used to selectively induce mycelium formation (Simonetti *et al.*, 1974; Shepherd *et al.*, 1980), also induces a specific catabolic pathway and binding protein (Biswas *et al.*, 1979; Singh *et al.*, 1979), the induction of which may not be essential for the expression of the hyphal phenotype (Shepherd *et al.*, 1980). In turn, regulation of the phenotype of released stationary-phase cells by pH may be superior to regulation by temperature, since the former leads to similar evagination kinetics and subsequent rates of growth in the diverging populations, whereas the latter leads to dramatically different evagination kinetics and rates of growth (Soll and Bedell, 1978; Mitchell and Soll, 1979a; Brummel and Soll, 1982). Therefore, the regulation of phenotype by a difference in pH affords an unusually simple and comparable situation for biochemical analyses of the two growth forms (for further discussion of this point, see Buffo *et al.*, 1984).

5. STATIONARY PHASE, THE CELL CYCLE, AND HYPHAL INDUCTION

Under most growth conditions, *C. albicans* appears to favor the budding growth form. Therefore, many researchers have approached phenotypic transition in this organism by investigating the specific conditions that are necessary for hypha formation. Chaffin and Sogin (1976) first presented evidence that cells in the exponential phase of growth at 25°C could not be induced to form hyphae after transfer to fresh medium at 37°C, whereas cells in stationary phase were readily induced. These results were subsequently confirmed (Soll and Bedell, 1978), but were then challenged by Mattia and Cassone (1979). It was first reported (Simonetti *et al.*, 1974) that log-phase cells growing at 25°C, when diluted into fresh medium containing GlcNAc at 37°C, formed hyphae in an imidazole but not in a phosphate buffer. Since imidazole buffer at the concentration employed in the original study dramatically decreases the growth rate of *C. albicans* (Herman and Soll, unpublished observation), the induction of hyphae may have been due to the transient cessation of growth or to a dramatic decrease in growth rate. However, in a more recent communication, Mattia and Cassone (1979) obtained hyphal induction at 37°C in log-phase cultures diluted into fresh medium containing either GlcNAc or serum in the absence of imidazole buffer. Unfortunately, the kinetics of growth were not monitored, leaving open the possibility that a transient cessation of cell growth or a depression in growth rate preceded hyphal formation.

These seemingly contradictory results appear to have been resolved in a recent analysis of the effects of starvation of log-phase cells on subsequent hyphal induction (Soll and Herman, 1983). In this study, single cells were monitored in a microscope perfusion chamber by time-lapse videotaping under controlled temperature and pH. If cells in the log phase of growth, at 25°C, are starved in a buffered salts solution for 0–10 min and then perfused with fresh nutrient medium at 37°C, pH 6.5, conditions conducive to hyphae formation, they will form an initial elongate daughter cell, but then revert to the budding form of growth, a phenotype referred to as *revertant* (Buffo *et al.*, 1984). However, if log-phase cells are starved for 20 min or longer, then perfused with fresh nutrient medium at 37°C, pH 6.5, they resume growth exclusively in the hyphal form. The manner in which mycelium formation occurs appears to depend on the point in the budding cycle at the initiation of starvation (Soll and Herman, 1983). The majority of singlets in the starved population evaginate on the average 90 min after release into fresh medium and then grow exclusively in the hyphal form. The majority of budded cells first form an evagination on the mother cell after an average period of 90 min, followed by an evagination on the daughter cell after an average subsequent period of 50 min. Evaginations on the mother cell form more frequently in a position adjacent to the bud and may reflect the positioning of the spindle plaque body (Byers, 1981). Evaginations are formed only on buds containing nuclei. A minority of starved budding cells resume growth by terminal expansion of the bud, tapering into an elongate mycelium. These cells appear to possess small buds at the time of starvation. In all cases, evaginations then grow for at least 100 min in the hyphal form (Soll and Herman, 1983).

Although several observations now support the relationship between the cessation of cell multiplication (by starvation or entrance into stationary phase) and acquisition of the capacity to form a hypha, the exact involvement of the cell cycle is not clear. If cells simply have to be in a particular phase of the cell cycle, then one would expect any cell population in log phase to contain a proportion of cells in this phase that are inducible, which is not the case (Chaffin and Sogin, 1976). It may not be fortuitous that stationary-phase cells, which are inducible, are homogeneously blocked in G_1 (Soll *et al.*, 1981b) and that the related budding yeast *Saccharomyces* must position itself at start, an entrance point to G_1, to enter the mating phase of its life cycle (Pringle and Hartwell, 1981). Therefore, the relationships among growth rate, the cell cycle, and the capacity to form a hypha deserve further attention. It will be especially interesting to test whether starved log-phase cells, which form hyphae on release into fresh medium at 37°C and pH 6.5, contain unreplicated nuclear DNA.

6. PHENOTYPIC COMMITMENT, SEPTUM FORMATION, AND FILAMENT-RING FORMATION

Since stationary-phase cells are pluripotent, one can define when they become committed to the alternate phenotypes by releasing them into medium conducive to one phenotype, then shifting them at various times to conditions conducive to the alternative phenotype. The average time at which a shift to the alternative environmental condition does not result in the alternative terminal phenotype is considered the average time of commitment. Shift experiments can be performed between high and low temperature (Evans *et al.*, 1975; Mitchell and Soll, 1979a; Chaffin and Wheeler, 1981) or between high and low pH (Mitchell and Soll, 1979a). In each of these methods, the former condition is conducive to hypha formation and the latter to bud formation. However, the pH-shift experiment has the advantage of identical evagination kinetics and similar initial growth rates under alternative sets of conditions (Soll *et al.*, 1981b; Brummel and Soll, 1982), making comparisons between the diverging populations more easily interpretable (Mitchell and Soll, 1979a). Using the pH-shift experiment, it has been demonstrated that cells at low pH (conducive to bud formation) become committed to the budding phenotype at the same time as initial evagination and that cells at high pH (conducive to hypha formation) become committed to the hyphal phenotype roughly 20–30 min after evagination (Mitchell and Soll, 1979a) (these results are also diagrammed in Figure 4). It has subsequently been demonstrated that the onset of septum formation in both budding and hypha-forming cells correlates with phenotypic commitment and that the position of the septum differs markedly in the diverging cell types (Mitchell and Soll, 1979b). As in *S. cerevisiae* (Cabib, 1975), the chitin-containing septum forms invariably at the mother–daughter cell junction in budding cells. In contrast, the germ-tube septum forms on the average 2 μm from the mother–daughter cell junction (Mitchell and Soll, 1979b; Soll and Mitchell, 1983) (these results are diagrammed in Figure 4).

It has recently been found that *C. albicans* forms a transient filament ring just prior to septum formation in both budding and hypha-forming cells (Soll and Mitchell, 1983). As in *Saccharomyces* (Byers and Goetsch, 1976), this ring is positioned invariably at the junction of mother cell and

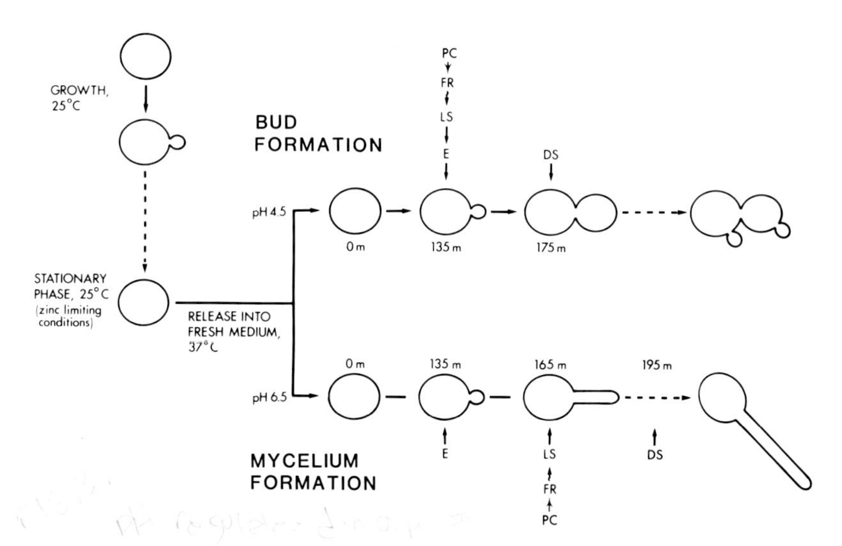

Figure 4. Temporal and spatial characterization of evagination (E), light (LS)- and dark (DS)-staining chitin septum, filament-ring formation (FR), and phenotypic commitment (PC) during pH-regulated dimorphism. Results are synopsized from Mitchell and Soll (1979a,b), Soll and Mitchell (1983), and Soll *et al.* (1981a). The timing of filament-ring formation was not as carefully defined as the other outgrowth parameters. Note the correlation of commitment, light-septum formation, and filament-ring formation. Light- and dark-septum formation reflect the intensity of staining by Calcofluor, a fluorescent dye specific for fibrillar chitin.

bud, the future location of the chitin ring and resulting septum (Figure 5A and B). A cross section of the ring includes, on the average, 12 filament cross sections just under the plasma membrane and equidistant from one another (Figure 5A and B). In hypha-forming cells, the ring is formed roughly 20–30 min after evagination and is positioned, on the average, 2 μm from the junction of the mother cell and daughter tube (Figure 5C and D), approximately the same average distance as the septum (Mitchell and Soll, 1979b). In both growth forms, the filament ring disappears when the primary septum grows centripetally, as is the case in *Saccharomyces* (Byers and Goetsch, 1976). It has been suggested (Soll and Mitchell, 1983) that the filament ring is involved in the localized activation of chitin synthetase, which appears to be distributed throughout the plasma membrane (Duran *et al.*, 1979).

The temporal correlation between phenotypic commitment, filament-ring formation, and septum formation in the alternate growth forms (diagrammed in Figure 4) may be no accident. If formation of the filament ring dictates septum formation, then the former is more likely to be involved in phenotypic commitment. Further investigation of this possibility is warranted, since the molecular events involved in phenotypic commitment must be fundamental to cell divergence.

Commitment to the budding phenotype is permanent throughout uninterrupted growth (Chaffin and Sogin, 1976; Mitchell and Soll, 1979a), but a brief period of starvation results in pluripotency (Soll and Herman, 1983). In contrast, commitment to hypha formation appears to occur each time a septum is formed and is limited to the single compartment distal to the most recently formed septum (Mitchell and Soll, 1979a), again indicating the more tenuous state of the hyphal form of growth.

7. BIOCHEMICAL AND PHYSIOLOGICAL COMPARISONS OF THE TWO GROWTH FORMS

The difficulty in assessing many of the biochemical and physiological comparisons of the two growth forms of *C. albicans* stems from three distinct problems: First, extreme differences in the two sets of environmental conditions employed in many studies to obtain homogeneous populations of the alternative phenotypes may result in physiological differences that are specific to the environmental differences, but are not basic to the difference in phenotypes. Second, temporal analyses of cells, including defined landmark events such as evagination, are rarely performed. This is especially complicating under conditions of outgrowth

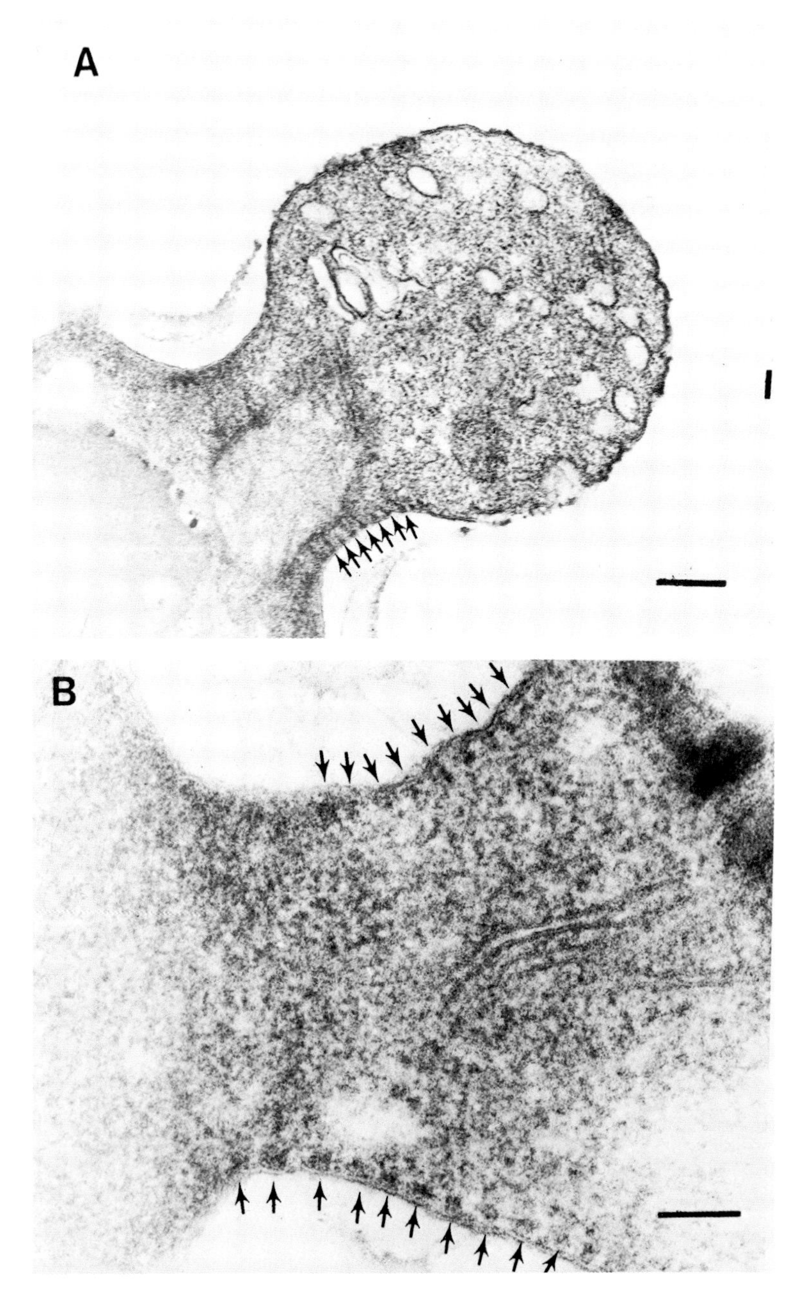

Figure 5. Electron micrographs of the filament ring in thin sections of *Candida albicans.* (A, B) Filament ring in budding cells; (C, D) filament ring in hypha-forming cells. Arrows

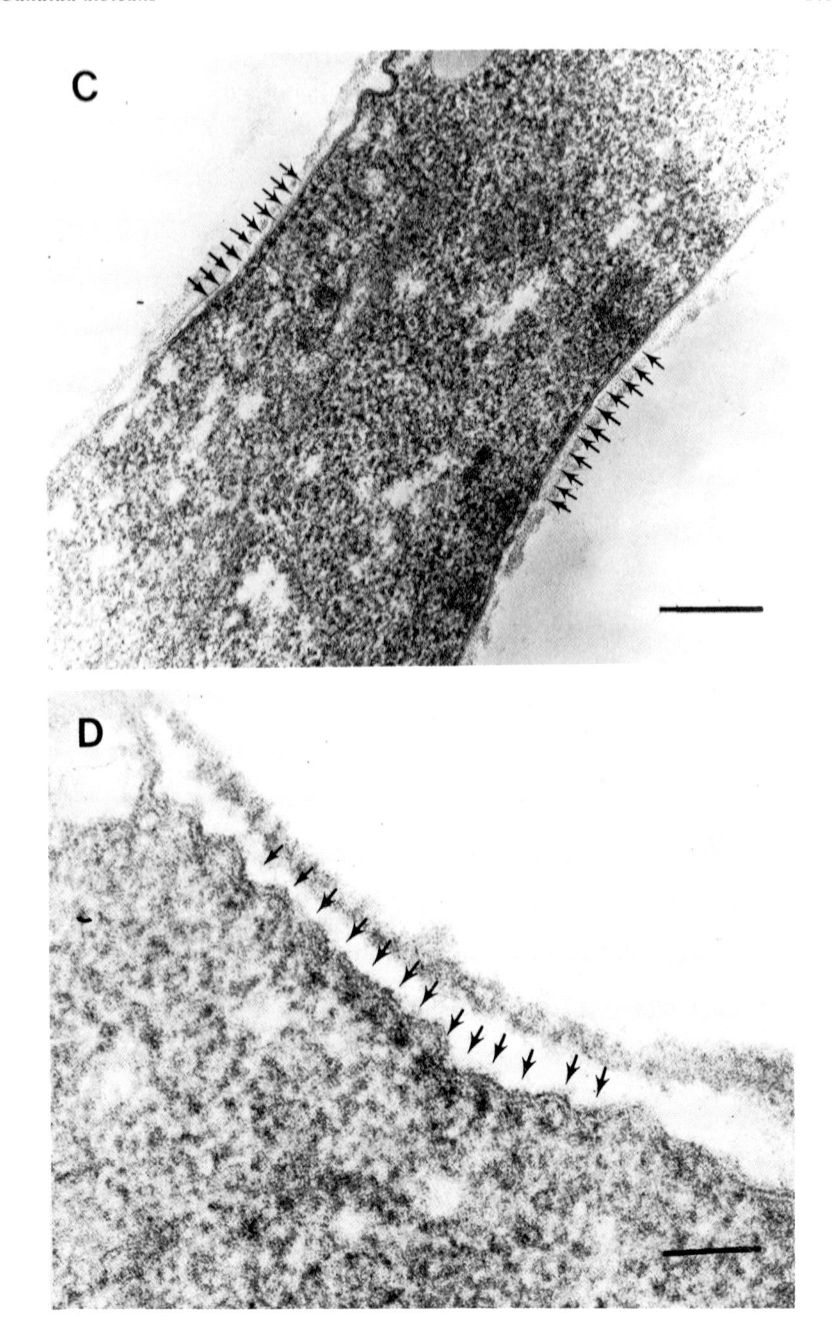

point to filament cross sections just under the plasma membrane. Scale bars: (A) 0.2 μm; (B) 0.1 μm; (C) 0.2 μm; (D) 0.05 μm.

(release from stationary phase), since a very detailed temporal program of gene expression accompanies this process in both growth forms (Brummel and Soll, 1982; Anderson and Soll, 1984; Finney *et al.*, 1985). Conversion induced by temperature differences can involve as much as a 2-fold difference in the timing of evagination in the diverging populations (Buffo *et al.*, 1984). Third, reversion of hyphae to budding cells in prolonged growth cultures, especially when the pH drops below 6.0, can result in a culture of mixed phenotype, a situation that is not conducive to biochemical analysis. In addition to these difficulties, the number of published studies is minimal, and most studies have uncovered qualitative rather than quantitative differences between the two growth forms. Nevertheless, several recent observations are worth considering.

7.1. Cyclic AMP

It was recently reported that the cellular level of cyclic AMP (cAMP) increases in germ-tube-forming populations but not in budding populations (Niimi *et al.*, 1980). On the other hand, the cGMP concentration does not increase in either population. Although these results imply that a difference in cAMP levels exists between hypha- and bud-forming populations, interpretation must be tempered by the fact that the former cells were grown at 40°C and the latter at 30°C. Chattaway *et al.* (1981) have also found an increase in cAMP content following release of stationary-phase cells into fresh medium at 37°C. In addition, there have been several reports that the addition of cAMP (Bhattacharya and Datta, 1977), dibutyryl-cAMP (Niimi *et al.*, 1980; Chattaway *et al.*, 1981), and the phosphodiesterase inhibitor theophylline (Chattaway *et al.*, 1981) enhances mycelium formation. Further work on the involvement of cAMP in *C. albicans* dimorphism is indeed warranted, especially since an increase in cAMP concentration has been implicated in the developmental program of gene expression in the slime mold *Dictyostelium discoideum* (Chung *et al.*, 1981), and as we shall see in the next section, a temporal program of gene expression accompanies outgrowth in *C. albicans.* Testing whether the level of cAMP varies between cell populations forming buds or mycelia at the same temperature and in the same basic medium but at different pHs should be an immediate objective.

7.2. Chitin Synthesis

As in the more carefully examined budding yeast *Saccharomyces* (Cabib, 1975), chitin is an important component of the *C. albicans* cell wall and of the septum in particular (Chattaway *et al.*, 1968; Horisberger and Vonlanthen, 1977; Braun and Calderone, 1978; Mitchell and Soll, 1979b). Chattaway *et al.* (1968) first presented evidence that the hyphal form of *C. albicans* contains roughly 3 times more chitin in wall preparations than the budding form. Subsequently, Braun and Calderone (1978) presented evidence that when yeast cells from agar-solidified medium are released into Sabouraud–dextrose broth and grown for 4 hr as budding yeasts, they incorporate [^{3}H]-GlcNAc into chitin at roughly 10 times the rate of cells that grow as hyphae when released into a buffered glucose solution containing biotin plus rabbit serum. In this study, it was also demonstrated that mycelia have roughly twice the chitin synthetase activity of budding cells. Although these results suggest a dramatic difference in chitin synthesis in the two growth forms under the conditions employed, it remains to be demonstrated that these differences also exist between the alternative phenotypes grown in the same medium and at the same temperature, but at different pH.

In recent years, a number of biochemical events related to chitin synthesis have been intensively studied in *C. albicans* (Singh and Datta, 1978, 1979a,b; Singh *et al.*, 1979; Chiew *et al.*, 1980; Shepherd *et al.*, 1980; Sullivan and Shepherd, 1982), including the inducibility of key enzymes in the pathway of UDP-GlcNAc synthesis, enzymes involved in the catabolism of GlcNAc, and the mechanism of GlcNAc uptake. So far, the results obtained indicate that the metabolism of G1cNAc, a known enhancer of germ-tube formation under select conditions (Simonetti *et al.*, 1974; however, see also Wain *et al.*, 1976a), as well as a precursor to chitin, is similar in bud- and hypha-forming populations [e.g., GlcNAc kinase induction is similar in the two growth forms (Shepherd *et al.*, 1980)]. Whether any differences exist between the two growth forms in the synthesis of the chitin precursor remains an important question, especially if the temporal and spatial differences in septum formation between the two forms prove to be basic in the establishment of alternate phenotypes (Mitchell and Soll, 1979b; Soll, 1984). It may be that temporal and spatial differences, rather than qualitative differences in GlcNAc and chitin synthesis, are basic to the establishment of alternate phenotypes in this case (Soll and Mitchell, 1983).

8. MACROMOLECULAR SYNTHESIS DURING OUTGROWTH IN THE TWO GROWTH FORMS OF *Candida*

Biochemical comparisons of the two phenotypes are by nature limited to one or a small number of molecular pathways or molecules. Such studies are focused by predictions of the possible molecular differences between the growth forms. Therefore, only a limited number of the thousands of gene products in the cell's genetic repertoire are examined, leaving open the possibility, or probability, that a number of extremely important gene products essential for the establishment and maintenance of the alternative phenotypes may go unnoticed. The new technologies of molecular genetics are well suited for examining this problem in *Candida,* and several laboratories have begun to employ them.

Unfortunately, very little is known about the metabolism of RNA during outgrowth. A single report by Wain *et al.* (1976b) demonstrated that the RNA content of cells growing in either form increases continuously throughout the cell cycle in synchronized cultures, but the RNA species were not determined. Recently, an analysis was made of the RNAs synthesized during outgrowth at 37°C of cells that had entered stationary phase under zinc-limiting or zinc-excess conditions (Anderson and Soll, 1984). It was discovered that [^{3}H]uridine began to be incorporated into RNA approximately 10 min after release from stationary phase in both cases. However, zinc-limited cells continued to incorporate at a very low rate for 70 subsequent min. At 80 min, the rate increased dramatically to a new level. In contrast, the rate of incorporation in zinc-excess cells increased to the maximum rate by 25 min. The difference between the two populations for the onset of maximum incorporation was found to be roughly 40 min (Anderson and Soll, 1984).

In contrast to incorporation into RNA, measurements of net RNA accumulation presented a very different picture (Anderson and Soll, 1984). During outgrowth of zinc-limited cells, the level of total cell RNA remained constant up to 110 min, then began to increase at a constant rate. In contrast, during outgrowth of zinc-excess cells, the level of total RNA remained constant up to 30 min, then increased at a low but constant rate between 30 and 90 min. At 90 min, the rate of accumulation increased to a maximum level. In this analysis of RNA synthesis (Anderson and Soll, 1984), it was concluded that incorporation kinetics indicated that new RNAs were indeed synthesized prior to evagination in both populations, but did not accurately represent the rates of RNA synthesis. The onset of net RNA accumulation correlated with evagination and hence probably reflected growth kinetics. In addition, the RNA synthesized prior to and after evagination in both populations was predominantly ribosomal (Anderson and Soll, 1984). No measurements of messenger RNA (mRNA) synthesis have been reported.

Although differences in the kinetics of RNA synthesis have been demonstrated between released populations of zinc-limited and zinc-excess cells, no significant differences have been observed between cells budding at low pH and cells forming hyphae at high pH (Anderson and

Soll, unpublished observations). As we shall see, this is not a surprising finding.

Interesting but conflicting results have recently been reported on the proteins synthesized during outgrowth (Manning and Mitchell, 1980b; Brummel and Soll, 1982; Brown and Chaffin, 1981; Syverson *et al.*, 1975; Finney *et al.*, 1985). When cells that have entered stationary phase under zinc-limiting conditions are released into fresh medium at 37°C and at either low pH (conducive to bud formation) or high pH (conducive to hyphae formation), they begin synthesizing protein after a 50-min lag period (Dabrowa *et al.*, 1970; Brummel and Soll, 1982; Anderson and Soll, 1984). At the time of evagination (approximately 140 min after release into fresh medium), and approximately 15–20 min later in hypha-forming cells, a dramatic increase in protein synthesis occurs. The pre-evagination period of protein synthesis has been designated phase II and the postevagination period of increased synthesis phase III (Brummel and Soll, 1982). The onset and subsequent increase in protein synthesis follow closely the onset and increase in RNA synthesis and therefore may reflect a direct coupling of the rate of protein synthesis to the rate of RNA synthesis (Anderson and Soll, 1984). These results are summarized in Figure 6.

Dabrowa *et al.* (1970) reported that in cytoplasmic extracts containing a limited number of proteins, one protein was specific to the budding phase and two proteins to the hyphal phase. Syverson *et al.* (1975), employing crossed immunoelectrophoresis with absorption *in situ*, presented evidence that each growth form had at least six antigens that were form-specific. With the advent of two-dimensional polyacrylamide gel electrophoresis (2D-PAGE), the resolution of proteins synthesized by either growth form increased dramatically. Manning and Mitchell (1980b) labeled cells with $^{35}SO_4$ for 3 hr at 24°C (conditions for bud formation) and for 6 hr at 37°C (conditions for hypha formation) and then separated total cellular protein by 2D-PAGE. They found that of the 200 identifiable polypeptides, several were labeled in the hyphal form that were not labeled in the budding form of the wild-type strain. However, variant analysis indicated that these polypeptides could be labeled in combination with the budding phenotype, leading these investigators to conclude that there were few if any phenotype-specific polypeptides. Manning and Mitchell (1980c) further generated antibodies to budding- and hyphal-cell extracts, then adsorbed labeled protein extracts of budding and hyphal forms with anti-hyphal- and anti-budding-phase immunoglobulins. Their results indicate that no identifiable antigens were specific to the hyphal form and that differences observed by 2D-PAGE may be due to protein modification. Brown and Chaffin (1981) labeled cells

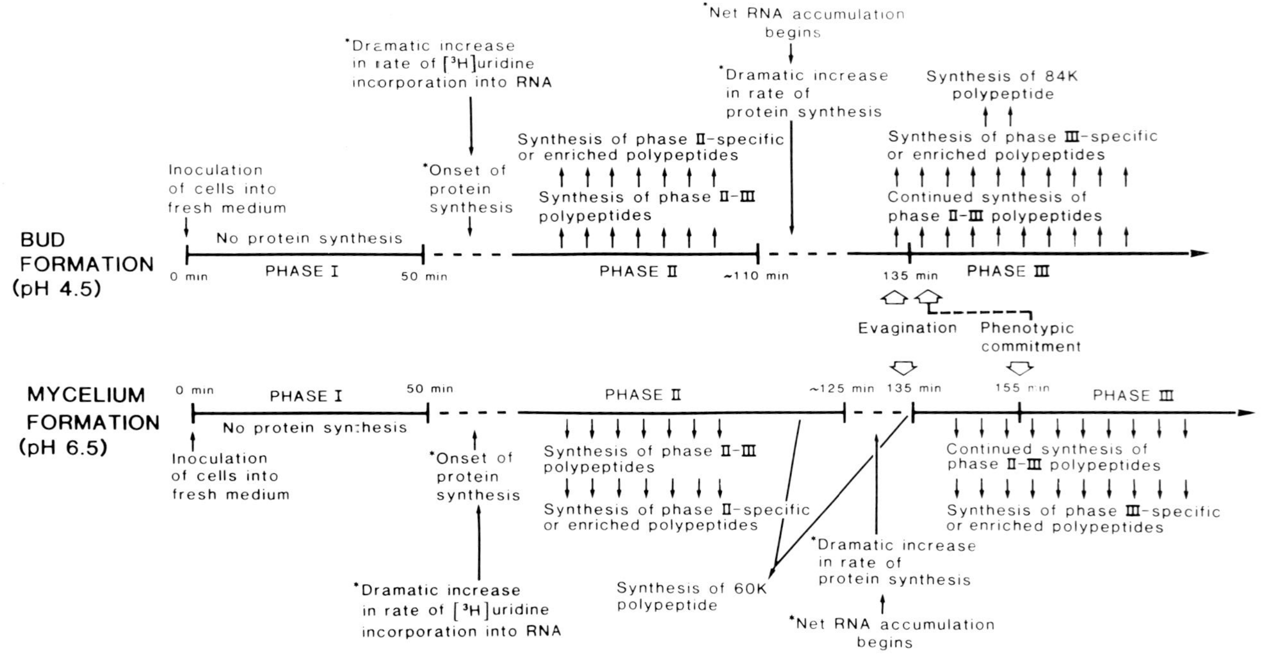

Figure 6. Diagram of the program of RNA and protein synthesis accompanying outgrowth in zinc-depleted stationary-phase cultures released into fresh medium at pH 4.5 to induce bud formation and at pH 6.7 to induce hypha formation. (*) Rough estimates. It should be noted that the RNA synthesis monitored by Anderson and Soll (1984) was predominantly ribosomal. No measurements of the kinetics of mRNA have been reported during pH-regulated dimorphism. Also, the very low but constant initial rate of [^{3}H]uridine incorporation into RNA (Anderson and Soll, 1984) has not been indicated in the figure. Although we have included the specific syntheses of phenotype-specific polypeptides, we have omitted syntheses of pH-specific polypeptides (for an explanation of these distinctions, see Anderson and Soll, 1984). Results are synopsized from Brummel and Soll (1982), Anderson and Soll (1984), Finney *et al.* (1985), and Soll *et al.* (unpublished observations).

with [^{35}S]methionine or [^{3}H]leucine for 20-min periods during outgrowth at low temperature (for bud formation) and at high temperature (for hypha formation) and identified roughly 230 polypeptides. They reported no temporal change in the pattern of synthesis during outgrowth in either growth form, but did find that budding cells synthesized 5 polypeptides that were not found in the hyphal phase; however, except for changes in labeling intensity, all polypeptides synthesized in the hyphal phase were synthesized in the budding phase. Recently, a temporal analysis of protein synthesis was performed during outgrowth in budding and hypha-forming populations employing both 1D-PAGE and 2D-PAGE (Brummel and Soll, 1982; Finney *et al.*, 1985). In this more detailed study (Finney *et al.*, 1984), stationary-phase cells were released into fresh medium at low pH (4.5) to induce bud formation or at high pH (6.7) to induce hypha formation, then pulse-labeled with [^{35}S]methionine between 50 and 100 min (the preevagination period, phase II), between 100 and 150 min (the evagination and phenotypic commitment period), and between 150 and 200 min (the postevagination period, phase III). Proteins were separated by 2D-PAGE, and 374 identifiable polypeptides were grouped in seven categories: (1) polypeptides labeled at roughly the same or similar intensities during the three pulse periods for cells evaginating at both low and high pH (237 polypeptides); (2) polypeptides not labeled during the initial pulse period, but labeled during the second or third pulse period, or both, at both low and high pH (37 polypeptides, phase III-specific); (3) polypeptides labeled at low levels during the first pulse period, but at significantly higher levels during the second or third pulse period, or both, at both low and high pH (23 polypeptides, phase III-enriched); (4) polypeptides labeled at relatively high levels during the first pulse period, but at lower or negligible levels during the second and third period at both low and high pH (18 polypeptides, phase II-specific or enriched); (5) polypeptides labeled at negligible or low levels at low pH, but at significant levels at high pH (2 polypeptides, high pH or hypha-specific); (6) polypeptides labeled at negligible or low levels at high pH, but at significant levels at low pH (4 polypeptides, low pH or bud-specific); (7) polypeptides labeled only during the second pulse (1 polypeptide, putative commitment protein); (8) polypeptides labeled in patterns that do not fit any logical or reproducible scheme (16 polypeptides); (9) polypeptides labeled at too low an intensity to accurately categorize (40 polypeptides). Four spots were categorized in two patterns each, but were only counted once in summing total spots analyzed (see Finney *et al.*, 1985). By examining the proteins synthesized by variant MD20, which forms buds at both low and high pH, these investigators further concluded that only 1 of the 2 polypeptides associated with hypha formation (category 5) was in fact hypha-specific, and only 1 of the 4 polypeptides associated with bud formation (category 6) was in fact bud-specific. The remaining polypeptides were specific to high or low pH, respectively (Finney *et al.*, 1985).

Employing a reticulocyte *in vitro* translation system, Finney *et al.* (in prep.) further demonstrated that translatable mRNA for the hypha-specific polypeptide exists only in hypha-forming cells and not in budding cells, indicating that regulation of at least one phenotype-specific polypeptide is at the level of transcription. The polypeptide that is specific to budding cells has a molecular weight just below 60,000, close to the molecular weight of a major cytoplasmic antigen released by *Candida* in both humans and animal models (Greenfield and Jones, 1981). Finally, the bud-specific polypeptide has a molecular weight close to 84,000, but is at the basic border of normal 2D gels and therefore must be confirmed by non-equilibrium 2D-PAGE.

The results so far obtained indicate that very few differences exist between the two growth forms for the kinetics of macromolecular synthesis (both RNA and protein) and for the repertoire of proteins synthesized during outgrowth (Manning and Mitchell, 1980b; Brown and Chaffin, 1981; Brummel and Soll, 1982; Anderson and Soll, 1984; Finney *et al.*, 1985). The combined results suggest that only a few major proteins differ between the budding and hyphal forms. However, caution must be used in interpreting the results obtained employing 2D-PAGE, since even though this method allows ready resolution of over 350 major polypeptides in *Candida* extracts, the genetic repertoire of *C. albicans* includes the potential for at least 10,000 polypeptides (Soll, 1984). Indeed, if regulatory proteins involved in establishing alternate phenotypes are synthesized transiently at the time of phenotypic commitment and at very low levels, they may be far beyond the resolution of normal 2D-PAGE. Another approach to this problem would be to test whether establishment of the alternative growth forms involves the appearance of transient or stable form-specific mRNAs. The technology necessary for examining this question is at hand.

9. GENETICS OF *Candida*

If differential gene expression proves to be involved in the establishment of alternate phenotypes in *Candida,* then genetic methods will be indispensable for future analyses of gene regulation. The lack of a known sexual phase in *Candida* makes this a more difficult but not insurmountable task.

Although a number of different measurements of DNA content have been published for *C. albicans,* three recent reports are in complete agreement. Whelan and Magee (1981) measured the DNA content of 17 independent isolates and obtained a range of 31–44 fg/cell with a mean of 35. Soll *et al.* (1981b) measured DNA in stationary-phase cells, presumably in G_1, and obtained a measure of 38 fg/cell. Recently, Riggsby *et al.* (1982) reported an average DNA content of 37 fg/cell. These figures are close to the reported DNA content of diploid *Saccharomyces* (Lauer *et al.*, 1977).

Although arguments concerning the ploidy of *C. albicans* still exist (see discussion in Riggsby *et al.*, 1982), it seems reasonable to conclude that most *Candida* strains are diploid. By analysis of the segregation of genetic markers in cell populations treated with low doses of irradiation to induce mitotic crossing over, it has been demonstrated that genetic heterozygosity exists at a number of gene loci (Whelan *et al.*, 1980, 1981; Whelan and Magee, 1981; Whelan and Soll, 1982; DeFever *et al.*, 1982), indicating that common *Candida* strains are diploid or at least aneuploid for the markers examined. By a number of indirect tests, including a comparison of *Candida* and *Saccharomyces* DNA content, UV survival, and chemical mutagenesis, Olaiya and Sogin (1979) concluded that *Candida* was diploid. Finally, Riggsby *et al.* (1982) recently examined ploidy by reassociation kinetics of denatured single-copy DNA. Their results again demonstrated a diploid genome. In addition, the latter investigators found that single-copy DNA composes approximately 85% of the total genome and that repetitive sequences compose approximately 15% (Riggsby *et al.*, 1982).

Although standard sexual methods for analyzing linkage do not exist, parasexual methods, as well as analyses of segregants after induced mitotic crossing over, have been successfully employed. Whelan and Soll (1982) demonstrated the linkage of a *MET* gene to two lethal genes (*LET1* and *LET2*) and have presented the inferred genotype of strain Ca526 to be *MET-LET1-LET2*-centriole. Recently, several laboratories have demonstrated the applicability of protoplast fusion in *Candida* and its potential for linkage analyses (Poulter *et al.*, 1981; Kakar and Magee, 1982; Pesti and Ferenczy, 1982; Sarachek and Rhoads, 1981).

So far, the genetic tools being developed for *C. albicans* have not been applied to problems of dimorphism. However, this will no doubt occur shortly and will constitute an important approach to the regulation of dimorphism, especially since developmental variants are relatively easy to obtain. A number of studies have been made of hypha-minus variants (e.g., Ogletree *et al.*, 1978; Manning and Mitchell, 1980a,b; Olaiya *et al.*, 1980), although the alternate variant phenotype, bud-minus or "divisionless" (e.g., Nickerson and Chung, 1954), appears to be far less common.

10. CONCLUSION

It should be clear that this chapter was not intended to include all the literature on *C. albicans* or even all the literature specifically on *Candida* dimorphism. Rather, it was my intention to consider a limited number of topics that are being actively investigated by laboratories at present and that it is to be hoped will coalesce in the next few years into an integrated picture of phenotypic regulation. It is therefore worthwhile to conclude by reconsidering a few of the problems that remain in analyses of *Candida* dimorphism and some of the basic questions that are at present unanswered.

I have stressed throughout this review the problems that have been inherent in most of the biochemical and physiological comparisons of the two phenotypes. The use of different media, sometimes undefined, and different temperatures, sometimes varying by as much as 13°C, to distinguish between the alternate phenotypes has led to dubious conclusions about real differences. This problem has haunted comparisons of alternate phenotypes in other dimorphic yeasts as well (e.g., see Ross and Orlowski, 1982). Indeed, many of the differences observed between the budding and the hyphal forms may very well be the result of the environment and may have nothing to do with the basic differences in phenotype. To compound this problem, it has recently been demonstrated that outgrowth involves a program of gene expression. Therefore, temporal analyses of outgrowth in the two growth forms must be performed. It is insufficient and sometimes misleading to compare populations outgrowing in the two phenotypes at only one time point, especially when the average time and the synchrony of evagination, as well as subsequent growth rates, vary due to medium composition or temperature. In addition, because of the clearly defined points of phenotypic commitment, one may be missing the most important events by comparing cells at the two terminal phenotypes rather than during establishment of those phenotypes.

At present, pH-regulated dimorphism appears to have the advantage of identical evagination kinetics for populations synchronously producing buds or germ tubes (Soll *et al.*, 1981b; Buffo *et al.*, 1984). In addition, the fact that the diverging populations are in the same medium at the same temperature should remove differences that are due to temperature or composition of the medium, leaving far fewer differences that in turn may be more likely basic to phenotype. However, one must still remain cautious, since differences due to pH and not to phenotype may still exist. This leads to the suggestion that any difference in phenotype should be documented by employing at least two independent methods for distinguishing between phenotypes, e.g., pH and temperature.

Finally, it should be clear from the literature reviewed in this chapter that several major questions concerning dimorphism in *C. albicans* are at present receiving concentrated attention, but remain unanswered. The role of differential gene expression in the establishment of alternative phenotypes must first be established. Are specific genes differentially expressed? If so, at what level of gene expression are they regulated? What is the molecular basis of phenotypic commitment for the alternative phenotypes? Can temporal and spatial differences in the synthesis of particular molecules and the formation of subcellular structures account for phenotypic differences in the absence of differential gene expression, a possibility rarely considered (Soll and Sonneborn, 1971)? What mechanisms are involved in the different modes of growth in elongating mycelia and expanding buds? Why do budding cells but not hyphae go through cell separation? What is different in wall formation in the two growth forms under comparable environmental conditions? Are the timing, location, and mode of chitin synthesis pivotal in the establishment of the alternative phenotypes? Are low-molecular-weight molecules such as MARS (Hazen and Cutler, 1979), cAMP (Niimi *et al.*, 1980; Chattaway *et al.*, 1981), or calmodulin (Hubbard *et al.*, 1982) involved in the establishment of alternate phenotypes? Many more basic questions can now be formulated concerning the regulation of phenotype in *C. albicans,* and that task will be left to the interested reader. The fact that so many detailed questions can be formulated and experimentally approached attests to the progress made in recent years both in the study of *C. albicans* and in related fields. With increased interest in *Candida* dimorphism, evidenced by the increase in the number of publications on the molecular biology, genetics, biochemistry, and biology of this organism, many of these questions will be answered in the next few years. These answers should not only be helpful in developing new strategies for treating *C. albicans,* but should also add to our understanding of the regulation of cell divergence and phenotypic commitment, two basic but poorly understood problems in the field of developmental biology.

REFERENCES

Anderson, J., and Soll, D. R., 1984, The effects of zinc on stationary phase phenotype and macromolecular synthesis accompanying outgrowth of *Candida albicans, Infect. Immun.* **46:**13–21.

Auger, P., and Joly, J., 1977, Factors influencing germ tube production in *Candida albicans, Mycopathologia* **61:**183–186.

Barlow, A. J. E., and Aldersley, T., 1974, Factors present in serum and seminal plasma which promote germ-tube formation and mycelial growth of *Candida albicans, J. Gen. Microbiol.* **82:**261–272.

Bedell, G., and Soll, D. R., 1979, The effects of low concentration of zinc on the growth and dimorphism of *Candida albicans:* Evidence for zinc resistant and zinc sensitive pathways for mycelium formation, *Infect. Immun.* **26:**348–354.

Bedell, G., Werth, A., and Soll, D. R., 1980. The regulation of nuclear migration and division during synchronous bud formation in released stationary phase cultures of the yeast *Candida albicans, Exp. Cell Res.* **127:**103–113.

Bell, G., and Chaffin, W. L., 1980, Nutrient-limited yeast growth in *Candida albicans:* Effect on yeast mycelial transition, *Can. J. Microbiol.* **26:**102–105.

Bhattacharya, A., and Datta, A., 1977, Effect of cAMP on RNA and protein synthesis in *Candida albicans, Biochem. Biophys. Res. Commun.* **7:**1438–1444.

Biswas, M., Singh, B., and Datta, A., 1979, Induction of *N*-acetylglucosamine catabolic pathway in yeast, *Biochim. Biophys. Acta* **585:**535–542.

Braun, P. C., and Calderone, R. A., 1978, Chitin synthesis in *Candida albicans:* Comparison of yeast and hyphal forms, *J. Bacteriol.* **135:**1472–1477.

Brown, L. A., and Chaffin, W. L., 1981, Differential expression of cytoplasmic proteins during yeast bud and germ tube formation in *Candida albicans, Can. J. Microbiol.* **27:**580–585.

Brummel, M., and Soll, D. R., 1982, The temporal regulation of protein synthesis during synchronous bud or mycelium formation in the dimorphic yeast *Candida albicans, Dev. Biol.* **89:**211–224.

Buffo, J., Herman, M., and Soll, D. R., 1984, A characterization of pH-regulated dimorphism in *Candida albicans, Mycopathologia* **85:**21–30.

Byers, B., 1981, Cytology of the yeast life cycle, in: *The Molecular Biology of the Yeast Saccharomyces: Life Cycle and Inheritance* (D. N. Strathern, E. W. Jones, and J. R. Broach, eds.), Cold Spring Harbor Laboratory, Cold Spring Harbor, New York, pp. 59–96.

Byers, B., and Goetsch, L., 1976, A highly ordered ring of membrane-associated filaments in budding yeast, *J. Cell Biol.* **69:**717–721.

Cabib, E., 1975, Molecular aspects of yeast morphogenesis, *Annu. Rev. Microbiol.* **29:**191:214.

Chaffin, W. L., and Sogin, S. L., 1976, Germ tube formation from zonal rotor fractions of *Candida albicans, J. Bacteriol.* **126:**771–776.

Chaffin, W. L., and Wheeler, D. E., 1981, Morphological commitment in *Candida albicans, Can. J. Microbiol.* **27:**131–137.

Chattaway, F. W., and O'Reilly, J., 1976, Induction of the mycelial form of *Candida albicans* by hydrolysates of peptides and seminal plasma, *J. Gen. Microbiol.* **96**:317–322.
Chattaway, F. W., Holmes, M. R., and Barlow, A. J. E., 1968, Cell wall composition of the mycelial and blastospore forms of *Candida albicans, J. Gen. Microbiol.* **51**:367–376.
Chattaway, F. W., Wheeler, P. R., and O'Reilly, J., 1981, Involvement of adenosine 3':5'-cyclic monophosphate in the germination of blastospores of *Candida albicans, J. Gen. Microbiol.* **123**:233–240.
Chiew, Y. Y., Shepherd, M. G., and Sullivan, P. A., 1980, Regulation of chitin synthesis during germ tube formation in *Candida albicans, Arch Microbiol.* **125**:97–104.
Chung, S., Landfear, S. M., Blumberg, D. D., Cohen, N. S., and Lodish, H. F., 1981, Synthesis and stability of developmentally regulated *Dictyostelium* mRNA's are affected by cell–cell contact and cAMP, *Cell* **24**:785–797.
Dabrowa, N., Howard, D. H., Landau, J. W., and Shechter, Y., 1970, Synthesis of nucleic acid and proteins in the dimorphic forms of *Candida albicans, Sabouraudia* **8**:163–169.
Dabrowa, N., Taper, S. S., and Howard, D. H., 1976, Germination of *Candida albicans* induced by proline, *Infect. Immun.* **13**:830–835.
DeFever, K., Whelan, W. L., Beneke, E. S., Rogers, A. L., Vaselenak, J., and Soll, D. R., 1982, Resistance to 5-fluorocytosine in *Candida albicans:* The frequency of partially resistant strains among clinical isolates, *Antimicrob. Agents Chemother.* **22**:810–815.
Duran, W., Cabib, E., and Bowers, B., 1979, Chitin synthetase distribution on the yeast plasma membrane, *Science* **203**:303–365.
Evans, E. G., Odds, F. C., Richardson, M. D., and Holland, R. T., 1974, Effect of growth medium on filament production in *Candida albicans, Sabouraudia* **12**:112–119.
Evans, E. G., Odds, F. C., and Holland, K. T., 1975, Optimum conditions for initiation of filamentation in *Candida albicans, Can. J. Microbiol.* **21**:338–342.
Finney, R., Langtimm, C., and Soll, D. R., 1985, The programs of protein synthesis accompanying the establishment of alternative phenotypes in *Candida albicans, Mycopathologia* (in press).
Gow, N. A., Gooday, G. W., Newsam, R. M., and Gull, K., 1980, Ultrastructure of the septum in *Candida albicans, Curr. Microbiol.* **4**:357–359.
Greenfield, R. A., and Jones, J. M., 1981, Purification and characterization of a major cytoplasmic antigen of *Candida albicans, Infect Immun.* **34**:469–477.
Hazen, R. C., and Cutler, J. E., 1979, Autoregulation of germ tube formation by *Candida albicans, Infect. Immun.* **24**:661–666.
Heinemann, H. S., Yunis, E. J., Siemienski, J., and Braude, A. I., 1961, Chlamydospores and dimorphism in *Candida albicans* endocarditis, *Arch. Intern. Med.* **108**:570–577.
Herman, M., and Soll, D. R., 1984, A comparison of volume growth during bud and mycelium formation in *Candida albicans:* A single cell analysis, *J. Gen. Microbiol.* **130**:2219–2228.
Horisberger, M., and Vonlanthen, M., 1977, Location of mannan and chitin on thin sections of budding yeasts with gold markers, *Arch. Microbiol.* **115**:1–7.
Hrmová, M., and Drobnica, L., 1981, Induction of mycelial type of development in *Candida albicans* by low glucose concentration, *Mycopathologia* **76**:83–96.
Hubbard, M., Bradley, M., Sullivan, P., Shepherd, M., and Forrester, I., 1982, Evidence for the recurrence of calmodulin in the yeasts *Candida albicans* and *Saccharomyces cerevisiae, FEBS Lett.* **137**:85–88.
Johnston, G. C., and Singer, R. A., 1978, RNA synthesis and control of cell division in the yeast *Saccharomyces cerevisiae, Cell* **14**:951–958.
Kakar, S. N., and Magee, P. T., 1982, Genetic analysis of *Candida albicans:* Identification

of different isoleucine-valine, methionine, and arginine alleles by complementation, *J. Bacteriol.* **151**:1247–1252.

Kott, E. J., Olson, U. L., Rolervic, L. J., and McClary, D. O., 1976, An alternate respiratory pathway in *Candida albicans, Antonie van Leeuwenhoek J. Microbiol. Serol.* **42**:33–48.

Land, G. A., McDonald, W. C., Stjernholm, R. L., and Friedman, L., 1975, Factors affecting filamentation in *Candida albicans:* Changes in respiratory activity of *Candida albicans* during filamentation, *Infect. Immun.* **12**:119–127.

Lauer, G. O., Roberts, T. M., and Klotz, L. C., 1977, Determination of the nuclear DNA content of *Saccharomyces cerevisiae* and implications of the organization of DNA in yeast chromosomes, *J. Mol. Biol.* **114**:507–526.

Lee, K. L., Buckley, H. R., and Campbell, H. R., 1975, An amino acid liquid synthetic medium for development of mycelial and yeast forms of *Candida albicans, Sabouraudia* **13**:148–153.

Lingappa, B. T., Prasad, M., and Lingappa, Y., 1969, Phenethyl alcohol and tryptophol: Autoantibodies produced by the fungus *Candida albicans, Science* **163**:192–194.

Mackenzie, D. W., 1964, Morphogenesis of *Candida albicans in vivo, Sabouraudia* **3**:225–232.

Manning, M., and Mitchell, T. G., 1980a, Strain variation and morphogenesis of yeast- and mycelial-phase *Candida albicans* in low sulfate, synthetic medium, *J. Bacteriol.* **142**:714–719.

Manning, M., and Mitchell, T. G., 1980b, Morphogenesis of *Candida albicans* and cytoplasmic proteins associated with differences in morphology, strain, or temperature, *J. Bacteriol.* **144**:258–273.

Manning, M., and Mitchell, T. G., 1980c, Analysis of cytoplasmic antigens of the yeast and mycelial phases of *Candida albicans* by two-dimensional electrophoresis, *Infect. Immun.* **30**:484–495.

Mardon, D. W., Balish, E., and Phillips, A. W., 1969, Control of dimorphism in a biochemical variant of *Candida albicans, J. Bacteriol.* **100**:701–707.

Mardon, D. W., Hurst, S. K., and Balish, E., 1971, Germ tube production by *Candida albicans* in minimal liquid culture media, *Can. J. Microbiol.* **17**:851–856.

Matile, P., Moor, H., and Robinow, C. F., 1969, Yeast cytology, in: *The Yeasts,* Vol. I (A. H. Rose and J. S. Harrison, eds.), Academic Press, New York, pp. 219–302.

Mattia, E., and Cassone, A., 1979, Inductibility of germ tube formation in *Candida albicans* at different phases of yeast growth, *J. Gen. Microbiol.* **113**:439–442.

Miller, S. E., and Finnerty, W. R., 1979, Age-related physiological studies comparing *Candida albicans* chlamydospores to yeast, *Can. J. Microbiol.* **25**:765–772.

Miller, S. E., Spurlock, B. O., and Michaels, G. E., 1974, Electron microscopy of young *Candida albicans* chlamydospores, *J. Bacteriol.* **119**:992–999.

Mitchell, L., and Soll, D. R., 1979a, Commitment to germ tube or bud formation during release from stationary phase in *Candida albicans, Exp. Cell Res.* **120**:167–179.

Mitchell, L., and Soll, D. R., 1979b, Septation during synchronous mycelium and bud formation in released stationary phase cultures of *Candida albicans, Exp. Mycol.* **3**:298–309.

Nickerson, W, J., and Chung, C. W., 1954, Genetic block in the cellular division mechanism of a morphological mutant of a yeast, *Am. J. Bot.* **41**:114–120.

Nickerson, W. J., and Mankowski, Z., 1953, Role of nutrition in the maintenance of the yeast-shape in *Candida, Am. J. Bot.* **40**:584–592.

Nickerson, W. J., and Van Rij, N. J., 1949, The effect of sulphhydryl compounds, penicillin, and cobalt on the cell division mechanism of yeast, *Biochim. Biophys. Acta* **3**:461–475.

Niimi, M., Niimi, K., Tokunagu, J., and Nakayama, H., 1980, Changes in cyclic nucleotide levels and dimorphic transition in *Candida albicans*, *J. Bacteriol.* **142:**1010–1014.
Odds, F. C., 1979, *Candida and Candidosis*, University Park Press, Baltimore.
Ogletree, F. F., Abdilal, A. T., and Ahearn, D. G., 1978, Germ-tube formation by atypical strains of *Candida albicans*, *Antonie van Leeuwenhoek J. Microbiol. Serol.* **44:**15–24.
Olaiya, A. F., and Sogin, S. J., 1979, Ploidy determination of *Candida albicans*, *J. Bacteriol.* **140:**1043–1049.
Olaiya, A. F., Steed, J. F., and Sogin, S. J., 1980, Deoxyribunucleic acid-deficient strains of *Candida albicans*, *J. Bacteriol.* **141:**1284–1290.
Persi, M. A., and Burnham, J. C., 1981, Use of tunnic acid as a fixative–mordant to improve the ultrastructural appearance of *Candida albicans* blastospores, *Sabouraudia* **19:**1–8.
Pesti, M., and Ferenczy, L., 1982, Protoplast fusion hybrids of *Candida albicans* sterol mutants different in nystatin resistance, *J. Gen. Microbiol.* **128:**123–128.
Poulter, R., Jeffery, K., Hubbard, M. J., Shepperd, M. G., and Sullivan, P. A., 1981, Parasexual genetic analysis of *Candida albicans* by spheroplast fusion, *J. Bacteriol.* **146:**833–840.
Pringle, J. R., and Hartwell, L. M., 1981, The *Saccharomyces cerevisiae* cell cycle, in: *The Molecular Biology of the Yeast Saccharomyces: Life Cycle and Inheritance* (J. N. Strathern, E. W. Jones, and J. R. Broach, eds.), Cold Spring Harbor Laboratory, Cold Spring Harbor, New York, pp. 97–142.
Riggsby, W. S., Torres-Bauza, L. J., Wills, J. W., and Townes, T. M., 1982, DNA content, kinetic complexity, and the ploidy question in *Candida albicans*, *Mol. Cell. Biol.* **2:**853–862.
Rogers, T. J., and Balish, E., 1980, Immunity to *Candida albicans*, *Microbiol. Rev.* **44:**660–682.
Ross, J. F., and Orlowski, M., 1982, Regulation of ribosome function in the fungus *Mucor:* Growth rate vis-à-vis dimorphism, *FEMS Microbiol. Lett.* **13:**325–328.
Saltarelli, C. G., 1973, Growth stimulation and inhibition of *Candida albicans* by metabolic by-products, *Mycopathol. Mycol. Appl.* **51:**53–63.
Sarachek, A., and Rhoads, D. P., 1981, Production of heterokaryons of *Candida albicans* by protoplast fusions: Effects of differences in proportions and regenerative abilities of fusion partners, *Curr. Genet.* **4:**221–222.
Scherwitz, C., Martin, R., and Ueberberg, H., 1978, Ultrastructural investigations of the formation of *Candida albicans* germ tubes and septa, *Sabouraudia* **16:**115–124.
Shannon, J. L., 1981, Scanning and transmission electron microscopy of *Candida albicans* chlamydospores, *J. Gen. Microbiol.* **125:**199–203.
Shannon, J. L., and Rothman, A. H., 1971, Transverse septum formation in budding cells of the yeast-like fungus *Candida albicans*, *J. Bacteriol.* **106:**1026–1028.
Shepherd, M. G., and Sullivan, P. A., 1976, The production and growth characteristics of yeast and mycelial forms of *Candida albicans* in continuous culture, *J. Gen. Microbiol.* **93:**361–370.
Shepherd, M. G., Moi Chin, C., and Sullivan, P. A., 1978, The alternate respiratory pathway of *Candida albicans*, *Arch. Microbiol.* **116:**61–67.
Shepherd, M. G., Yin, C. Y., Ram, S. P., and Sullivan, P. A., 1980, Germ tube induction in *Candida albicans*, *Can. J. Microbiol.* **26:**21–26.
Simonetti, N., Strippoli, V., and Cassone, A., 1974, Yeast–mycelial conversion induced by *N*-acetyl-D-glucosamine in *Candida albicans*, *Nature (London)* **250:**344–346.
Singh, B., and Datta, A., 1978, Glucose repression of the inducible catabolic pathway for *N*-acetylglucosamine in yeast, *Biochem. Biophys. Res. Commun.* **84:**58–64.

Singh, B., and Datta, A., 1979a, Induction of *N*-acetylglucosamine catabolic pathway in spheroplasts of *Candida albicans, Biochem. J.* **178:**427–431.

Singh, B., and Datta, A., 1979b, Regulation of *N*-acetylglucosamine uptake in yeast, *Biochim. Biophys. Acta* **557**248–258.

Singh, B., Biswas, M., and Datta, A., 1979, Inducible *N*-acetylglucosamine binding protein in yeasts, *J. Bacteriol.* **144:**1–6.

Soll, D. R., 1985, The role of zinc in *Candida* dimorphism, in: *Current Topics in Medical Mycology,* Vol. 1 (M. R. McGinnis, ed.), Springer-Verlag, New York (in press).

Soll, D. R., 1984, The cell cycle and commitment to alternate cell fates in *Candida albicans,* in: *The Microbial Cell Cycle* (P. Nurse and E. Streiblova, eds.), CRC Press, Boca Raton, Florida, pp. 143–162.

Soll, D. R., and Bedell, G. W., 1978, Bud formation and the inducibility of pseudo-mycelium outgrowth during release from stationary phase in *Candida albicans, J. Gen. Microbiol.* **108:**173–180.

Soll, D. R., and Herman, M., 1983, Growth and inducibility of mycelium formation in *Candida albicans:* A single cell analysis using a perfusion chamber, *J. Gen. Microbiol.* **129:**2809–2824.

Soll, D. R., and Mitchell, L., 1983, Filament ring formation in the dimorphic yeast *Candida albicans, J. Cell Biol.* **96:**486–493.

Soll, D. R., and Sonneborn, D. R., 1971, Zoospore germination in *Blastocladiella emersonii:* Cell differentiation without protein synthesis?, *Proc. Natl. Acad. Sci. U.S.A.* **68:**459–463.

Soll, D. R., Stasi, M., and Bedell, G., 1978, The regulation of nuclear migration and division during pseudo-mycelium outgrowth in the dimorphic yeast *Candida albicans, Exp. Cell Res.* **116:**207–215.

Soll, D. R., Bedell, G. W., and Brummel, M., 1981a, Zinc and the regulation of growth and phenotype in the infectious yeast *Candida albicans, Infect. Immun.* **32:**1139–1147.

Soll, D. R., Bedell, G. W., Thiel, J., and Brummel, M., 1981b, The dependency of nuclear division on volume in the dimorphic yeast *Candida albicans, Exp. Cell Res.* **133:**55–62.

Speller, C. D., 1980, *Antifungal Chemotherapy,* John Wiley, New York.

Sullivan, P. A., and Shepherd, M. G., 1982, Gratuitous induction by *N*-acetyl-glucosamine of germ-tube formation and enzymes for *N*-acetylglucosamine utilization in *Candida albicans, J. Bacteriol.* **151:**1118–1122.

Syverson, R. E., Buckely, H. R., and Campbell, C. C., 1975, Cytoplasmic antigens unique to the mycelial or yeast phase of *Candida albicans, Infect. Immun.* **12:**1183–1188.

Szawathowski, M., and Hamilton-Miller, J. M., 1975, Anaerobic growth and sensitivity of *Candida albicans, Microbios Lett.* **5:**61–66.

Taschdjian, L. L., Burchall, J. J., and Kozinn, P. J., 1960, Rapid identification of *Candida albicans* by filamentation on serum and serum substitutes, *Am. J. Dis. Child.* **99:**212–215.

Vaughan, V. J., and Weinberg, E. D., 1978, *Candida albicans* dimorphism and virulence: Role of copper, *Mycopathologia* **64:**39–42.

Wain, W. H., Brayton, A. R., and Cawson, R. A., 1976a, Variations in the response to *N*-acetyl-D-glucosamine by isolates of *Candida albicans, Mycopathologia* **58:**27–29.

Wain, W. H., Price, M. F., Brayton, A. R., and Cawson, R. A., 1976b, Macromolecular synthesis during the cell cycles of yeast and hyphal phases of *Candida albicans, J. Gen. Microbiol.* **97:**211–217.

Whelan, W. L., and Magee, P. T., 1981, Natural heterozygosity in *Candida albicans, J. Bacteriol.* **145:**896–903.

Whelan, W. L., and Soll, D. R., 1982, Mitotic recombination in *Candida albicans:* Recessive lethal alleles linked to a gene required for methionine biosynthesis, *Mol. Gen. Genet.* **187**:477–485.

Whelan, W. L., Partridge, R. M., and Magee, P. T., 1980, Heterozygosity and segregation in *Candida albicans, Mol. Gen. Genet.* **180**:107–113.

Whelan, W. L., Beneke, E. S., Rogers, A. L., and Soll, D. R., 1981, Segregation of 5-fluorocytosine-resistant variants by *Candida albicans, Antimicrob. Agents Chemother.* **19**:1078–1081.

Yamaguchi, H., 1975, Control of dimorphism in *Candida albicans* by zinc: Effect on cell morphology and composition, *J. Gen. Microbiol.* **86**:370–372.

Yamaguchi, H., Kanda, Y., and Oswoni, M., 1974, Dimorphism in *Candida albicans.* II. Comparison of fine structure of yeast like and filamentous phase growth, *J. Gen. Appl. Microbiol.* **20**:101–110.

Chapter 8

Exophiala werneckii

James L. Harris

1. INTRODUCTION AND BRIEF HISTORY OF *Exophiala werneckii* AS A PATHOGEN

Exophiala werneckii (Horta) von Arx is the etiological agent of tinea nigra, a superficial, asymptomatic fungus infection of the stratum corneum characterized by brown to black, nonscaly macules (Rippon, 1982). The disease was originally described in Brazil in 1891. Horta isolated the pathogen in 1921 and named it *Cladosporium werneckii* Horta (Rippon, 1982). The painless cosmetic condition is easily treated topically with keratolytic lotion or ointments. It is noteworthy, in light of the mild nature of the disease, that misdiagnosis of the lesions as malignant melanoma has occasionally resulted in drastic and unwarranted surgical procedures (Graham and Barros-Tabita, 1971; Rippon, 1982). Although difficulty in inducing experimental infections has been reported (Graham and Barros-Tabita, 1971), Rippon (1982) states that lesions can be easily produced in abraded skin of human volunteers.

As a pathogen, *E. werneckii* has understandably received little attention, but it merits serious consideration as a model organism for morphogenetic studies among the dimorphic fungi. The fungus is easily grown on simple, defined media (Hardcastle and Szaniszlo, 1974) and can be manipulated without appreciable hazard to investigators. Neverthe-

James L. Harris • Mycobacteriology/Mycology Section, Bureau of Laboratories, Texas Department of Health, Austin, Texas 78756; Department of Microbiology, The University of Texas at Austin, Austin, Texas 78712.

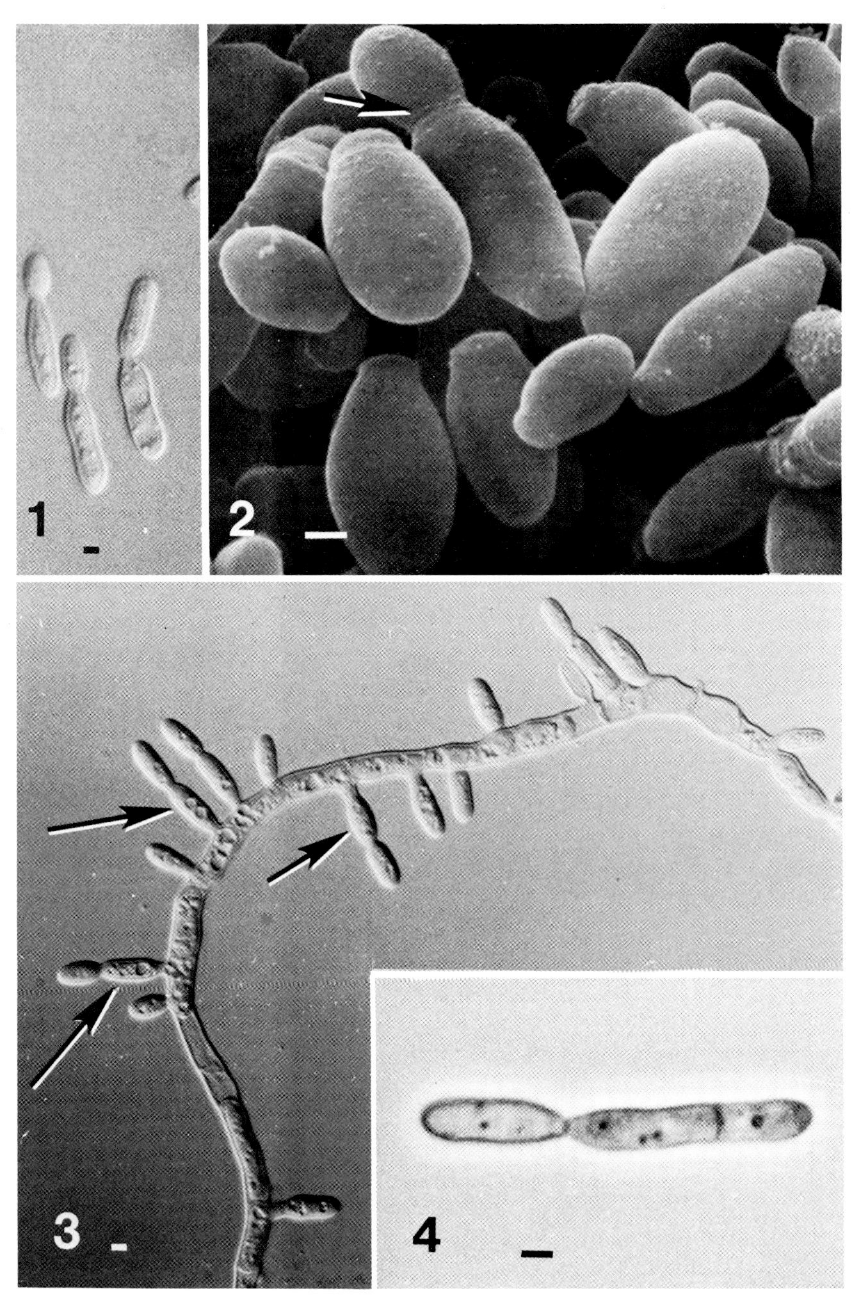

Figure 1. Three yeast cells with apical buds in progressive stages of development, left to right. Characteristic middle constriction is shown in the mother cells. Nomarski optics light micrograph. Scale bar: 1 μm. (Courtesy of C. R. Cooper, Jr.)

less, this organism remains incompletely studied; nothing is known about the biochemistry of its morphogenesis, and it has received only minimal ultrastructural attention.

2. TAXONOMIC POSITION OF THE ORGANISM

McGinnis (1979) lists ten names that he considers to be in synonymy with *E. werneckii*. The organism was first moved to the genus *Exophiala* in 1970 (von Arx, 1970). Other names have since been proposed, but McGinnis (1979) returned the fungus to the genus *Exophiala* on verifying its annellidic pattern of conidiogenesis. Carrion (1950) noted that under various growth conditions, *E. werneckii* exhibits several distinctive morphologies. The traditionally heavy emphasis on morphology in fungal classification and the ability of *E. werneckii* to grow in several forms explains the long history of taxonomic confusion of this imperfect fungus. With the discovery of sympodial conidiogenesis in an isolate from the neotype culture, Nishimura and Miyaji (1984) have proposed yet another genus name, *Hortaea*.

3. MORPHOLOGICAL FORMS OF *Exophiala werneckii*

The characteristic appearance of isolates on common mycological media is as a two-celled yeast in which either or both cells may act as an annellide, capable of generating conidia at, or near, the apex (Figure 1). After several conidia have been produced, annellations mark the somewhat constricted and elongated conidiophore surface (Gustafson *et al.*, 1975; Cole, 1978; McGinnis, 1979; Cole and Samson, 1983). Scanning electron micrographs (Figure 2) most clearly show the annellations (Cole and Samson, 1983). *Exophiala werneckii* also grows as a filamentous fungus, and the *in vitro* conversion from yeasts to hyphae has been well-

Figure 2. Scanning electron micrograph of yeast cells. (→) Annellides. Scale bar: 1 μm. (From Cole and Samson, 1983.)

Figure 3. Hyphal form of *E. werneckii* produced in enriched medium of Hardcastle and Szaniszlo (1974). Several intermediate cells (→) are shown growing out of the hypha and functioning as annellides. Nomarski optics light micrograph. Scale bar: 1 μm. (Courtesy of C. R. Cooper, Jr.)

Figure 4. Yeast cell giving rise to a hypha. One septum has formed in the hypha. Phase-contrast light micrograph. Scale bar: 1 μm. (Courtesy of C. R. Cooper, Jr.)

documented by light microscopy (Figure 3) (Hardcastle and Szaniszlo, 1974). Microscopic examination of scrapings of infected stratum corneum reveals an *in vivo* morphology of both branched filaments and budding cells (Rippon, 1982).

Various dimorphic fungal pathogens that exist in host tissue as blastospores are known to follow one or more of three developmental patterns in converting from the saprophytic (hyphal) phase to the pathogenic (yeast) phase (Howard, 1962). One conversion sequence includes formation of an intermediate phase cell from a hypha that, in turn, gives rise to yeasts. Under appropriate *in vitro* conditions, *E. werneckii* hyphal cells produce an interconverting lateral hyphal bud that, acting as an annellide, forms yeast cells (annelloconidia) by budding (Hardcastle and Szaniszlo, 1974). Several interconverting lateral hyphae are shown in Figure 3. In contrast, a yeast cell may convert directly to hyphal growth under certain conditions. Elongation of a yeast cell followed by septum formation and continued apical growth would produce a hyphal morphology. The initial stages of this process are illustrated in Figure 4.

A paper by Gustafson *et al.* (1975) presents the only published internal-ultrastructure data on *E. werneckii,* and it emphasizes aspects of annellidic bud formation (Figure 5). The authors suggests that because the generative apex constricts with each successive bud, there may be some finite number of buds possible from a single apex, and once this number is produced, a new bud site may form in older cells.

Thin sections of *E. werneckii* demonstrate no unusual fungal cell ultrastructure (Figures 5–7). The walls of the organism are thick, and this may account for the difficulties encountered in successful preparation of this fungus for transmission-electron-microscopic observations (Gustafson, personal communication; Harris, unpublished data). Septal regions do not stain the same as other wall regions (Figures 6 and 7), indicating compositional differences between these sites.

4. CONTROL OF MORPHOLOGY

Romano (1966) outlines three factors of morphological control in dimorphic fungi: temperature, nutrition, and the combined actions of temperature and nutrition. From the few studies of morphogenic control of *E. werneckii,* it is apparent that both temperature and nutrition influence its morphogenesis.

In a study of antigenic relationships among dematiaceous fungi, including *E. werneckii,* Nielson and Conant (1967) grew isolates on a cys-

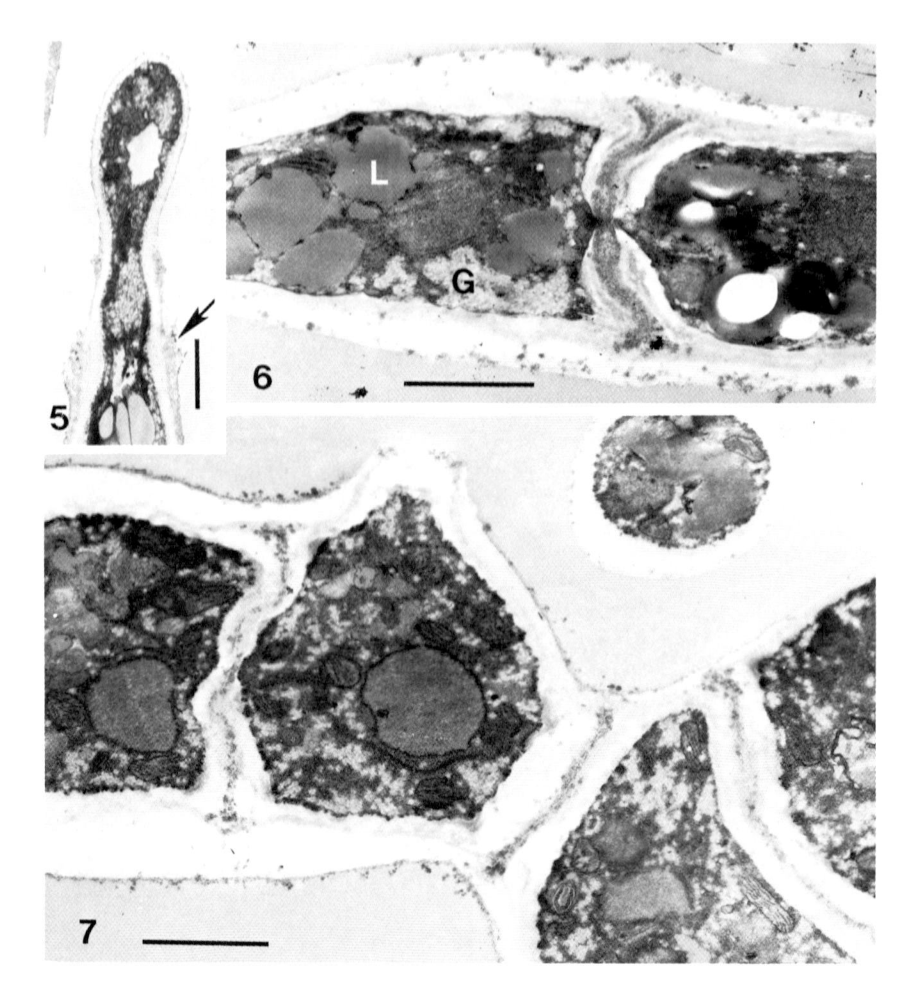

Figure 5. Generative apex of a budding yeast cell showing the annellidic scars in cross section. (←)Transmission electron micrograph. Scale bar: 1 μm. (From Gustafson *et al.*, 1975.)

Figure 6. Septum of *E. werneckii* showing pore. Differences in electron density of septum wall and side wall indicate a compositional distinction between them. Internal structure of the cells is typical. Apparently, both glycogenlike material (G) and lipid (L) may occur as storage compounds. Granular material in the outer wall layer may represent some of the melanin that is characteristic of these organisms. Transmission electron micrograph. Scale bar: 1 μm.

Figure 7. Multiple bud sites on *E. werneckii*. Presence of damage in the walls reflects the poor embedding quality of this fungus even in low-viscosity media. Transmission electron micrograph. Scale bar: 1 μm.

teine–starch medium to obtain yeast growth. Although they indicated that certain of the fungi in the study required repeated transfers before yeast growth was obtained, it is not clear that such transfers were necessary for their isolates of *E. werneckii.* Because typical clinical isolates grow initially in the yeast morphology on a variety of media, it is doubtful that a sequence of transfers was required for induction of a yeast phase.

Houston *et al.* (1969) examined several parameters influencing dimorphism in *E. werneckii,* including various liquid and solid culture media, temperature, and gaseous environment. Their study indicated nutrition to be the major control of dimorphism in this fungus. Reducing conditions, provided by sulfhydryl groups or a carbon dioxide atmosphere, were shown to promote yeast growth. They noted that early growth on Sabouraud dextrose agar is yeastlike and that yeast growth persists even on the periphery of aging colonies in which most of the central, older growth shifts to hyphal production. The most extensive and controlled study of dimorphism in *E. werneckii* is that of Hardcastle and Szaniszlo (1974). Recognizing the importance of the density and physiological state of the inoculum in conversion experiments, these authors established some of the cultural parameters that influence yeast-to-mold and mold-to-yeast morphogenesis. Studies were conducted in liquid shake culture on Czapek–Dox (CD) medium and in CD broth supplemented with 1% yeast extract (CDY). By measuring average particle volumes, they were able to relate cell growth rate to morphological conversion. True hyphal conversion occurs in slow-shaking (40 rpm) cultures of 10^4 yeast cells/ml grown in CDY at 25°C, with visible changes in these cells appearing as early as 9 hr. Unbudded yeasts form hyphae directly, but mother cells that have initiated a budding sequence prior to transfer to the yeast-extract-supplemented medium will remain as yeasts while the newly formed buds initiate hyphal growth (see Figure 4). A 10-fold increase of inoculum density to 10^5 cells/ml results in production of moniliform hyphae in CDY medium. The effect of increasing the inoculum size could be viewed as merely a decrease in the available nutrient per propagule, but experiments suggest that this morphological response may be due to the increased concentration of endogenous factors that unavoidably accompany a larger inoculum. For example, when yeast-phase cells produced in CDY medium are inoculated at a density of 10^5 cells/ml into fresh CDY and incubated at 25°C, a yeast population is maintained. If the inoculum concentration is 10^4 cells/ml, pleomorphic budding forms result. In contrast, when an inoculum consisting of yeasts grown in CD medium is introduced into CDY medium, hyphal forms result. Hardcastle and Szaniszlo (1974) interpreted this to be possible evidence for a factor in yeast extract, or induced by the presence of yeast extract, that inhibits yeast-to-hyphal transition of CDY-grown inoculum. If the former is the case, the factor apparently is taken up slowly enough by the CD-grown inoculum that the cells are induced to convert to filamentous forms before the factor reaches its effective inhibiting threshold within the cells.

The physical parameter of temperature is known to influence growth forms in *E. werneckii.* When CD medium is inoculated with either 10^4 or 10^5 cells/ml and incubated at 25° or 30°C, moniliform hyphal growth results (Hardcastle and Szaniszlo, 1974). These moniliform hyphae are apparently identical ultrastructurally to those induced to form in yeast-extract-supplemented cultures receiving heavy inocula (Hardcastle and Gustafson, unpublished observations).

Strains of *E. werneckii* are variable in their response to incubation at elevated temperature. At 37°C, yeastlike growth in unsupplemented sucrose–salts medium was reported by Houston *et al,* (1969). However, the isolate studied by Hardcastle and Szaniszlo (1974) failed to grow at 37°C on all of several types of standard laboratory media, and only seven of more than two dozen cultures investigated by McGinnis (1979) grew at 37°C on Sabouraud dextrose agar. In contrast, in a recent study published by Mok (1982), 46 isolates of *E. werneckii* demonstrated slow but steady growth even at 42°C. The influence of nutrients on growth of certain fungi at different temperatures has been demonstrated (Barnett and Lilly, 1948; Fries, 1953) and may explain the variations among these results.

Differences in cell-wall chemistry have been revealed in comparative studies of morphological forms of several dimorphic fungi (Kanetsuna, 1981; San-Blas and San-Blas, 1984). Besides compositional differences, physical orientation of fibrillar components appears to influence their cellular morphology. Kanetsuna (1981) suggested that in dimorphic fungi, apical growth may result from preferential growth of longitudinally oriented inner-wall fibrils. The yeast-wall composition of *E. werneckii* has been extensively studied (Lloyd, 1970, 1972), but no corresponding data for hyphal forms are available. Fibril orientation patterns have not been observed for any morphology of this fungus. The relative chemical complexities of the yeast and hyphal walls are not known. One might expect appreciable differences in the chemical complexities and fibril arrangement of two growth forms. The initial steps of yeast-to-hyphal transition may be analogous to bud emergence that is then followed by a period of apical growth and the arrest of mother–daughter cell septum formation. For hyphal forms to produce yeasts, a functional annellide may first have to be synthesized with the ability to repeatedly generate complete septa between itself and a succession of annelloconidia.

REFERENCES

Barnett, H. L., and Lilly, V. G., 1948, The interrelated effects of vitamins, temperature and pH upon vegetative growth of *Sclerotinia camelliae, Am. J. Bot.* **35**:297–302.

Carrion, A. L., 1950, Yeast-like dematiaceous fungi infecting the human skin, *Arch. Dermatol. Syphilol.* **6**:966–1009.

Cole, G. T., 1978, Conidiogenesis in the black yeasts, in: *Proceedings of the Fourth International Conference on the Mycoses: The Black and White Yeasts,* Scientific Publication No. 356, Pan American Health Organization, Washington, D.C., pp. 66–78.

Cole, G. T., and Samson, R., 1983, Conidium and sporangiophore formation in pathogenic microfungi, in: *Fungi Pathogenic for Humans and Animals,* Part A, *Biology* (D. Howard, ed.), Marcel Dekker, New York, pp. 437–524.

Fries, L., 1953, Factors promoting growth of *Coprinus fimentarius* under high temperature conditions, *Physiol. Plant.* **6**:551–563.

Graham, J. H., and Barros-Tabita, C., 1971, Dermal pathology of superficial fungus infections, in: *Human Infection with Fungi, Actinomycetes and Algae* (R. D. Baker, ed.) Springer-Verlag, New York, pp. 211–382.

Gustafson, R. A., Hardcastle, R. V., and Szaniszlo, P. J., 1975, Budding in the dimorphic fungus *Cladosporium werneckii, Mycologia* **67**:942–951.

Hardcastle, R. V., and Szaniszlo, P. J., 1974, Characterization of dimorphism in *Cladosporium werneckii, J. Bacteriol.* **119**:294–302.

Houston, M. R., Meyer, K. H., Thomas, N., and Wolf, F. T., 1969, Dimorphism in *Cladosporium werneckii, Sabouraudia* **7**:195–198.

Howard, D. H., 1962, The morphogenesis of the parasitic forms of dimorphic fungi, *Mycopathol. Mycol, Appl.* **18**:127–139.

Kanetsuna, F., 1981, Ultrastructural studies on the dimorphism of *Paracoccidioides brasiliensis, Blastomyces dermatitidis* and *Histoplasma capsulatum, Sabouraudia* **19**:275–286.

Lloyd, K. O., 1970, Isolation, characterization and partial structure of peptidogalactomannans from the yeast form of *Cladosporium werneckii, Biochemistry* **9**:3446–3453.

Lloyd, K. O., 1972, Molecular organization of a covalent peptido-phospho-polysaccharide complex from the yeast form of *Cladosporium werneckii, Biochemistry* **11**:3884–3890.

McGinnis, M. R., 1979, Taxonomy of *Exophiala werneckii* and its relationship to *Microsporum mansonii, Sabouraudia* **17**:145–154.

Mok, W. Y., 1982, Nature and identification of *Exophiala werneckii, J. Clin. Microbiol.* **16**:976–978.

Nielson, H. S., and Conant, N. F., 1967, Practical evaluation of antigenic relationships of yeast-like dematiaceous fungi, *Sabouraudia* **5**:283–294.

Nishimura, K., and Miyaji, M., 1984, *Hortaea,* a new genus to accommodate *Cladosporium werneckii,* Japanese, *J. Med. Mycol.* **25**:139–146.

Rippon, J. W., 1982, *Medical Mycology: The Pathogenic Fungi and the Pathogenic Actinomycetes,* W. B. Saunders, Philadelphia.

Romano, A. H., 1966, Dimorphism, in: *The Fungi: An Advanced Treatise,* Vol. 2 (G. C. Ainsworth and A. S. Sussman, eds.), Academic Press, New York, pp. 188–209.

San-Blas, G., and San-Blas, F., 1984, Molecular aspects of fungal dimorphism, *CRC Crit. Rev. Microbiol.* **11**:101–127.

Von Arx, J. A., 1970, *The Genera of Fungi Sporulating in Pure Culture,* J. Cramer, Lehre, Germany, pp. 171, 180.

Chapter 9

Polymorphism of *Wangiella dermatitidis*

Philip A. Geis and Charles W. Jacobs

1. INTRODUCTION

Wangiella dermatitidis exhibits a polymorphism consisting of three well-defined morphologies, together with various forms characteristic of transitions among them (Figure 1). The organism may exist as moniliform or true hyphae, characterized by apical growth and production of blastoconidia. Alternatively, it may be found as unicellular budding yeasts, characterized by intermittent polar growth associated with bud formation and secondary isotropic (spherical) growth. Third, it may form enlarged, thick-walled cells, characterized by isotropic growth and, eventually, by the formation of internal septa. This third morphology, the multicellular form, resembles the sclerotic bodies produced by etiological agents of chromoblastomycosis (Rippon, 1982).

Although the various aspects of morphological development have been investigated, the development of multicellular forms from the yeast morphology has received the most attention. This transition is of interest because it is a simple form of vegetative cellular differentiation that is under cell-cycle control. Multicellular-form development can be induced by cultivation of yeasts in very acidic medium or long-term incubation on solid medium (Szaniszlo *et al.*, 1976), by inoculation into animals (Marlowe, 1977; Nishimura and Miyaji, 1983), or as a consequence of

Philip A. Geis • Sharon Woods Technical Center, Procter and Gamble Company, Cincinnati, Ohio 45241. **Charles W. Jacobs** • Division of Biological Sciences, University of Michigan, Ann Arbor, Michigan 48109.

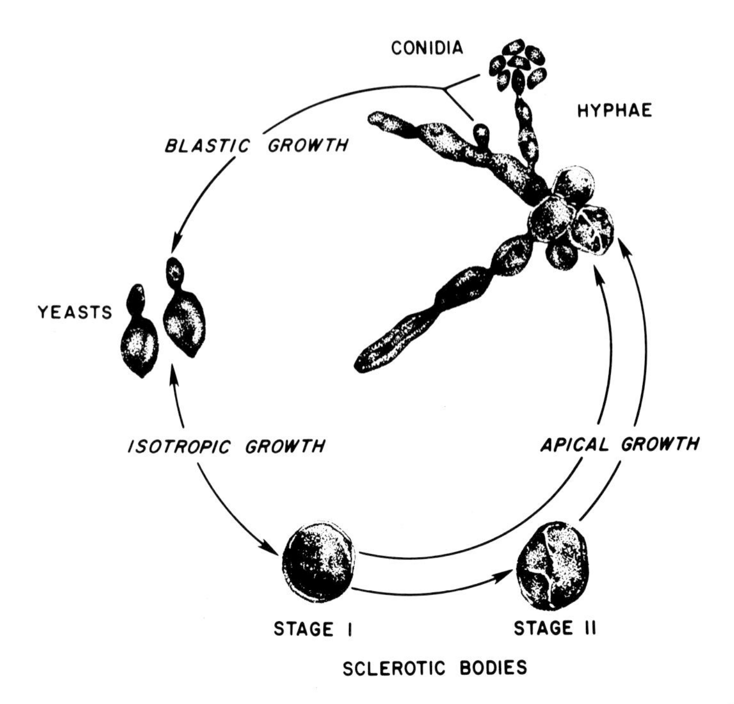

Figure 1. Transitions among the three major vegetative morphologies of *Wangiella dermatitidis*. (Courtesy of P. J. Szaniszlo.)

infection in humans (McGinnis, 1983). The study of the yeast-to-multicellular-form transition has been facilitated by the derivation and isolation of temperature-sensitive, morphological mutants that grow as yeasts at 25°C and rapidly and quantitatively initiate multicellular (Mc)-form development at 37°C (Roberts and Szaniszlo, 1978). These Mc mutant strains define at least two genetic complementation groups (Schafer *et al.*, 1984) and are especially useful because they allow the investigator to grow wild-type, budding yeasts under the identical conditions that allow the development of multicellular forms and thus separate the events involved in multicellular-form development from those that result from temperature shifts.

In addition to its polymorphism, *W. dermatitidis* has a number of synonyms, which were summarized by McGinnis (1977) and DeHoog (1977). The confused state of the nomenclature of this organism and other dematiaceous fungi renders attempts at historical reviews of morphogenesis impossible. Although the morphogenesis of black yeasts termed *Fonsecaea dermatitidis* and *Philalophora dermatitidis* has been studied (Butterfield and Jong, 1976; Silva, 1957), the taxonomic uncertainties mentioned make the relevance of these observations unclear. This review deals primarily with investigations of strain ATCC 34100, which was classified as *W. dermatitidis* (McGinnis, 1977) and *Exophiala mansonii* (DeHoog, 1977), and of mutant strains derived from it.

2. YEAST CELL

2.1. Morphology

Development of *W. dermatitidis* yeasts is characterized primarily by polarized, site-specific cell-wall synthesis that results in bud formation and secondarily by isotropic growth that results in a general increase in cell volume. Yeast cells in rapidly growing cultures are generally thin-walled and hyaline to brown. They are usually globose to ovoid or slightly ellipsoidal and in the unbudded state measure about 5×7 μm. Budding usually occurs near the poles of ellipsoidal cells, and successive buds can arise in annellidic or phialidic succession from a single site or multiple sites on the cell surface (Figure 2). The yeast cells and buds are uninucleate (Grove *et al.*, 1973; Roberts *et al.*, 1979; Jacobs and Szaniszlo, 1982) and, in exponential-phase cultures of strain ATCC 34100, disassociate soon after nuclear division to yield homogeneous unicellular populations or, in other strains, infrequently remain attached to form toruloid chains or pseudohyphae (Carrion, 1950; Reiss and Mok, 1979).

Exponential-phase yeast cells appear, by phase-contrast microscopy, to have relatively thin cell walls and a number of cytoplasmic inclusions (Oujezdsky *et al.*, 1973; Roberts and Szaniszlo, 1978). Ultrastructural studies have shown that the walls of these yeasts are about 75–125 nm thick and are almost electron-transparent when stained with uranyl acetate and lead citrate (Grove *et al.*, 1973; Oujezdsky *et al.*, 1973). The outer surface is delimited by a thin, electron-dense layer and a thin capsule that appears fibrillar in electron-microscopic preparations (Figure 2). The inner surface is delimited by the plasma membrane, which has prominent lomasomes and plasmalemmasomes (Grove *et al.*, 1973). Interior to the plasma membrane are irregular glycogen deposits, often thicker in cross section than the cell wall. The cytoplasm is filled with ribosomes, and mitochondria are abundant. The single nucleus with its nucleolus is prominent, and numerous vesicles are distributed throughout the cytoplasm and are sometimes found associated with a rudimentary Golgi apparatus. Large, electron-dense bodies are frequently observed in the cytoplasm (Oujezdsky *et al.*, 1973; Grove *et al.*, 1973).

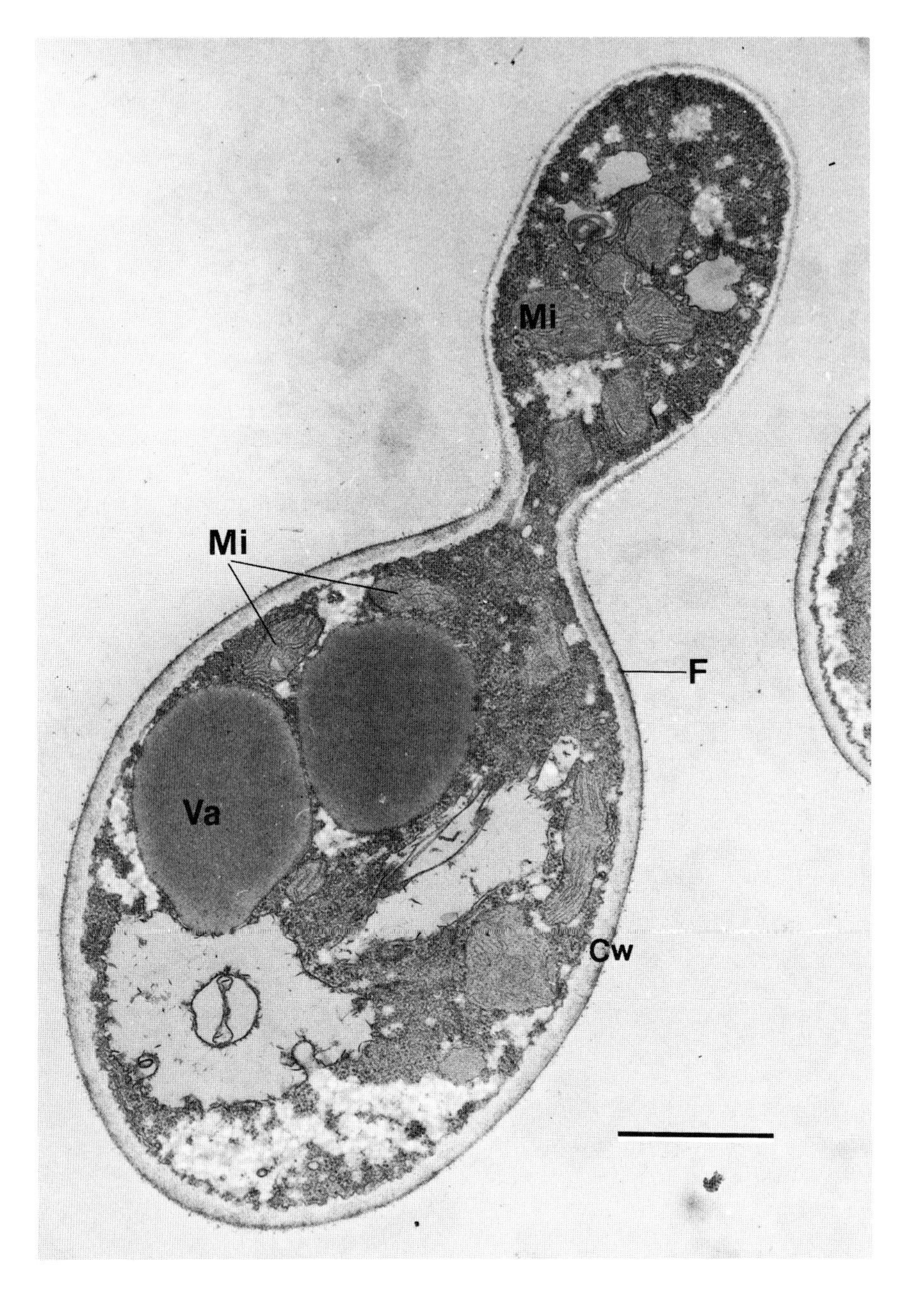

Figure 2. Budded yeast cell. (Cw) Cell wall; (F) fibrillar cell-wall layer; (Mi) mitochondrion; (Va) vacuole. Scale Bar: 1 μm. (Courtesy of J. L. Harris.)

2.2. Yeast-Cell Division

Yeasts of *W. dermatitidis* reproduce by forming one bud each cell cycle. The wall of the nascent bud is continuous with the inner layer of the mother cell wall (Grove *et al.*, 1973), and ribosomes, mitochondria, and other cellular inclusions are prominent within the developing bud. When the bud reaches a diameter approximately two thirds to three quarters that of the mother cell, the nucleus migrates into the neck between the mother cell and bud. Mitosis occurs rapidly (Roberts and Szaniszlo, 1980) within the intact nuclear membrane (Grove *et al.*, 1973). The two daughter nuclei segregate into the mother cell and daughter bud, the septum is completed across the neck, and the two cells separate, The newly formed daughter is generally smaller than the mother cell.

2.3. Yeast-Cell Cycle

Elucidation of the yeast-phase cell cycle of *W. dermatitidis* was prompted because multicellular-form development appeared to result from inhibition of the cell-cycle event of bud emergence (Szaniszlo *et al.*, 1976; Roberts and Szaniszlo, 1978, 1980; Roberts *et al.*, 1979). The temperature-sensitive mutant strains Mc2 and Mc3 commit to multicellular-form development within one cell cycle after exposure to the restrictive temperature (Roberts and Szaniszlo, 1978; Jacobs and Szaniszlo, 1982), suggesting that multicellular-form development in these strains results from a cell-cycle defect.

Flow microfluorimetric analysis facilitated the initial characterization of the yeast-phase cell cycle (Roberts and Szaniszlo, 1980). This technique revealed that the cell cycle consists of four phases: G_1, S (the period of DNA synthesis), G_2, and M (mitosis). The durations of each of these phases in exponential-phase cultures, under standard conditions of incubation, were determined and used as the basis for a preliminary cell-cycle model (Roberts and Szaniszlo, 1980). Studies of synchronously dividing cells (Roberts *et al.*, 1980) and asynchronously dividing cells (Roberts and Szaniszlo, 1980) determined that bud emergence in *W. dermatitidis* usually occurs in G_2. Subsequent investigations placed this event at about 0.69 of the cell cycle in the wild-type and mutant Mc2 and Mc3 strains (Figure 3) (Jacobs and Szaniszlo, 1982). Bud emergence is not dependent on DNA synthesis, and cells that are inhibited in the latter event accumulate as budded forms (Roberts and Szaniszlo, 1980). These observations suggest that the cell cycle of *W. dermatitidis* is basically similar to that of *Saccharomyces cerevisiae* (Pringle and Hartwell, 1981). Consequently, Roberts and Szaniszlo (1980) presented a two-sequence model of the cell cycle, one sequence controlling DNA synthesis and nuclear

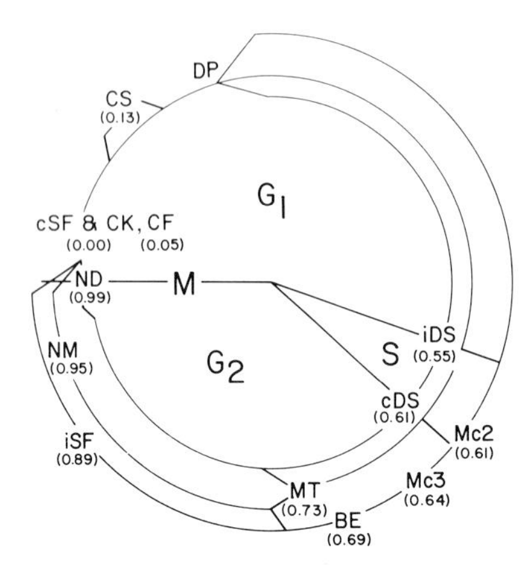

Figure 3. Yeast-phase cell cycle of *Wangiella dermatitidis.* (cSF) Completion of septum formation; (CK) cytokinesis; (CF) appearance of Calcofluor-stainable material in the septum; (CS) cell separation; (DP) divergence of pathways; (iDS) initiation of DNA synthesis; (cDS) completion of DNA synthesis; (Mc2) execution point; (Mc3) execution point; (BE) bud emergence; (MT) microtubule function; (iSF) initiation of septum formation; (NM) nuclear migration; (ND) nuclear division. (From Jacobs and Szaniszlo, 1982; Szaniszlo *et al.,* 1983.)

division, the other controlling bud formation and nuclear migration. Further investigations, including studies of the effects of the microtubule inhibitors nocodazole {methyl-5-[2-(thienylcarbonyl)-1-*H*-benzimidazol-2-yl]-carbamate} and MBC [methyl-(benzimidazol-2-yl)-carbamate], provided further data that indicated that the *W. dermatitidis* cell cycle is composed of at least three independent sequences: the two previously described plus a third that includes events leading to microtubule function (Figure 3).

3. HYPHA

Hyphal growth of *W. dermatitidis* is characterized primarily by apical extension and secondarily by budding growth associated with the production of blastoconidia and phialo- or annelloconidia (Grove *et al.,* 1973; Oujezdsky *et al.,* 1973; Cole, 1978; Hironaga *et al.,* 1981). Hyphae are thin-walled structures of relatively constant diameter. Thin sections of hyphal walls, stained with OsO_4 and poststained with uranyl acetate and lead citrate, appear in electron micrographs to consist of several layers (Figure 4). Septa arise from the inner layers of the cell wall and are simple, with a septal pore and Woronin bodies. Often the septal pore is closed by a pore plug. Walls of hyphal branches are continuous with the entire hyphal wall, but lateral hyphal buds are produced from the inner layers of the cell wall by blastic growth. Conidia arise from the apices of relatively undifferentiated conidiophores that are derived from hyphal branches or are generated directly from the hyphal wall (Oujezdsky *et al.,* 1973; Cole, 1978).

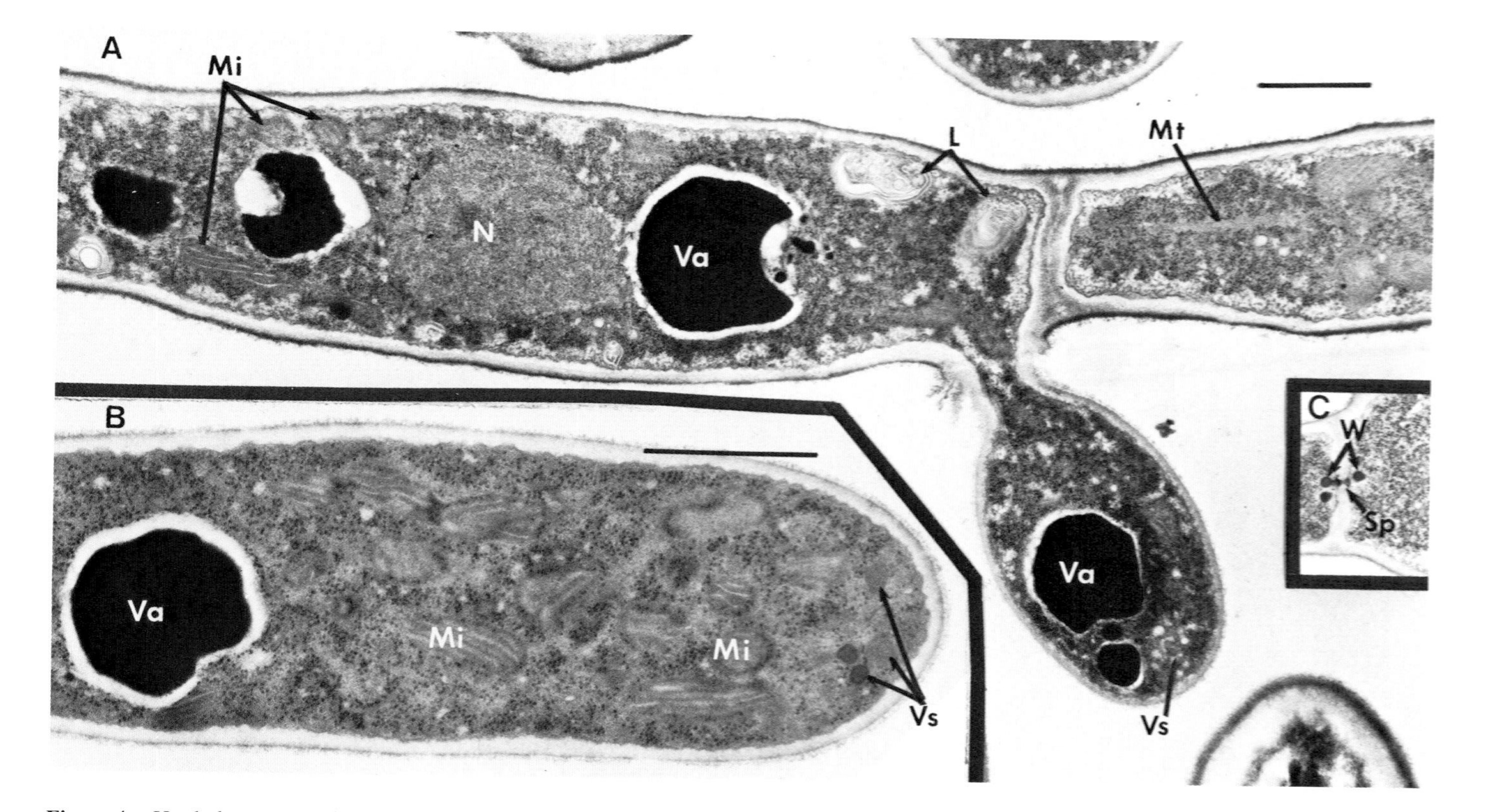

Figure 4. Hyphal segments: (A) Hypha width blastoconidium; (B) hyphal tip; (C) septal region. (L) Lomasome; (Mi) mitochondrion; (Mt) microtubules; (N) nucleus; (Sp) septal pore; (Va) vacuole; (Vs) vesicles; (W) Woronin body. Scale bar: 1 μm. (Courtesy of S. N. Grove.)

4. MULTICELLULAR FORM

Development of multicellular forms can be conveniently, if arbitrarily, divided into two stages. Stage I is characterized by isotropic cell-wall growth and the absence of budding or apical growth. As cellular growth continues, the cell enlarges (Roberts and Szaniszlo, 1978; Jacobs and Szaniszlo, 1985) and becomes multinucleate (Roberts *et al.,* 1979). In stage II development, the growth that characterized stage I development continues, and the cell forms transverse septa that generate the multicellular or muriform morphology (Szaniszlo *et al.,* 1976; Roberts and Szaniszlo, 1978).

4.1. Stage I

Transmission electron micrographs of acid-induced stage I cells, fixed in OsO_4 and stained with uranyl acetate and lead citrate, are readily distinguished from those of yeast-phase cells (Szaniszlo *et al.,* 1976). The cell walls are thickened with respect to those of yeasts and appear to be composed of a number of layers. The outermost layer stains darkly, and the inner layers stain less darkly to not at all (Szaniszlo *et al.,* 1976). The cytoplasm of these cells contains ribosomes and mitochondria, as well as numerous vesicles and vacuoles, some lipid bodies, and, occasionally, small electron-dense bodies. One to several nuclei are prominent in electron micrographs of wild-type, acid-induced stage I cells (Szaniszlo *et al.,* 1976) in stage I cells of strain Mc3 (J. L. Harris, personal communication), and at the level of light microscopy in stage I cells of the Mc strains (Roberts *et al.,* 1979). Electron micrographs indicate that stage I cells generated by incubating the mutant strain Mc3 at 37°C (Figure 5) are identical to those generated by incubation of wild-type cells at low pH (J. L. Harris, personal communication).

4.2. Stage II

Stage II development is characterized by continued isotropic cell-wall growth and the formation of transverse septa (Figure 6). Stage II cells have extremely thickened, multilayered, hyperpigmented cell walls (Geis, 1981; Szaniszlo *et al.,* 1976). The outer layers of the wall slough as the cells age and enlarge. The characteristic septa of these forms appear to be of two kinds: simple septa with septal pores, Woronin bodies, and often pore plugs, and complete septa, composed of several layers with no apparent cytoplasmic continuity between the cells they delimit. The com-

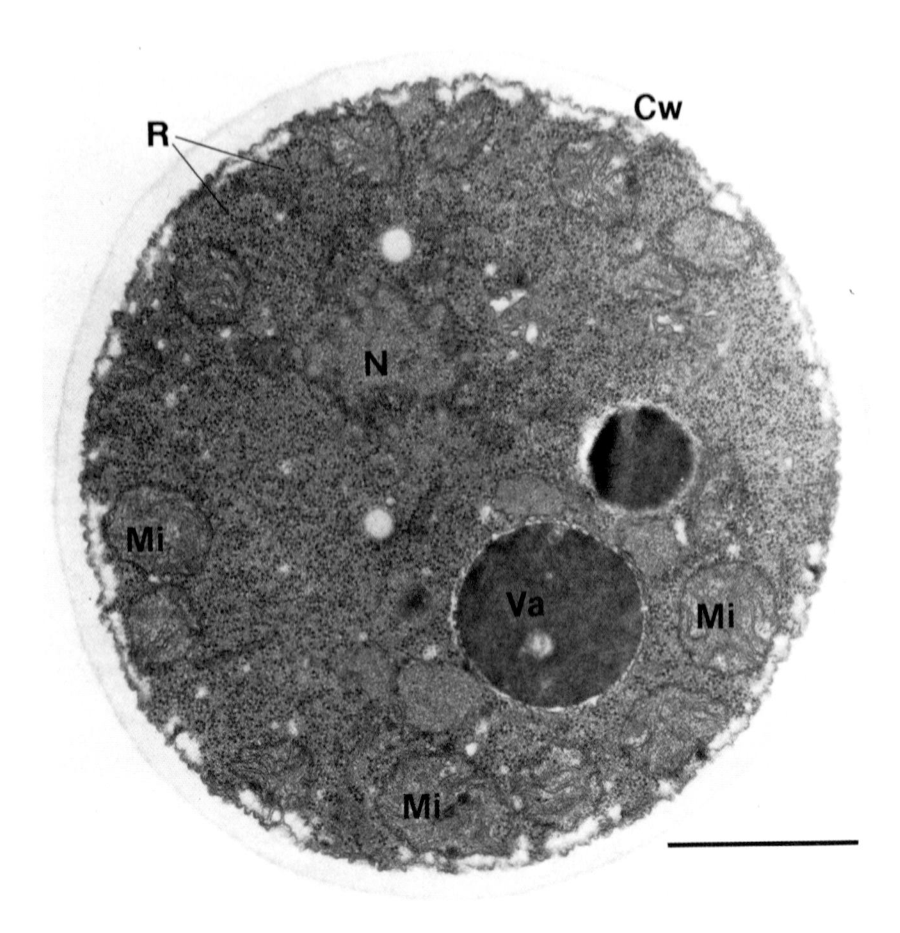

Figure 5. Multicellular-form development: Stage I cell. (Cw) Cell wall; (Mi) mitochondrion; (N) nucleus; (R) ribosomes; (Va) vacuole. Scale bar: 1 μm. (Adapted from Cooper *et al.*, 1984.)

plete septa are thought to evolve from primary simple septa via a maturation process (Szaniszlo *et al.*, 1976). The cytoplasm of wild-type, acid-induced stage II forms contains large lipid and glycogen deposits, in addition to the inclusions observed in yeasts and stage I cells. The cytoplasm of stage II forms induced by incubation of strain Mc3 at 37°C for 24–48 hr contains smaller lipid deposits and almost no glycogen; otherwise, the cells are similar to the acid-induced forms (J. L. Harris, personal communication).

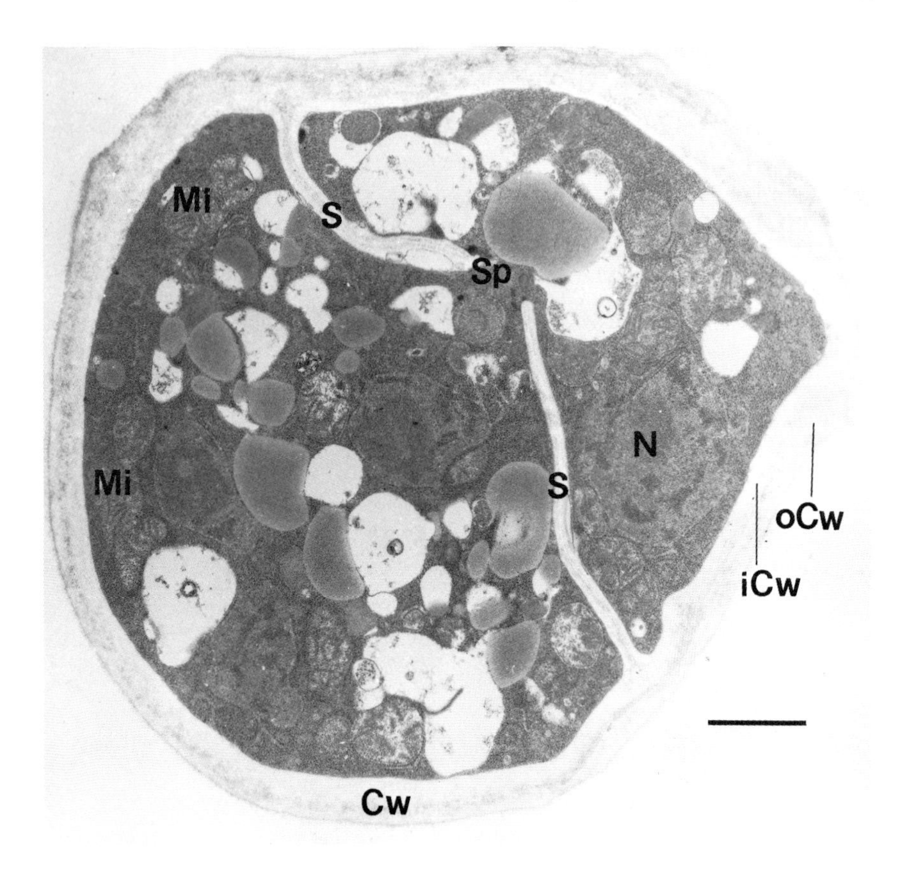

Figure 6. Multicellular-form development: Stage 2 cell. (Cw) Cell wall; (iCw) inner cell-wall layer; (oCw) outer cell-wall layer; (Mi) mitochondrion; (N) nucleus; (S) internal septum; (Sp) septal pore. Scale bar: 1 μm. (Adapted from Szaniszlo *et al.*, 1983.)

5. TRANSITIONS BETWEEN MORPHOLOGIES

5.1. Hyphae to Yeasts

Yeasts can be generated from hyphae via blastoconidia or phialo/annelloconidia. The blastoconidia are ultrastructurally identical to yeast cells (Grove *et al.*, 1973), and the phialo/annelloconidia are morphologically similar to both yeasts and blastoconidia (Oujezdsky and Szaniszlo, 1974; Cole, 1978). It appears that all three cell types are physiologically similar in that when inoculated into fresh medium, they develop into budding yeasts (Oujezdsky *et al.*, 1973) or give rise to yeasts by a budding process (Cole, 1978).

5.2. Yeasts to Multicellular Forms

5.2.1. Stage I

Stage I forms have been induced by three different methods. Long-term (2–4 weeks) incubation of the wild-type strain on solid medium yields significant quantities of stage I cells (Oujezdsky *et al.*, 1973). Incubation of the wild-type strain in acidic medium yields stage I cells within a few days (Szaniszlo *et al.*, 1976). Finally, incubation of strains Mc2 and Mc3 at 37°C induces stage I development within one cell cycle [about 5.5 hr (Jacobs and Szaniszlo, 1985)]; stage I development of strain Mc1 at 37°C begins after only a few cell divisions (Roberts and Szaniszlo, 1978). After incubation of the wild-type strain for 4–7 days on solid medium, or 48 hr in acidified broth, cells exhibit thicker cell walls, larger glycogen storage areas, and fewer ribosomes than do logarithmic-phase yeast cells (Oujezdsky *et al.*, 1973; Szaniszlo *et al.*, 1976). These thick-walled cells appear to accumulate large lipid deposits in the cytoplasm, which is consistent with the observations of Calderone (1976) that the lipid content of *W. dermatitidis* increases with the age of the culture. Poorly characterized, electron-dense bodies are prominent in most cells (Oujezdsky *et al.*, 1973; Szaniszlo *et al.*, 1976).

After 3–4 weeks of incubation on solid medium (Oujezdsky *et al.*, 1973) or 2–3 days of incubation in acidified broth (Szaniszlo *et al.*, 1976), the wild-type stage I cells have undergone significant changes in morphology as observed by light and electron microscopy. By phase-contrast microscopy, the cells appear to have extremely thick walls and several refractile inclusions. By electron microscopy, the cell wall appears to have several layers; the glycogen storage areas are almost nonexistent in cells grown for long periods of time, but are prominent in the acid-grown cells, and most of the cytoplasm is occupied by large lipid bodies.

Stage I development in strain Mc3 grown at 37°C in liquid medium is morphologically and ultrastructurally similar to stage I development in wild-type cells. After 6–12 hr at 37°C, the cells appear by light microscopy to be enlarged with slightly thickened walls (Roberts and Szaniszlo, 1978), By electron microscopy, early stage I Mc3 cells appear similar to those induced in acidic medium or by long-term incubation, in that ribosomes, mitochrondria, nuclei, and vacuoles are prominent. They differ from the aged or acid-induced forms primarily in that their lipid bodies are smaller and their polysaccharide storage areas are practically nonexistent (J. L. Harris, personal communication). After 24–72 hr at 37°C, the cells exhibit extremely thickened cell walls and numerous refractile inclusions (Roberts and Szaniszlo, 1978). Electron micrographs indicate once again that Mc3 cells in this phase of stage I development differ from their aged or acid-induced counterparts primarily in the size of their lipid bodies and their lack of large polysaccharide storage areas (J. L. Harris, personal communication).

5.2.2. Stage II

Continued incubation of stage I forms under the conditions which induced their formation from yeasts will yield stage II forms (Szaniszlo *et al.*, 1976; Roberts and Szaniszlo, 1978). Stage II development is essentially a continuation of stage I development, and is marked by the formation of transverse septa. Stage II development may be blocked in strain Mc3 if high-density inocula (about 10^7 cells/ml) are used (Geis, 1981), and occurs at a very low level in aged wild-type cultures (Szaniszlo *et al.*, 1976). Results such as these have been interpreted to mean that stage II development requires relatively active metabolism and can be blocked by specific nutrient-limiting conditions late in the developmental cycle (P. J. Szaniszlo, personal communication).

5.3. Stage I Forms to Yeasts

Stage I forms, generated by growth on solid medium for less than 2 weeks, will outgrow into the yeast morphology on transfer to fresh medium (Oujezdsky *et al.*, 1973). Stage I forms of strain Mc3, generated by growth at 37°C for 6–24 hr, also outgrow into the yeast morphology when incubated at 25°C (Roberts, 1979; Jacobs, 1983; Jacobs, Roberts, and Szaniszlo, 1985).

5.4. Stage I and II Forms to Hyphae

Yeasts cannot generate hyphae directly. Stage I cells from cultures grown for at least 3 weeks on solid medium (Oujezdsky *et al.*, 1973) or stage II forms (Szaniszlo *et al.*, 1976) can do so on transfer to fresh medium. The cells produce numerous ribosomes and mitochondria prior to hyphal outgrowth. True hyphae develop at the distal end of a series of two or more moniliform transition cells. The thin wall of the transition cell arises from the inner layer of the thick wall of stage I or II forms, and the septa of the transition cells resemble those of hyphae in that they are simple, with a septal pore and Woronin bodies. Often the septal pore is closed by a pore plug. The series of moniliform transition cells may give rise to a true hypha, which is distinguished from the moniliform transitional cells by its uniform diameter and lack of constrictions in the septal region.

6. CELL-WALL ALTERATIONS DURING MULTICELLULAR-FORM DEVELOPMENT

The mutant strain Mc3, by virtue of its rapid multicellular-form development and retention of viability at the restrictive temperature, has been extremely useful in studies of the dynamics of cellular differentiation. A series of studies concerning the composition and spatial distribution of the cell wall have been performed using this mutant strain and its wild-type parent.

6.1. Quantitative Analyses of Cell Walls

Analysis of cell walls of yeasts and multicellular forms indicated that although their compositions are qualitatively identical, there are major quantitative differences (Figure 7) (Geis, 1981; Szaniszlo *et al.*, 1983). The cell walls of wild-type yeasts and those of strain Mc3, incubated at 25°C, are identical in composition. However, significant differences in the quantitative compositions of multicellular-form walls of strain Mc3 and of wild-type yeasts occur when both are grown at 37°C (Table I). In addition, small differences exist in the amounts of certain cell-wall components in wild-type cells grown at 25 or 37°C.

In multicellular-form walls, the concentrations of total neutral sugar (glucose, mannose, and galactose) and inorganic ash are about half those in yeast walls. Conversely, the concentration of melanin is 5-fold and that of *N*-acetylglucosamine (GlcNAc) 6-fold greater in multicellular-form walls than in yeast walls (Table I). The concentrations of lipid and protein are similar in the two forms.

↑ CHITIN (10X)
↑ MELANIN (5X)
↓ GLUCOSE (0.5X)
↓ ASH (0.5X)

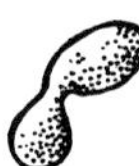

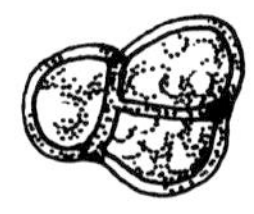

Figure 7. Relative changes in cell-wall composition that occur during morphogenesis.

Table I
Major Cell-Wall Components of Yeast (Y) and Multicellular (M) Morphologies for Wild-Type (Wt) and Mc3 Strains[a]

Strain and treatment	Neutral sugar	Lipid	Melanin	Protein	*N*-Acetyl-glucosamine	Ash	Total recovery
Wt Y (25°C)	72.9	3.0	4.3	8.3	2.1	3.4	94.0
Mc3 Y (25°C)	71.7	2.0	4.4	9.9	1.9	3.3	93.2
Wt Y (37°C)	73.7	2.9	5.7	8.5	3.2	3.1	97.1
Mc3 M (37°C)	43.0	2.2	24.8	10.8	11.8	1.7	94.3

[a]Averages of analyses of multiple, independently derived wall samples for each morphology (Geis, 1981).

6.2. Cell-Wall Polymers

Spectroscopic, cytological, and chemical techniques have shown the polymeric constituents of the cell walls of the yeast and multicellular forms to be qualitatively identical (Table II). However, the spatial location or amount of each is altered during morphogenesis.

6.2.1. Melanin

The pentaketide pathway is employed for melanin synthesis by *W. dermatitidis* (Geis *et al.*, 1984), and a significant part of this synthesis appears to take place in intimate association with the cell wall (Geis, 1981). Isolation of melanin-deficient *(Mel)* mutants of both the wild-type and Mc3 strains has shown that melanin is not necessary for either yeast growth or multicellular-form development (Geis, 1981).

Table II
Polysaccharides Detected and Localized in the Cell Walls of Yeast and Multicellular Morphologies[a]

Polysaccharide	Yeast	Multicellular
α-Mannan	Outer layer	Outer layer
α-Glucan	Not detected	Not detected
β-Glucan	Generalized	Generalized
Chitin	Bud scars (?)	Inner layer
Chitosan	Not detected	Not detected

[a]Conclusions based on solubility, cytochemical, lectin-interaction, and infrared spectroscopic data (Geis, 1981; P. A. Geis and C. R. Cooper, unpublished data).

6.2.2. Mannans

The mannans of both yeast and multicellular-form walls are α-linked polymers concentrated in the outer cell-wall layers of both morphologies (Geis, 1981). As alkali-soluble extracts, mannans of both forms are similar in apparent molecular size and reactivity with concanavalin A (Con A). Although an α-mannan-rich cell-wall layer is shed from the surface of developing multicellular forms, additional α-mannan is apparently synthesized and the mannan-rich outer wall layer is maintained (Geis, 1981). Despite their relative abundance in the cell walls, there is no evidence that mannans play a direct role in morphological development.

6.2.3. Glucans

Glucans were detected in the cell walls of both yeasts and multicellular forms by spectroscopic analysis. Although α-glucans were not detected, β-glucans are distributed throughout the walls of both cell types, as indicated by aniline blue staining (Geis, 1981). Alkali-soluble and alkali-insoluble glucans appear to be present in greater amounts. The acute sensitivity of *Mel* mutants to Zymolyase, a preparation consisting primarily of $(1 \rightarrow 3)$ glucanases (Kitamura and Yamamoto, 1972), indicates that this linkage may be of structural importance to the cell wall (Jacobs, 1983). However, no systematic study of the types of glucan linkages has been undertaken, although a β-glucan synthetase and its product have recently been described (Kang *et al.*, 1984; Szaniszlo *et al.*, 1985).

6.2.4. Chitin

Much of the cell-wall GlcNAc in *W. dermatitidis* is present as chitin, which can be detected spectroscopically and chemically in yeast and multicellular-form walls (Geis, 1981; Szaniszlo *et al.*, 1983). Multicellular forms have about 10-fold more cell-wall chitin than yeasts grown at 25°C and about 6-fold more than yeasts grown at 37°C. In multicellular forms, chitin seems to be embedded in the matrix of the inner cell wall and in the septum as revealed by fluorescence staining and light microscopy (Geis, 1981; Jacobs, Cooper, and Szaniszlo, in prep.) and gold-labeled chitinase (Figure 8) (J. L. Harris, personal communication). Inhibiting chitin synthesis during multicellular-form development causes cell lysis; chitin seems to play an important role in stabilizing cells during the developmental process (Geis, 1981; Cooper *et al.*, 1984).

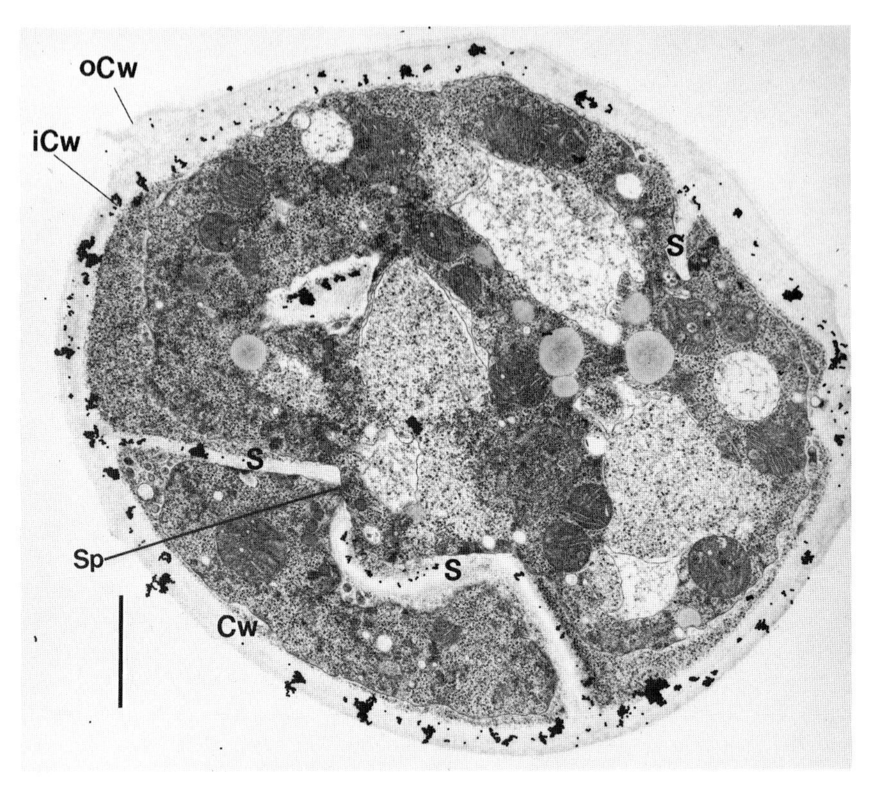

Figure 8. Stage 2 cell exposed to colloidal-gold-labeled chitinase. (Cw) Cell wall; (iCw) inner cell-wall layer; (oCw) outer cell-wall layer; (S) internal septum; (Sp) septal pore. Scale bar: 1 μm. (Courtesy of J. L. Harris.)

6.2.5. Galactose-Containing Polymers

The outer layer that is shed from the cell wall during multicellular-form development is a galactomannan–protein complex (Geis, 1981). Although the galactose content of both yeast and multicellular-form walls is relatively low, multicellular-form walls contain about twice as much as yeast walls. Cells in both stage I and stage II of multicellular-form development have a higher affinity than do yeasts for fluorescently labeled, galactose-specific agglutinin from castor bean *(Ricinis communis)* (Jacobs, Cooper, and Szaniszlo, in prep.). However, the significance of galactose in multicellular-form development is not yet known.

6.3. Dynamics of Polysaccharide Synthesis during Development

6.3.1. *Rates of Polysaccharide Syntheses*

When multicellular-form development is induced by shifting strain Mc3 to 37°C, the rate of glucan synthesis increases through the first 3- to 6- hr period and then drops dramatically, whereas the rate of chitin synthesis does not change during the first 6 hr, but then increases exponentially (Figure 9A). In contrast, the rates of both chitin and glucan syntheses in wild-type cells increase during the first 3 hr after the shift to 37°C and then stabilize (Figure 9B). The increase in the rate of chitin synthesis is consistent with the same time as the increased affinity of stage I cell walls for colloidal-gold-labeled chitinase (J. L. Harris, personal communication). The rates of chitin and insoluble-glucan incorporation during stage I development suggest that there may be a common mode of

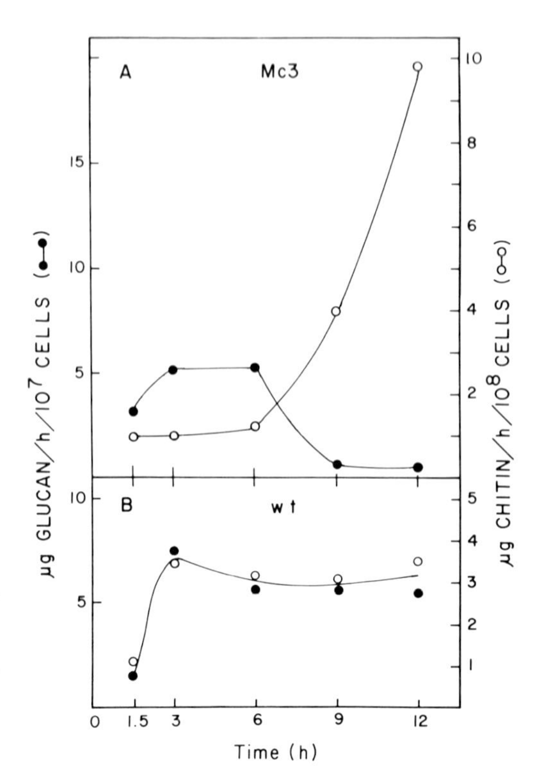

Figure 9. Rates of chitin and acid/alkali-insoluble glucan incorporation into cell walls of developing multicellular forms (A) and yeasts (B) at 37°C. The rates were calculated from chemical data of relative chitin and glucan contents. (Adapted from Szaniszlo *et al.*, 1983.)

regulation that reciprocally affects the incorporation of these two materials.

6.3.2. Spatial Distribution of Cell-Wall Polymers

The spatial distribution of several cell-wall polymers has been studied using fluorescent probes. In yeasts, Calcofluor, which preferentially stains chitinaceous regions of the cell wall (Roberts *et al.,* 1983; Cooper *et al.,* 1984) although it has other affinities (Maeda and Ishida, 1967; Holan *et al.,* 1981), and fluorescently labeled Con A (F-Con A), which is indicative of mannan, strongly stain bud and birth scars and the mother cell–bud juncture; the Calcofluor has a weak affinity for the remainder of the cell wall, but the F-Con A has a high affinity for developing buds. During stage I and stage II development, Calcofluor and F-Con A, as well as fluorescently labeled castor bean agglutinin that has little affinity for yeasts, each strongly stain the cell wall. Also, the galactomannan-protein outer wall layer that sloughs from the surface of the cell during stage I and stage II development (Geis, 1981) has a high affinity for F-Con A and fluorescent castor bean agglutinin (Jacobs, Cooper, and Szaniszlo, in prep.). Thus, cell-wall synthesis that seems highly localized during budding growth is apparently delocalized during multicellular-form development.

6.4. Effect of Polysaccharide Synthetase Inhibitors

Polyoxins and tunicamycins (analogues of UDP-GlcNAc) and aculeacin (an analogue of UDP-glucose) have been used to prove the developmental role of polysaccharide synthesis. The results of such experiments must be interpreted with caution, since nucleotide sugars have many roles in the cell and can be involved in glycosylation of proteins or as primers for elongation of nonhomologous polysaccharides (as in the inhibition of mannan synthesis by tunicamycin). With this caveat in mind, there are several interesting effects of these three analogues on multicellular-form development.

6.4.1. Polyoxins

Polyoxins are well known as chitin-synthesis inhibitors (Endo *et al.,* 1970). Polyoxin AL and purified fractions of polyoxins B and D arrest multicellular-form development early in stage I, block chitin synthesis, inhibit the increase in Calcofluor affinity, cause cell lysis, and induce a high degree of cell death (Geis, 1981; Cooper *et al.,* 1984). In yeasts, they inhibit cell separation, induce formation of chains or clusters of cells, and cause formation of aberrant, incurvate septa in yeast cells (Szaniszlo *et al.*, 1983; Cooper *et al.*, 1984). Since the major effect of polyoxins in *W. dermatitidis* is to block chitin synthesis, it appears that chitin is an important structural polymer involved in normal septum formation and in stabilizing the cell wall during multicellular-form development.

6.4.2. Aculeacin A

During multicellular-form development of strain Mc3, Aculeacin A, an inhibitor of glucan synthesis, induces cell death after about 6–9 hr of incubation at 37°C. This is near the end of the increased levels of glucan synthesis (Figure 9). As in the case of exposure to polyoxins, wild-type cells form chains or clusters (Szaniszlo *et al.*, 1983). Interestingly, multicellular-form development can be induced in strain Mc3 at the permissive temperature in the presence of aculeacin A (C. R. Cooper, personal communication). Whether this is an effect of inhibition of glucan synthesis or of other glycosylations is not known. What does seem clear is that pertubation in glucose metabolism is detrimental to multicellular-form development of strain Mc3 at 37°C.

6.4.3. Tunicamycins

Tunicamycins inhibit yeast-cell growth and division at 25°C and cause cell death and lysis in both wild-type yeasts and developing multicellular forms at 37°C (Wang, 1982). However, the broad specificity of the tunicamycins makes it difficult to interpret the results, because they inhibit both glycosylation of proteins and mannan synthesis (Kuo and Lampen, 1974; Tkacz and Lampen, 1975), and although they are analogues of UDP-GlcNAc, they appear to have little effect on chitin synthesis *in vivo* (Kuo and Lampen, 1974; Katoh *et al.*, 1978). The lack of a differential effect against yeasts and developing multicellular forms suggests that mannan synthesis and protein mannosylation are necessary for cellular growth in both forms. Developmental regulation by mannosylation of specific proteins may be significant, but would not be detected in experiments such as these.

6.5. Relevance of Cell-Wall Carbohydrate Polymers to Differentiation

The synthesis of mannans and glucans is necessary for the continued maintainance of the cell wall. The greatly increased and delocalized incorporation of chitin during multicellular-form development is necessary for stabilization of the cell wall and for stage I and II development. Stage I wall development seems to occur in two steps. The first step can occur in the absence of exogenous substrate (R. L. Roberts, personal communication) and results in discrete ruptures in the outer mannan-rich cell-wall layer. The second, substrate-requiring, step is initiated 9–12 hr after induction of multicellular-form development. Here, the cell wall is weakened by the decreased incorporation of the skeletal β-glucans and greatly increased incorporation of the nonstructural, polyphenolic melanin. However, the concurrent substantial increase in chitin incorporation into the inner cell-wall layers reinforces and maintains the structure of the cell wall and allows development to proceed.

7. INTEGRATION OF THE YEAST-CELL CYCLE AND MULTICELLULAR-FORM DEVELOPMENT

7.1. "Start"

Observations of cells from late log phase and early stationary phase suggest that there is a "Start" event in the cell cycle of *W. dermatitidis.* "Start" is the control point in the cell cycle, early in G_1 and soon after cell separation, at which cells are blocked if any of a number of conditions are unsuitable for completion of the cell cycle. Factors that are known to cause *S. cerevisiae* to be arrested at "Start" include nutrient limitation, inhibition of growth, mating pheromone, and dysfunction of events governed by certain *cdc* mutations (Pringle and Hartwell, 1981). Cells blocked at "Start" by nutritional factors are usually smaller than those in balanced growth (Johnston *et al.,* 1977) and cannot initiate DNA synthesis, bud emergence, or any other sequential cell-cycle functions.

In *W. dermatitidis,* cells that have reached growth-limiting conditions are uniformly small and unbudded (Figure 10), uninucleate with a single complement of DNA, and arrested in the G_1 phase of the cell cycle (Roberts and Szaniszlo, 1980). They initiate neither DNA synthesis nor budding growth until inoculated into fresh medium. However, just as "Start" may serve as a departure point for sequences leading to mitotic, budding growth or conjugation in *S. cerevisiae,* "Start" in *W. dermatitidis* may be the departure point for sequences leading to mitotic, budding growth or to the formation of thick-walled stage I cells that eventually gain competence to germinate into hyphae. These observations suggest that budding growth is arrested at "Start" by nutritional limitation in stationary-phase cultures, but that slow metabolism and cellular growth continue, with subsequent alterations of the cell's capacity for growth when

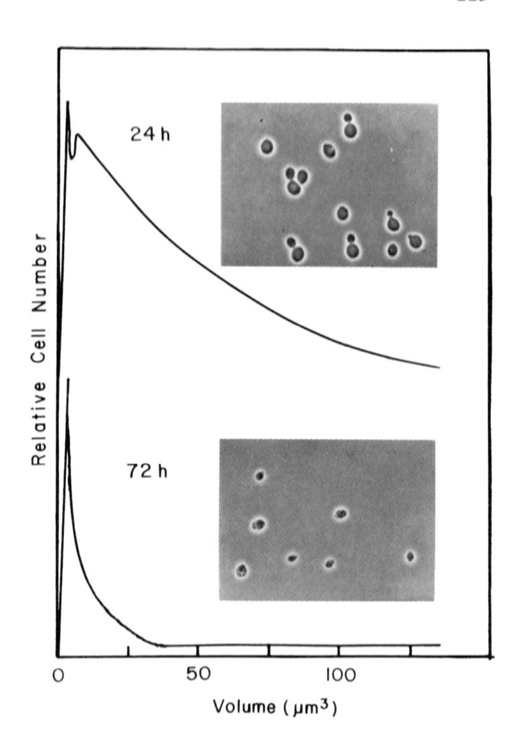

Figure 10. Morphology and size distributions of exponential-phase yeasts (24 hr) and stationary-phase yeasts of *W. dermatitidis*. The size-distribution data were obtained with a Coulter Channelizer.

the nutritional limitation is relieved. Thus, "Start"could be a point of morphological divergence for *W. dermatitidis*.

7.2. Divergence of Control Sequences

At some time after the cells pass "Start," three control sequences diverge (see Figure 3). One sequence contains the events of DNA synthesis and nuclear division, whereas a second contains events leading to bud emergence and yeast septum formation. Microtubule function is necessary for the completion of the third sequence of independent events of nuclear migration and nuclear division. The temperature-sensitive blocks in strains Mc2 and Mc3 seem to be departure points for morphological development as either budding yeasts or multicellular forms. The blocks seem to occur late in the S or early in the G_2 phase of the cell cycle, prior to bud emergence and microtubule function.

7.3. Convergence of Sequences

Just after mitosis, the divergent control sequences converge, allowing cytokinesis and cell separation to occur. Since these two events do not occur unless bud emergence, nuclear migration, mitosis, and all their prerequisite events have taken place (Roberts and Szaniszlo, 1978), they are dependent on all the control pathways that are described in the previous section. Cytokinesis and septum formation seem to be completed at about the same time (Figure 3), which leads to the possibility that centripetal growth of the septum may be the driving force behind cytokinesis. Some events related to maturation of the septum seem to occur after completion of septum formation (Figure 3).

7.4. Cell Separation

Pseudohyphae are probably chains of yeast cells that have failed to undergo cell separation. Although morphologically similar to moniliform hyphae at the level of light microscopy, they lack the simple septa with septal pores and Woronin bodies that are characteristic of the moniliform hyphae of *W. dermatitidis* (Oujezdsky *et al.,* 1973). Although rare in homogeneous exponential-phase cultures, pseudohyphae and clusters of yeasts that have not undergone cell separation are sometimes observed. The yeastlike mode of growth of pseudohyphae and their presence in some cultures suggest that cell separation is not an obligatory step in the yeast-cell cycle.

8. NATURE OF THE MUTATIONS IN Mc STRAINS AND THEIR RELEVANCE TO MORPHOLOGICAL DEVELOPMENT

The mutations in strains Mc1, Mc2, and Mc3 all generate identical morphological forms, but by different mechanisms (Roberts and Szaniszlo, 1978). The mutation in strain Mc1 does not induce multicellular-form development for several cell cycles; this may be the result of any number of phenomena. A mutant gene product may be involved that is not directly involved in budding. At the restrictive temperature, the faulty gene product of strain Mc1 may prevent additional synthesis or activation of proteins that are required for bud emergence; budding could continue by use of preexisting active protein (conversely, budding could continue if the mutant gene product blocked the normal inactivation of proteins that regulate bud emergence). Alternatively the mutant gene in strain Mc1 may produce a protein that is directly involved in budding. If this protein was temperature sensitive and its activity slowly decayed after the temperature shift to 37°C, several cell cycles could pass before budding ceased. Similarly, if no synthesis of the protein took place at the restrictive temperature, budding could continue until the level of preexisting protein was insufficient to support activity. Strains Mc2 and Mc3 have been shown by parasexual analysis to harbor temperature-sensitive mutations in different genes, *mcm2* and *mcm3*, respectively (Schafer *et al.*, 1984). The mutation in *mcm2* causes considerable cell death after several hours at 37°C, but *mcm3* causes little death. These latter mutations may be in structural genes, because they seem to be expressed almost immediately on shifting the incubation temperature from 25 to 37°C.

The morphologically significant events governed, at least indirectly, by the *mcm* mutations include inhibition of bud emergence and polar cell-wall synthesis, stimulation of isotropic growth, repression of the increase in rate of chitin incorporation, and, later, decrease in the rate of insoluble glucan incorporation and exponential increase in the rate of chitin synthesis. All these events seem to be affected by one or more events that occur at a specific point in the cell cycle and that have an execution point before bud emergence.

9. POSSIBLE ROLES OF THE DEFECTIVE GENE PRODUCTS

Current models of fungal cell-wall growth suggest that the cell-wall synthetases and hydrolases and their specific activators and inhibitors are synthesized on the endoplasmic reticulum, packaged into vesicles in the Golgi apparatus, and delivered to the desired sites on the cell envelope by an intracellular transit system (Farkaš, 1979). Although there is disagreement on some specifics, such as the intracellular locations of the inactive chitin synthetase and its activator (Duran *et al.*, 1975; Bartnicki-García *et al.*, 1979), the concept of the model is widely accepted. During polarized growth, such as hyphal extension and branching, and yeast bud formation, synthesis of specific cell-wall polymers is directed toward discrete sites on the cell envelope. During isotropic growth, however, the cell expands uniformly, and little directed synthesis of the packaged components is necessary.

Since the phenotypes of the mutants are complex and seem to be caused by single-gene mutations, it is unlikely that they are in the structural genes for polysaccharide synthetases. A single-gene mutation that affects the incorporation of both chitin and insoluble glucan, as well as other events that determine the orientation of cell-wall synthesis, is likely to be conditionally defective in the function of the polarization director. Dysfunction of the polarization director could prevent delivery of specific components of cell-wall synthesis to discrete loci on the cell envelope and, thus, immediately prohibit bud emergence. If delivery of these components became random, because the orientation of the cell was disrupted, then isotropic growth and delocalized synthesis of normally localized polysaccharides such as chitin could occur. Finally, the normal rates of polysaccharide synthesis observed in yeast cells could be altered because of temporal and spatial changes in the mechanism of activation. All these situations seem to be consistent with events observed during stage I development in *W. dermatitidis.*

9.1. Nature of the Polarization Director

Although the identity of the proposed polarization director is unknown, some of its characteristics are known:

1. *The polarization director localizes site-specific synthesis of certain cell-wall polymers.* One requirement inherent in the definition of the polarization director is that it direct the site-specific cell-wall synthesis in both apical extension and budding growth.

2. *The polarization director persists.* Yeast cells of the wild-type strain are slightly ellipsoidal [average ratio of long to short axes is 1.34 ± 0.01 (Jacobs and Szaniszlo, 1985)]. In addition, the distal end of a newly detached bud is generally more rounded than the proximal end, and the birth scar on the proximal end can be visualized using Calcofluor or fluorescein-labeled Con A (Jacobs, Cooper, and Szaniszlo, in prep.). Using these criteria, the first bud from a new cell generally emerges antipodally (opposite) to the birth scar. Subsequent buds usually form either at or near the site of the previous bud, or near the antipode, along the long axis of the ellipsoid. Thus, the polarization director must have elements that persist between one bud and the next and that indicate the distal end of nonparous cells. The designation of the budding sites is flexible, however, because buds sometimes emerge along the short axis of the ellipsoid. This indicates that the polarization director must involve structures that define antipodes on the cell envelope and remain intact throughout the cell cycle, but are not immutably fixed in place.

3. *The polarization director in the Mc mutants is rapidly inactivated and reactivated by temperature shifts.* According to the calculated execution points, only those cells of first-cycle arrest mutants that are within about 20 min of bud emergence at the time of temperature upshift can accomplish this event (Jacobs and Szaniszlo, 1982, 1985). Similarly, on downshift from the restrictive to the permissive temperature, budding resumes quickly after restoration of the permissive conditions (Jacobs, Roberts, and Szaniszlo, 1985). These observations are consistent with the hypothesis that cell division proceeds almost immediately on downshift to the permissive temperature.

9.2. Candidates for the Polarization Director

Linear organelles that could extend between antipodes of the cell have been suggested as candidates for the polarization director (Byers and Goestch, 1974, 1975; Farkaš, 1979; Hartwell, 1974; Sloat and Pringle, 1978; Sloat *et al.*, 1981). Chief among these organelles are microtubules and microfilaments, which make up the cytoskeletal system. Microtubules have been associated by many investigators with the movement of organelles such as mitochondria, nuclei, vacuoles, and vesicles (see Stephens and Edds, 1976). Microfilaments of actin are contractile and probably provide the driving force for some intracellular movement.

9.2.1. Microtubules

Both intra- and extranuclear microtubules have been observed in *W. dermatitidis* (Grove *et al.*, 1973; J. L. Harris, personal communication). These seem to be similar to the microtubules of other higher fungi, in that the microtubule-dependent events of nuclear migration and mitosis are insensitive to colchicine, but sensitive to methylbenzimidazole carbamate and its derivatives (Jacobs and Szaniszlo, 1982; Jacobs, 1983). However, their role in selecting the site for bud emergence is doubtful, because if microtubule function is inhibited, yeast cells accumulate as multiply budded forms with unmigrated, premitotic nuclei (Jacobs and Szaniszlo, 1982). Similarly, *S. cerevisae* cells that lack microtubules can initiate and completely develop buds (Jacobs, unpublished data). If microtubules were the polarization director in *W. dermatitidis,* inhibition of microtubule function would induce development of multicellular forms. Since this is not the case, and since multicellular forms undergo the microtubule-dependent event of nuclear division, the case for microtubules being the polarization director is weak.

9.2.2. Microfilaments

The role of microfilaments in development of *W. dermatitidis* has not yet been probed. However, concentrations of actin are strongly correlated with areas of cell-wall growth in *S. cerevisiae* (Adams and Pringle, 1984), *S. uvarum* (Kilmartin and Adams, 1984), and *Schizosaccharomyces pombe* (P. Nurse, personal communication). This is true even in cells in which the microtubules have been disrupted (Jacobs, unpublished data). This correlation warrants investigation of the role of actin and other microfilament structures in the regulation of fungal dimorphism.

9.2.3. Other Hypotheses

Jacobs and Szaniszlo (1982) suggested that the polarization director could be a set of plasma membrane loci, defined by one or more proteins that are anchored to the cell envelope by glycosidic linkages. The polarization director could function by serving as recognition sites at which vesicles could fuse with the plasma membrane as well as by serving as attachment sites for cytoskeletal elements that would allow the proper orientation of mitosis. If the loci contained the elements of an ion pump (Jaffe and Nuccitelli, 1977), they could generate polarity through the cell by means of an electrical current that flows from one pole to the other.

10. CONCLUSIONS

The development of multicellular forms from yeast is the best-studied aspect of polymorphism in *W. dermatitidis*. However, this organism is also one of the few that exhibit continuous polar growth, intermittent polar growth, and isotropic growth and can yield cultures that exhibit each homogeneously. The mechanisms by which the organism regulates the temporal and spatial synthesis and composition of its cell wall (and hence its morphology) present an intriguing puzzle. For the development of the multicellular form, many of the cell-cycle events associated with development have been determined, and the chemical architecture responsible for the cell-wall development and maintenance is known. However, the identity of the lesions responsible for multicellular-form development, as well as the mechanisms by which these control morphological development, remain to be revealed. It is to be hoped that the development of the parasexual system, as well as techniques of molecular biology, will be able to aid in identifying the roles of the thermolabile gene products in both yeasts and developing multicellular forms of the Mc strains. Such investigation may be the key to understanding cellular differentiation and regulation of polarity in this organism, in other fungi, and in eukaryotic cells in general.

REFERENCES

Adams, A. E. M., and Pringle, F. R., 1984, Relationship of actin and tubulin distribution to bud growth in wild-type and morphogenetic-mutant *Saccharomyces cerevisiae, J. Cell. Biol.* **98:**934–945.

Bartnicki-García, S., Ruiz-Herrera, J., and Bracker, C. E., 1979, Chitosomes and chitin synthetase, in: *Fungal Walls and Hyphal Growth* (J. H. Burnett and A. P. J. Trinci, eds.), Cambridge University Press, Cambridge, England, pp. 149–168.

Butterfield, W., and Jong, S. C., 1976, Effect of carbon source on conidiogenesis in *Fonsecaea dermatitidis*, agent of chromomycosis, *Mycopathologia* **58**:59–62.
Byers, B., and Goetsch, L., 1974, Duplication of spindle plaques and integration of the yeast cell cycle, *Cold Spring Harbor Symp. Quant. Biol.* **38**:123–131.
Byers, B., and Goetsch, L., 1975, Behavior of spindles and spindle plaques in the cell cycle and conjugation of *Saccharomyces cerevisiae*, *J. Bacteriol.* **124**:511–523.
Calderone, R. A., 1976, Endogenous respiration and fatty acids of *Phialophora dermatitidis*, *Mycologia* **68**:99–107.
Carrion, A. L., 1950, Yeast-like dematiaceous fungi infecting human skin, *Arch. Dermatol. Syphilol.* **61**:966–1009.
Cole, G. T., 1978, Conidiogenesis in the black yeasts, in: *Proceedings of the Fourth International Conference on the Mycoses: The Black and White Yeasts*, Scientific Publication No. 356, Pan American Health Organization, Washington, D.C., pp. 66–78.
Cooper, C. R., Harris, J. L., Jacobs, C. W., and Szaniszlo, P. J., 1984, Effects of polyoxin AL on cellular development in *Wangiella dermatitidis*, *Exp. Mycol.* **8**:349–363.
DeHoog, G. S., 1977, *Rhinocladiella* and allied genera, in: *Studies in Mycology*, Vol. 15, *The Black Yeasts and Allied Hyphomycetes* (G. W., DeHoog and E. J. Hermanides-Nijof, eds.), Centraalbureau voor Schimmelcultur, Baarn, The Netherlands, pp. 1–118.
Duran, A., Bowers, B., and Cabib, E., 1975, Chitin synthetase zymogen is attached to the yeast plasma membrane, *Proc. Natl. Acad. Sci. U.S.A.* **72**:3952–3955.
Endo, A., Kakiki, K., and Misato, T., 1970, Mechanisms of action of the antifungal agent polyoxin D, *J. Bacteriol.* **104**:189–196.
Farkaš, V., 1979, Biosynthesis of cell walls of fungi, *Microbiol. Rev.* **43**:117–144.
Geis, P. A., 1981, Chemical composition of the yeast and sclerotic cell walls of *Wangiella dermatitidis*, Ph.D. dissertation, University of Texas, Austin, Texas, pp. 1–183.
Geis, P. A., Wheeler, M. H., and Szaniszlo, P. J., 1984, Pentaketide metabolites of melanin synthesis in the dematiaceous fungus *Wangiella dermatitidis*, *Arch. Microbiol.* **137**:324–328.
Grove, S. W., Oujezdsky, K. B., and Szaniszlo, P. J., 1973, Budding in the dimorphic fungus *Phialophora dermatitidis*, *J. Bacteriol.* **115**:323–329.
Hartwell, L. H., 1974, *Saccharomyces cerevisiae* cell cycle, *Bacteriol. Rev.* **38**:164–198.
Hironaga, M., Watanabe, S., Nishimura, K., and Miyaji, M., 1981, Annellated conidiogenous cells in *Exophiala dermatitidis*, agent of phaeohyphomycosis, *Mycologia* **73**:1181–1183.
Holan, Z., Pokorny, R., Beran, K., Gemperle, A., Tuzar, Z., and Baldrian, J., 1981, The glucan–chitin complex in *Saccharomyces cerevisiae*. V. Precise location of chitin and glucan in bud scar and their physico-chemical characterization, *Arch. Microbiol.* **130**:312–318.
Jacobs, C. W., 1983, Events associated with cellular development and differentiation in *Wangiella dermatitidis*, Ph.D. dissertation, University of Texas, Austin, Texas, pp. 1–178.
Jacobs, C. W., and Szaniszlo, P. J., 1982, Microtubule function and its relation to cellular development and the yeast cell cycle in *Wangiella dermatitidis*, *Arch. Microbiol.* **133**:155–161.
Jacobs, C. W., and Szaniszlo, P. J., 1985, Altered development in a temperature sensitive morphological mutant of *Wangiella dermatitidis*, *Mycologia* **77**:142–148.
Jacobs, C. W., Roberts, R. L., and Szaniszlo, P. J., 1985, Reversal of multicellular form development in a conditional morphological mutant of the fungus *Wangiella dermatitidis*, *J. Gen. Microbiol.*, in press.
Jaffe, L. F., and Nuccitelli, R., 1977, Electrical controls of development, *Annu. Rev. Biochem.* **6**:445–476.

Johnston, G. C., Singer, R. A., and McFarlane, E. S., 1977, Growth and cell division during nitrogen starvation of the yeast *Saccharomyces cerevisiae, J. Bacteriol.* **132:**723–730.

Kang, M. S., Szaniszlo, P. J., and Cabib, E., 1984, Fungal β-(1 → 3) glucan synthetases; stimulation by nucleotides, inhibition by papulocandin and cooperative effects, *Fed. Proc. Abstr. ASBC/AAE Am. Meet.* **84:**1697.

Katoh, Y., Kuninaka, A., Yoshino, H., Takatsuki, A., Yamasaki, M., and Tamura, G., 1978, Chemical composition of giant cells induced by tunicamycin and normal mycelium of *Penicillium citrinum, Agric. Biol. Chem.* **42:**1833–1840.

Kilmartin, J., and Adams, A. E. M., 1984, Structural rearrangements of tubulin and actin during the cell cycle of the yeast *Saccharomyces, J. Cell Biol.* **98:**922–933.

Kitamura, K., and Yamamoto, T., 1972, Purification and properties of an enzyme, zymolyase, which lyses viable yeast cells, *Arch. Biochem. Biophys.* **153:**403–406.

Kuo, S. C., and Lampen, J. O., 1974, Tunicamycin—an inhibitor of yeast glycoprotein synthesis, *Biochem. Biophys. Res. Commun.* **58:**287–295.

Maeda, H., and Ishida, N., 1967, Specificity of binding hexopyranosylpolysaccharides with fluorescent brightener, *J. Biochem.* **62:**276–278.

Marlowe, J. D., 1977, The development of the sclerotic cell in agents of chromoblastomycosis, an ultrastructural study, M. A. thesis, University of Texas, Austin, Texas, pp. 1–139.

McGinnis, M. R., 1977, *Wangiella,* a new genus to accommodate *Hormiscium dermatitidis, Mycotaxon* **5:**353–363.

McGinnis, M. R., 1983, Chromomycosis and phaeohyphomyxosis: Concepts, diagnosis and mycology, *J. Am. Acad. Dermatol. (St. Louis)* **8:**1–16.

Nishimura, K., and Miyaji, M., 1983, Defence mechanisms of mice against *Exophiala dermatitidis* infection, *Mycologia* **81:**9–21.

Oujezdsky, K. B., and Szaniszlo, P. J., 1974, Conidial ontogeny in *Phialophora dermatitidis, Mycologia* **66:**537–542.

Oujezdsky, K. B., Grove, S. N., and Szaniszlo, P. J., 1973, Morphological and structural changes during the yeast-to-mold conversion of *Phialophora dermatitidis, Mycologia* **66:**537–542.

Pringle, J. R., and Hartwell, L. H., 1981, The *Saccharomyces cerevisiae* cell cycle, in: *The Molecular Biology of the Yeast Saccharomyces: Life Cycle and Inheritance* (J. N. Strathern, E. W. Jones, and J. R. Broach, eds.), Cold Spring Harbor Monographs, Cold Spring Harbor, New York, pp. 97–142.

Reiss, N. R., and Mok, W. Y., 1979, *Wangiella dermatitidis* isolated from bats in Manaus, Brazil, *Sabouraudia* **17:**213–218.

Rippon, J. W., 1982, *Medical Mycology: The Pathogenic Fungi and the Pathogenic Actinomycetes,* W. B. Saunders, Philadelphia, pp. 1–842.

Roberts, R. L., 1979, Characterization of temperature-sensitive multicellular mutants of *Wangiella dermatitidis,* Ph.D. dissertation, University of Texas, Austin, Texas, pp. 1–167.

Roberts, R. L., and Szaniszlo, P. J., 1978, Temperature-sensitive multicellular mutants of *Wangiella dermatitidis, J. Bacteriol.* **135:**622–632.

Roberts, R. L., and Szaniszlo, P. J., 1980, Yeast-phase cell cycle of the polymorphic fungus *Wangiella dermatitidis, J. Bacteriol.* **144:**721–731.

Roberts, R. L., Lo, R. J., and Szaniszlo, P. J., 1979, Nuclear division in temperature-sensitive multicellular mutants of *Wangiella dermatitidis, J. Bacteriol.* **137:**1456–1458.

Roberts, R. L., Lo, R. J., and Szaniszlo, P. J., 1980, Induction of synchronous growth in the yeast phase of *Wangiella dermatitidis, J. Bacteriol.* **141:**981–984.

Roberts, R. L., Bowers, B., Slater, M. L., and Cabib, E., 1983, Chitin synthesis in cell division cycle mutants of *Saccharomyces cerevisiae, Mol. Cell. Biol.* **3**:922–930.

Schafer, R. C., Cooper, C. R., and Szaniszlo, P. J., 1984, Complementation of two multicellular genes from *Wangiella dermatitidis* by spheroplast fusion, *Abstr. Annu. Meet. Am. Soc. Microbiol.*, 1984, p. 293.

Silva, M., 1957, The parasitic phase of the fungi of chromoblastomycosis: Development of the sclerotic cell *in vitro* and *in vivo, Mycologia* **49**:318–331.

Sloat, B. F., and Pringle, J. R., 1978, A mutant of yeast defective in cellular morphogenesis, *Science* **200**:1171–1173.

Sloat, B. F., Adams, A., and Pringle, J. R., 1981, Roles of the CDC24 gene product in cellular morphogenesis during the *Saccharomyces cerevisiae* cell cycle, *J. Cell Biol.* **89**:39–40.

Stephens, R. E., and Edds, K. T., 1976, Microtubules: Structure, chemistry and function, *Physiol. Rev.* **56**:709–776.

Szaniszlo, P. J., Hsieh, P. H., and Marlowe, J. D., 1976, Induction and ultrastructure of the multicellular (sclerotic) morphology in *Phialophora dermatitidis, Mycologia* **68**:117–130.

Szaniszlo, P. J., Geis, P. A., Jacobs, C. W., Cooper, C. R., and Harris, J. L., 1983, Cell wall changes associated with yeast-to-multicellular form conversion in *Wangiella dermatitidis*, in: *Microbiology*, Vol. 83 (D. Schlessinger, ed.), American Society of Microbiology, Washington, D.C., pp. 239–244.

Szaniszlo, P. J., Kang, M. S., and Cabib, E., 1985, Stimulation of $\beta(1 \rightarrow 3)$glucan synthetase of various fungi by nucleoside triphosphates: A generalized regulatory mechanism for cell wall biosynthesis, *J. Bacteriol.* **161**:1188–1194.

Tkacz, J. S., and Lampen, J. O., 1975, Tunicamycin inhibition of polyisoprenyl *N*-acetylglucosaminyl pyrophosphate formation in calf liver microsomes, *Biochem. Biophys. Res. Commun.* **65**:248–257.

Wang, J.-Y., 1982, Effects of tunicamycin and polyoxin AL on morphogenesis and viability of *Wangiella dermatitidis*, M.A. thesis, University of Texas, Austin, pp. 1–104.

Part IV

Fungi with Isotropically Enlarged Tissue Morphologies

Chapter 10

Dimorphism in *Chrysosporium parvum*

Milan Hejtmánek

L'un et l'autre nous cherchons la verité pour elle, non pour avoir raison, ni pour faire du bruit. Entre nos arguments inverses elle se trouve cernée. L'avenir dira qui s'est le plus approché d'elle.

R. Sabouraud

1. INTRODUCTION

The hyphomycetes *Chrysosporium parvum* var. *parvum* and *C. parvum* var. *crescens* cause a disease called adiaspiromycosis, which is of worldwide distribution. Although it affects primarily the lungs of rodents and other mammals, there are reports, though rare, of its occurrence in man, with only 14 human cases being known (Otčenášek *et al.*, 1982). The first finding of the parasitic (adiasporic) stage of *C. parvum* var. *crescens* in a granuloma of the human lung was associated with another principal disease (Doby-Dubois *et al.*, 1964). The definition of disseminated granulomatous pulmonary adiaspiromycosis as a new nosological entity in human medicine is based on a Czechoslovak case (Kodousek *et al.*, 1970b, 1971). The clinical, pathological, and epidemiological aspects of this disease, together with the ecology and geographic distribution of its

Milan Hejtmánek • Department of Biology, Medical Faculty, Palacky University, 775 00 Olomouc, Czechoslovakia.

causative agent, are dealt with in reviews by Jellison (1969), Dvořák *et al.* (1973), Kodousek (1974), and Otčenášek *et al.* (1982).

Of the two varieties, *C. parvum* var. *crescens* should in particular attract the attention of developmental mycologists. Its ability to produce by isotropic growth giant spherical cells with thick cell walls (the adiaspores) is generally unparalleled in fungi and provides a useful model for developmental research.

1.1. Taxonomy

The causative agents of adiaspiromycosis are referred to under various names that reflect their taxonomic history. The first identification of the fungus responsible for this disease was by Kirschenblatt (1939), who found it in small rodents and described it using the taxonomically nonvalid binomial *Rhinosporidium pulmonale.* Subsequently, the fungus was redescribed by Emmons and Ashburn (1942) as *Haplosporangium parvum* and by Ciferri and Montemartini (1959), who established the new form-genus *Emmonsia* with the single species *E. parva.* Emmons and Jellison (1960) more recently added another species, *E. crescens.* The morphological similarity of *Emmonsia, Chrysosporium,* and other related fungi prompted Carmichael (1962) and Padhye and Carmichael (1968) to transfer both species of *Emmonsia* to the genus *Chrysosporium* under the names *C. parvum* and *C. parvum* var. *crescens.* According to McGinnis (1980), this is the best classification. Boisseau-Lebreuil (1981), in discussing the taxonomic criteria for the discrimination between the two taxons, is of the same opinion. Chandler *et al.* (1980) used the names *C. parvum* var. *parvum* and *C. parvum* var. *crescens,* which will be employed in this review. The genus *Chrysosporium* is the anamorph of some species of *Arthroderma* and other members of the Gymnoasaceae (McGinnis, 1980). The teleomorphs of *C. parvum* var. *parvum* and *C. parvum* var. *crescens* are unknown.

2. MORPHOLOGY

Chrysosporium parvum is a temperature-dependent dimorphic fungus. Its dimorphism is expressed phenotypically by the mycelial and adiasporic stages. The mycelial stages of both varieties are generally agreed to have the same morphology, whereas the adiasporic stages differ in this respect (Boisseau-Lebreuil, 1981). When growing on agar media of various compositions at temperatures below 30°C, the fungus becomes mycelial and forms unicellular, uninucleate conidia (aleuriospores). On

Sabouraud's glucose agar, the colonies of *C. parvum* var. *crescens* are initially flat or with slight elevations, but later become furrowed to a larger or smaller extent. The coloring of the colony surface is white or cream to brownish.

Otčenášek and Zlatanov (1975) describe powdered, floccose, and fluffy strains of relatively unique micromorphology. The conidia of 13 strains had smooth or rough surfaces and, as measured by these authors, reach a mean length ($\pm$S.D.) of 3.43 ± 0.07 to 4.41 ± 0.16 μm and a mean width of 3.13 ± 0.07 to 4.08 ± 0.16 μm. The morphological variability of the colonies is not markedly influenced by the host species or geographic origin of the strains.

At 37°C, *C. parvum* var. *crescens* (at 40°C for var. *parvum*) enters the adiasporic stage. This stage is characterized by the presence of adiaspores [= adiaconidia in the terminology of McGinnis (1980)], with no conidia or mycelium yet being formed. The adiaspores are thick-walled cells of a generally spherical shape, several tens of micrometers in diameter in var. *parvum* and several hundreds of micrometers in var. *crescens* (Figure 1).

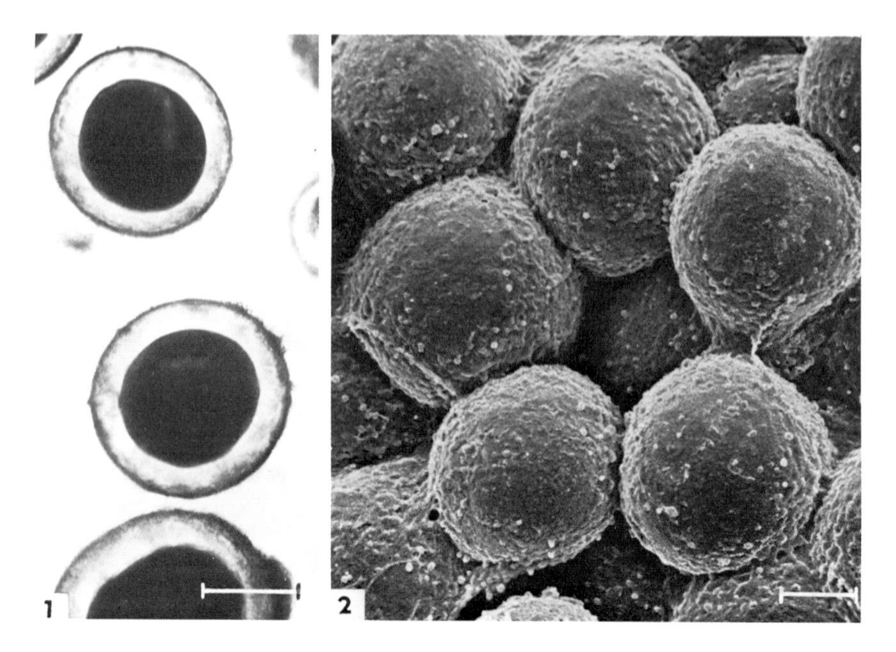

Figure 1. Thick-walled adiaspores of *C. parvum* var. *crescens* in agar culture. Lugol preparation. Scale bar: 100 μm.

Figure 2. Granulomas caused by *C. parvum* var. *crescens* on the pancreas of experimentally infected mouse. Scanning electron micrograph. Scale bar: 100 μm.

Table I
Comparison of the Mycelial and Adiasporic Stages in *C. parvum* var. *parvum* and *C. parvum* var. *crescens*[a]

Characteristics	var. *parvum*	var. *crescens*
Mycelial stage		
In vitro		
Size of conidia	2–4 × 2.5–4.5 μm	2–4 × 2.5–4.5 μm
Number of nuclei in conidium	One	One
Number of nuclei in hyphal tips	Numerous	Numerous
Number of hyphae germinating from one adiaspore	1–3	Numerous
Temperature stopping hyphal growth	40°C	30°C
In vivo		
Absent		
Adiasporic stage		
In vitro		
Temperature suitable for adiasporogenesis	40°C	35–37°C
Size of adiaspores	25 μm (10–20 μm)	120 μm (200–480 μm)
Thickness of adiaspore wall	2–4 μm	10–80 μm
Number of nuclei in adiaspore	One or several	Numerous
In vivo		
Largest adiaspores	46 μm	700 μm
Number of nuclei in adiaspore	One or several	Numerous

[a]Based on data of Emmons and Jellison (1960), Emmons (1964), Dvořák *et al.* (1973), Vanbreuseghem *et al.* (1978), Chandler *et al.* (1980), Boisseau-Lebreuil (1981), and Hejtmánek (unpublished).

The term *adiaspore* signifies a fungal spore enlarging without multiplication at elevated temperature (Emmons and Jellison, 1960). On agar medium, the adiaspore population developing from the inoculum of the mycelial stage forms wrinkled, elevated, glabrous, and compact colonies that do not grow into the medium and do not show flat extension. They are gray or brown. Large inocula of the mycelial stage give rise to larger adiasporic colonies than do small inocula. Morphologically, the adiasporic stage corresponds to the parasitic stage of the fungus. The two stages of both varieties are compared in Table I.

3. GROWTH RATE

The comparative study of Boisseau-Lebreuil (1975b) on the influence of temperature within the range of 5–40°C on the growth and morphology of colonies in 22 strains confirms the existence of (1) "nonthermophilic" strains showing maximum growth rates at 20–25°C, complete growth inhibition at 30°C, and production of adiaspores at 35°C and (2) "thermophilic" strains showing maximum growth rates at 25°C, complete growth inhibition at 40°C, and formation of small adiaspores at 40°C. No significant difference was found by Ciferri and Montemartini (1959) between the assimilation of 14 various nitrogen sources by 3 thermophilic strains (growth optimum at about 35°C) and 4 nonthermophilic strains (temperature optimum around 20°C).

The colonies of 13 strains of *C. parvum* var. *crescens* reached a diameter of 45–55 mm after 20 days on modified Sabouraud's glucose agar (SGA) at 28°C (Otčenášek and Zlatanov, 1975). The growth rate of one wild-type strain of this variety growing on Sabouraud's glucose agar at 26°C was 139 μm/hr, which corresponds to the colony diameter of 47 mm in 14 days. The growth rates of mutants derived from this strain amounted to 32.8–98.7% of the wild-type growth rate (Vacková-Janečková and Hejtmánek, 1983).

The adiaspores grow isotropically by volume enlargement (Table II).

Table II
Dynamics of Adiaspore Enlargement in *C. parvum* var. *crescens*

Age (days)	In mice[a]	On SGA at 37°C[b]	On SGA with 0.25 M glucose in four strains at 37°C[c]
4	—	10	—
5	16	—	—
7	30	22	9.28 ± 0.7 to 37.9 ± 8.7
12	60	79	—
14	—	—	11.20 ± 0.5 to 60.8 ± 5.8
15	90	—	—
16	—	109	—
17	100	—	—
20	110	—	—
21	—	—	14.30 ± 3.0 to 99.00 ± 10.9
25	150	—	—
28	—	—	12.80 ± 1.6 to 113.10 ± 4.6
30	170	142	—
35	—	—	11.80 ± 2.3 to 90.70 ± 5.2
36	180	—	—
42	225	—	—
80	310	—	—
120	350	—	—
570	380	—	—

[a]According to Šlais (1976); most frequent diameter values.
[b]According to Hamáček *et al.* (1971); maximal diameter values.
[c]According to Weigl and Hejtmánek (1973); mean diameter values ± S.E. × 3.

A conidium of the var. *crescens* with a diameter of about 4 μm and with a wall thickness of less than 1 μm can develop into an adiaspore up to 700 μm in diameter with a wall as thick as 80 μm. This represents a volume increase of 5.3×10^6 times. A positive correlation was found between the growth rate of the mycelial and the adiasporic stages in some cases (Hejtmánek and Bártek, 1976). Significant differences were observed in the growth rate and size of the adiaspores between individual strains of *C. parvum* var. *crescens* (Dvořák, *et al.,* 1973; Weigl and Hejtmánek, 1973). Boisseau-Lebreuil (1970) states that adiaspore size is dependent on rodent host species, e.g., 87 μm (25–150 μm) for *Pitymys subterraneus,* 287 μm (100–475 μm) for *Apodemus sylvatica,* and 336 μm (200–475 μm) for *Clethriomys glareolus.*

When *C. parvum* var. *crescens* grows in 1 liter of glucose asparagine medium at 28°C for 2 weeks, 16–20 g of moist mycelial biomass is obtained, whereas culture at 37°C for 4 weeks yields only 1.0–1.5 g of "purified" adiaspores (Kashkin, 1980). No information is available on the dynamics of growth of the smaller *C. parvum* var. *parvum* adiaspores.

4. ADIASPORE–HOST INTERACTIONS

Both fungus varieties are present in warm-blooded animals only as adiaspores. The histopathological effect of adiaspores on the host organism (Kodousek, 1974; Boisseau-Lebreuil, 1975a; Watts *et al.,* 1975; Šlais, 1976; Chandler *et al.,* 1980) is expressed in the development of granulomas. The adiaspore of *C. parvum* var. *crescens* enveloped in granulation tissue forms a typical granuloma (adiaspiroma) (Figure 2) 0.5–1.0 mm in diameter. Electron microscopy of experimental adiaspiromycosis in mice has shown that 2–4 days after inoculation, a tissue reaction occurs characterized by a massive appearance of various forms of migrating cells, granulocytes, heparinocytes, epitheloid histiocytes, cells of resorptive type, and multinuclear giant cells (Malínský *et al.,* 1972). In naturally infected animals, adiaspiromycotic granulomas mostly occur in the lungs as solitary or multiple nonnecrotic granulomas. In contrast, experimental adiaspiromycosis of mice, guinea pigs, and other animals induced by intraperitoneal inoculation of conidia and mycelial fragments exhibits granulomas in the liver, spleen, and pancreas and on the diaphragm, kidney, omentum, peritoneum, and other organs (Hejtmánek and Kodousek, 1972a,b; Hejtmánek, 1976c). One granuloma usually contains one adiaspore, and rarely two or three.

Mice respond with the development of granulomas not only to viable but also to fixed adiaspores of *C. parvum* var. *crescens* and to fragments of their walls to extracted with HCl, NaOH, ethanol, and chloroform. Conversely, intraperitoneal injection of dead conidia or mycelial fragments into mice does not result in granulomas. The conclusions of these experiments (Hejtmánek and Kodousek, 1985) are that (1) the cell wall of the adiaspores is of decisive importance for the processes of tissue reaction and formation of the adiaspiromycotic granuloma; (2) the composition of the granulomas containing chemically processed wall material from adiaspores is, in histological terms, deprived of some components of the migrating cells, probably due to poorer antigenic activity; and (3) the granulomas are formed around the rather large cell-wall fragments, while no development of granulomas is provoked by the small fragments. The fragments can be phagocytosed like other nonviable, degenerated elements of the fungus (Malínský *et al.*, 1972). The conidia of *C. parvum* var. *crescens* passing through the digestive tract of the animals remain alive and do not show any pathogenic effect (Hejtmánek, 1973; Kodousek and Hejtmánek, 1975).

5. STRUCTURE AND CYTOCHEMISTRY

The available information on the structure of the adiaspores of *C. parvum* var. *crescens* will serve as the basis for a review of structure and cytochemistry because similar data from var. *parvum* are still missing. A fully differentiated adiaspore is covered by a thick cell wall, and its cytoplasm contains numerous nuclei and nucleoli, much endoplasmic reticulum, many ribosomes, lysosomes, peroxisomes, and vacuoles, glycogen arranged in clusters, and the equivalent of Golgi structures (Kodousek *et al.*, 1972b,c).

5.1. Adiaspore Wall

The adiaspore wall contains chitin and proteins (Blank, 1957). It is periodic-acid–Schiff-stain-positive, which proves the presence of polysaccharides. When preoxidized with acid $KMnO_4$ it is stained by alcian blue and Halle–Muller's method for bound colloidal iron. According to optical density, three layers can be distinguished in the wall by phase-contrast and fluorescence microscopy (Kodousek *et al.*, 1970a). When stained with hematoxylin and eosin, the wall of a mature adiaspore appears to be composed of two layers; Gridley's method and Gomori's methenamine silver method reveal three layers (Watts *et al.*, 1975; Chandler *et al.*, 1980).

The wall of a differentiated adiaspore consists of three cytochemically different layers (Ždárská and Šlais, 1972): The outer layer (thickness 2–3 μm, Gomori-positive, Grocott-negative) contains mainly proteins with arginine, tyrosine, and tryptophan, and traces of hydrophilic lipids. The external 1- to 2-μm portion of the middle layer (7–10 μm thick, Gomori-negative, Grocott-positive) and the whole inner layer (20–25 μm, Grocott-positive) consist of neutral mucosubstances. The ground substance of the internal 6- to 8-μm portion of the middle layer is also a neutral mucosubstance. The networklike structure of this layer consists of proteins with arginine, tyrosine, and tryptophan. By means of transmission electron microscopy, three layers are distinguished in the cell wall of an adiaspore present in a granuloma: outer (thin, very high contrast), middle (also thin, but very pale), and inner (the thickest, of medium density). All three layers are almost amorphous, but some specimens show signs of a lamellar pattern in the outer layer and of a fibrillar structure in the inner layers. In some places, the external layer forms relatively large thickenings that are visible even by light microscopy and that suggest buds on the adiaspore surface. The central portions of these "buds" are filled with a gray substance having a finely filamentous ultrastructure in a meshlike pattern (Malínský *et al.*, 1972). The walls of adiaspores grown on agar medium are somewhat different and consist of an outer thin layer of high electron density ("scleroderma"), an electron optically light interlayer (very thin), and a thick inner layer with two sublayers (Kodousek *et al.*, 1972b,c). Freeze–etching demonstrated the inner face of the adiaspore wall to be coated with isolated particles about 10 nm in diameter and with short wall ridges 80–120 nm long. A longitudinal split is evident in some of the ridges (Hejtmánek *et al.*, 1974).

5.2. Plasmalemma

Invaginations in the plasmalemma are complementary to the wall ridges on the inner face of the adiaspore wall. The outer face of the plasmalemma is very densely coated with small globules. The plasmalemma is not entirely flat, forming small infoldings on the cellular surface (Malínský *et al.*, 1972).

5.3. Adiaspore Content

Numerous nuclei (1.1–1.7 μm in diameter) occupy the peripheral portion of the cytoplasm of a mature adiaspore. Toward the center of the adiaspore, the number of vacuoles in the cytoplasm appears greater. A mature adiaspore often contains one large central vacuole, the protoplast lying at the cell wall. The nuclei divide by mitosis; no spindles or centrioles have been found. An immature adiaspore of 15 μm diameter contains 14–16 nuclei, whereas nuclei of a 48-μm adiaspore may number as many as 25 (Hejtmánek *et al.*, 1968). The number of nuclei increases as the adiaspore grows and may reach several hundred (Emmons *et al.*, 1971).

Using histochemical methods, Žďárská and Šlais (1972) proved that the networklike structure on the periphery of the cytoplasm is basophilic and contains proteins with arginine, tyrosine, tryptophan, SH and SS groups, hydrophilic lipids, and alkaline and acid phosphatases. The network contains minute spherical particles of different sizes (gram-positive, Ziehl–Neelsen-positive) with a positive reaction for proteins and SS and SH groups and with a negative reaction to both neutral and acid mucosubstances. The central portion of the cytoplasm shows a positive reaction for hydrophobic lipids in the contents of the vacuoles occupying the meshes of networklike structure. The network in this portion gives a feebly positive reaction for proteins and alkaline and acid phosphatases and a negative reaction for hydrophilic lipids. The network contains numerous glycogen granules and protein granules.

Electron-microscopic studies (Malínský *et al.*, 1972; Kodousek *et al.*, 1972a,b; Hejtmánek *et al.*, 1974) confirmed the presence in adiaspores of the aforementioned structures as well as endoplasmic reticulum, ribosomes, mitochondria with cristae or tubuli or both, lysosomes, peroxisomes, and structures probably equivalent to Golgi structures. The nuclei in the adiaspores contain nucleoli, and the nuclear envelope is composed of two unit membranes with numerous pores.

The following enzyme activities were found in the cytoplasmic content of the adiaspores developing on agar medium: (1) hydrolytic enzymes: alkaline and acid phosphatase, nonspecific esterase, and aminopeptidase; (2) respiratory enzymes: lactic dehydrogenase, malic dehydrogenase, succinic dehydrogenase, isocitric dehydrogenase, glucose-6-phosphate dehydrogenase, diaphorase, and peroxidase. The degree of positivity in various dehydrogenase reactions is used as a test of adiaspore viability (Kodousek and Hejtmánek, 1971, 1972a; Kodousek *et al.*, 1972a).

5.4. Structure of Hyphae and Conidia

The cell wall of *C. parvum* var. *crescens* hyphae contains polysaccharide of the chitin type. Woronin bodies are found on both sides of septa. The cytoplasm comprises mitochondria, glycogen granules, vacuoles, lipid bodies, and granular endoplasmic reticulum (Zíková *et al.*, 1973). Numerous nuclei, which can be easily visualized by a fluorescence technique (Hejtmánek and Hejtmánková, 1976), are present in the hyphal tips. The conidia have one nucleus each. In some strains, the conidial surface is smooth; in others, it is rough (Otčenášek and Zlatanov, 1975). The enzyme activities given above for adiaspores have also been demonstrated in mycelial cells and conidia.

6. BIOCHEMICAL AND IMMUNOCHEMICAL ASPECTS

The conversion of *C. parvum* var. *crescens* from one stage to another is accompanied by changes in the spectrum and relative antigen content of the fungal cells and also by antigens excreted into the culture medium (Kashkin, 1980). The enzyme activity is changed as well (Kashkin, 1980). Electrophoretic analysis revealed up to 23 fractions from mycelial cells differing in electrophoretic mobility, 14 of which are present regularly but 9 only sporadically. The adiaspore cell-sap proteinogram showed 18 fractions, 11 or 12 of which occur regularly and 6 or 7 only infrequently. The mycelial and adiasporic stages differ in the number of cytoplasmic isoenzymes participating in energy metabolism. The mycelial stage shows higher activity and a greater number of malate dehydrogenase isoforms. The activity of succinate dehydrogenase (SDH) is greater in the adiasporic stage. Three of seven SDH isoforms from the adiaspore are also present in the mycelial stage. In adiaspore culture filtrates, SDH activity (and spectrum) is also higher than in the mycelial cells. Cells in both stages do not differ in the store of catalase and peroxidase isoforms. However, adiaspores excrete both catalase isoenzymes into the medium, and their activity is higher than in the medium of the mycelial stage.

The activities of esterases and of acid and alkaline phosphatases are higher in the mycelial stage than in adiaspores. Conversion of mycelial cells to adiaspores is associated with a decrease of intracellular and extracellular amylase. It was also found (Kashkin, 1980) that mycelial and adiasporic stages differ in the content of "phase-specific" isoenzymes, which are active only in a certain stage of fungus development. A greater quantity of isoenzymes was observed in the culture filtrate of the adiasporic stage, and their activity was found to be higher than those from the mycelial stage.

By means of electrophoresis, 7–10 antigens were detected in mycelial cell sap and 7 in adiaspore cell sap. Most of these antigens are common to both stages. Extracellular antigens of the adiasporic stage contain 11 to 13 components, among which are antigens detected in the extracts of adiaspores (6 or 7 components) and antigens revealed only in the culture filtrate (6 or 7 components). Immunoelectrophoretic comparison of different antigen preparations of both stages shows that culture filtrates of the adiasporic stage contain a greater number of antigens. These antigens have higher immunogenicity than those of the fungal-cell extracts. Some antigens, like the isoenzymes, may be detected only in culture filtrates, whereas others are phase-specific and found only in mycelial or adiasporic stage (Kashkin, 1980).

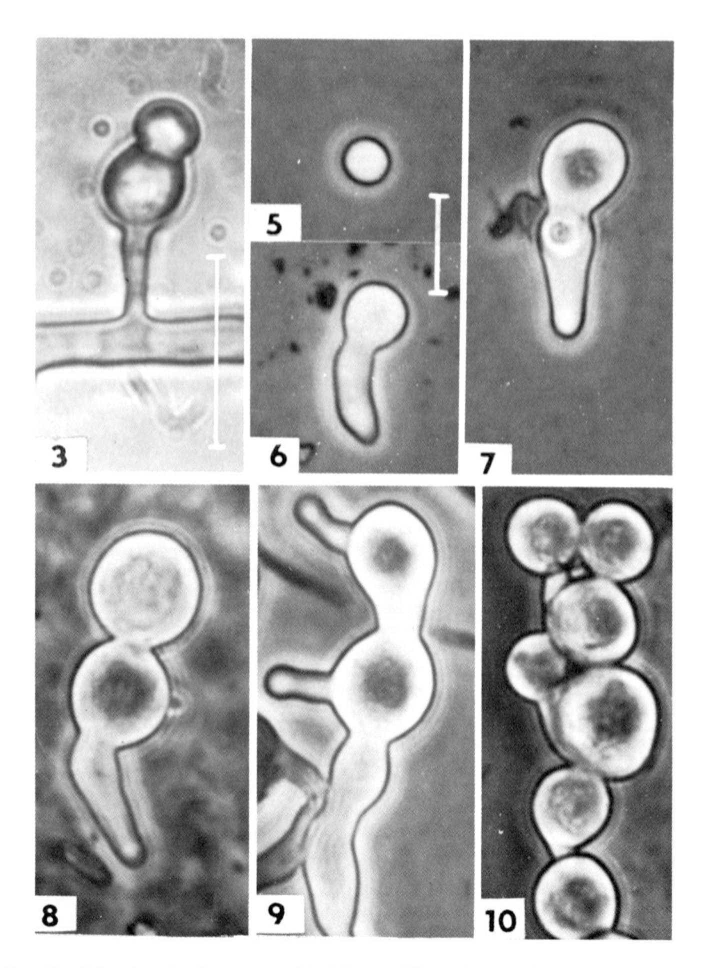

Figure 3. Conidia developing on pedicel in a slide culture of *C. parvum* var. *crescens*. Native preparation. Scale bar: 10 μm.

Figures 5–10. Spherical cells developing by swelling of conidium (5), by repeated swellings of germ hypha (6–8), and by swellings and differentiation of hyphal cells (9,10) in *C. parvum* var. *crescens*. Phase-contrast, native preparation. Scale bar: 10 μm.

7. CONIDIOGENESIS

The term "aleuriospore," as applied to *C. parvum,* is regarded as obsolete (McGinnis, 1980). Evidence based on light microscopy suggests that conidia of *C. parvum* var. *crescens* developing below 30°C have a thallic origin. Conidia either are attached directly to the sides or ends of hyphae or they may develop on short or longer pedicels (Figure 3). The distal portion of the pedicel is frequently swollen. A single conidium or short chains of two or three conidia develop on this swelling (Otčenášek and Zlatanov, 1975). The origin of the conidial wall, where conidial loci are to be found, and whether the conidiogenous cell is developmentally of a determinate or proliferative type (Kendrick, 1971; Cole and Samson, 1979) have not been established. Therefore, an exact conclusion cannot be drawn about the nature of the conidium until relevant data on the ultrastructure of the cell wall of developing conidia and on the dynamics of conidiogenesis become available.

8. DEVELOPMENT OF THE ADIASPORE

Dowding (1947) and Emmons (1964) observed that adiaspores are formed by conidial development of aerial mycelium and by the differentiation of some hyphal cells as well. This was later confirmed by others (e.g., Hamáček *et al.,* 1971; Hejtmánek and Kodousek, 1971, 1972b).

8.1. Development from Conidia

Conidia of *C. parvum* var. *crescens,* inoculated on Sabouraud's agar medium or in liquid medium, exhibit early phases of adiasporogenesis by the following sequence (Figures 4–8): (1) Conidia enlarge by swelling. (2) The enlarged conidia germinate uni- or bilocularly. (3) The nonseptate germ hypha continues swelling at its basal end. The apex of the germ hypha grows longitudinally, swelling subapically. In this developmental stage, the thallus does not contain any septa, being composed of three morphologically distinguishable parts: the most swollen part (the oldest, corresponding to the conidium), the medium swollen part (subapical), and the hyphal tip. (4) The most swollen part is delimited by a septum (septa). This gives rise to the adiaspore precursor cell, or trophocyte (Hejtmánek and Kodousek, 1971, 1972b), which is spherical (6–20 μm in diameter), thin-walled, and delimited from the other cells. By further isotropic growth and septation, germ hypha (about 10–15 μm long) may

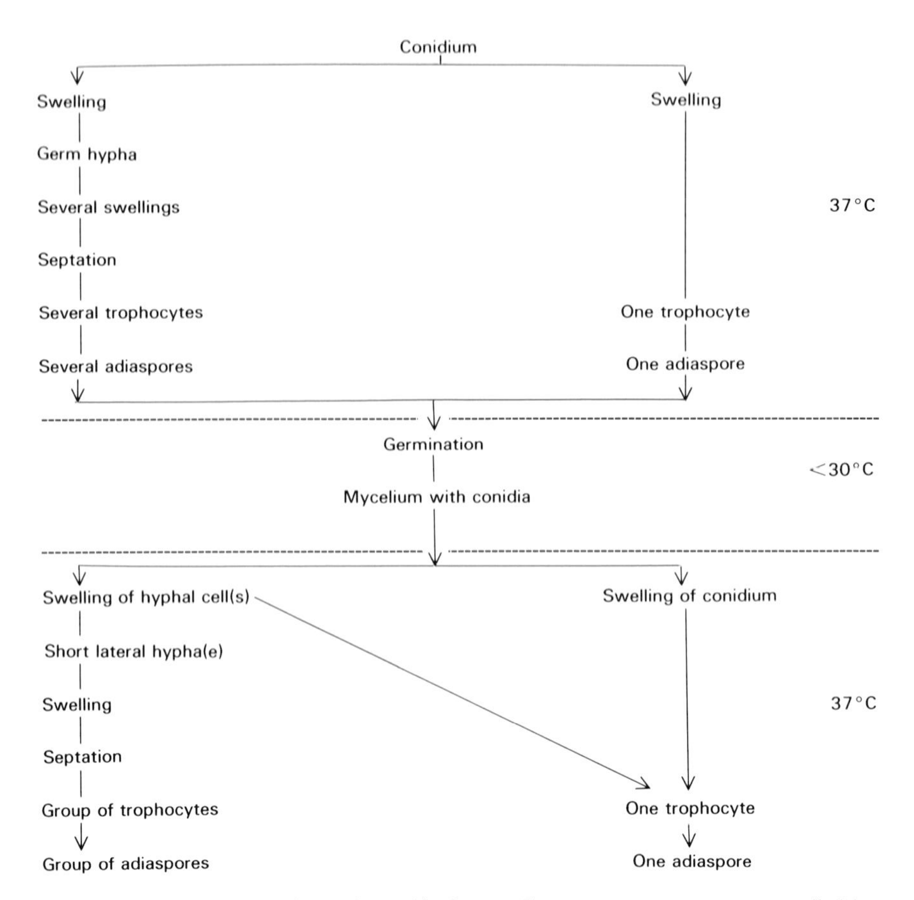

Figure 4. Development of the dimorphic fungus *C. parvum* var. *crescens* controlled by temperature.

form a group of trophocytes that gradually differentiate into adiaspores. As their enlargement continues, their walls thicken. Some adiaspores are connected by relatively short hyphae. This connection is fragile, and adiaspore dehiscence leaves SEM-visible scars on the hyphae (Hejtmánek, 1976a,b). Individual adiaspores are also differentiated from single conidia through isotropic growth without signs of germination in the host organism, and on conidiophores of mycelial colonies growing on the agar medium at 37°C. Under optimum conditions, differentiation of a conidium into an adiaspore requires 2–4 weeks. Adiaspore enlargement can go on for 3 months or more (Šlais, 1976).

8.2. Development from Hyphal Cells

Hyphal cells of *C. parvum* var. *crescens* growing on agar or liquid media at temperatures less than 30°C can also differentiate into adiaspores, if transferred to 37°C. Both the terminal and intercalary cells of the mycelium swell (Figures 9 and 10), while the adjacent cells usually die. Single hyphal cells can have one, two, or more swellings. The swollen parts are at first not delimited by septa, and some even produce short lateral hyphae. As the swollen parts become larger, septa are differentiated and spherical trophocytes delimited (see above). Continuing enlargement and isotropic deposition of wall material of trophocytes give rise to thick-walled adiaspores. However, not all cells of the mycelium differentiate in this way; other mycelial cells degenerate gradually and lose their cytoplasm.

8.3. Conversion of Colony and Inoculum

When a colony of *C. parvum* var. *crescens* growing on agar medium at less than 30°C for 10–14 days is transferred to 37°C, mycelial growth stops, and some days later conversion signs begin to appear. Conversion starts at the margins of the colony and advances toward the center. The original white fluffy colony that has many conidia is gradually converted into a brown, glabrous, irregularly wrinkled colony consisting of budding-like ("yeast") cells, trophocytes, and adiaspores of various sizes. This remarkable morphological heterogeneity is presumably caused by processes of adiaspore development from conidia and hyphal cells that are not synchronous and proceed at different rates. Colony conversion takes 3 or more weeks depending on its size.

If an adiasporic colony developing at 37°C is transferred to 25°C, the mycelium resumes growth and conidium formation. The reversible conversion processes require physiologically adequate growth media (Hejtmánek, unpublished data).

The population of cells developing at 37°C on agar medium inoculated with mycelium and conidia shows various developmental stages of adiaspores, even after several weeks of cultivation and transfer to new agar medium. These include the swelling phase, budding-like cells, trophocytes of various sizes, and thick-walled adiaspores of various dimensions and with varying wall thicknesses. This phenomenon was reported to be caused only by enlargement of the original aleuriospores in which the adiasporogenesis is inhibited by crowding (Emmons *et al.*, 1971). A similar heterogeneity can, however, be seen during cultivation in fresh liquid medium. The following seems to be a plausible conclusion: Adiasporogenesis in a mixed conidial and mycelial inoculum is not a synchronous process, and so it does not reach the final stage, i.e., adiaspore, in all the adiasporogenic cells. Therefore, the variance of the adiaspore mean diameter is rather great and adiaspore size in a cell population is best given in mode values. No information about the parameters allowing adiasporogenic cell detection prior to the phase of swelling and about synchronization of the processes of adiasporogenesis is available. Neither have the parameters of fully differentiated, i.e., mature, adiaspores been defined with sufficient precision, obviously because of their quantitative nature. This is unfortunate, since the enlargement of *C. parvum* var. *crescens* cells by isotropic growth and their conversion into adiaspores is undoubtedly one of the important pathogenic factors of adiaspiromycosis (Hejtmánek and Křivanec, 1977).

8.4. Blastic and Thallic Development

The processes of adiasporogenesis in *C. parvum* var. *crescens* show signs of both blastic and thallic development (for a review, see Cole and Samson, 1979):

1. Adiasporogenesis of conidia on agar medium or in liquid medium shows signs of the blastic process, since a marked isotropic enlargement of the spore occurs before it is delimited by a septum (or septal) and differentiated from a part of the cell (i.e., the germ hypha).
2. Adiasporogenesis in hyphal cells corresponds to thallic development in cases of the adiaspore differentiating from one whole hyphal cell. This cell corresponds to the spore initial delimited by a septum (or septa) before adiasporogenesis has started. Two or more adiaspores can, however, differentiate out of one long hyphal cell. Their initials are then represented by a severalfold enlargement of one hyphal cell.
3. A spherically enlarged hyphal cell can produce a short lateral hypha that swells and is delimited by a septum. The new cell gives rise to a spherical cell by further isotropic growth and enlargement into an adiaspore. This secondary adiaspore is thus of blastic origin and develops similarly to budding.

Adiaspore development evidently comprises both thallic and blastic "episodes" that are easy to distinguish since—as stated by Cole and Samson (1979)—a clear differentiation of blastic and thallic development based on septation alone is not possible (see also Ingold, 1981). The adiaspore appears both in structure and development to be most similar to a chlamydospore, which can be defined as a thick-walled, thallic, terminal or intercalary propagule (Kendrick, 1971) that is usually nondeciduous and released only after lysis of the adjacent cell(s) (Cole and Samson, 1979). Development at the molecular level can thus be accounted for by the hypothesis of growth units located on the cell surface (Bartnicki-García, 1973), the hypothesis of the activation of a latent chitin synthase in the plasma membrane (Farkaš, 1978), and the hypothesis of physical movement of synthases, hydrolases, and precursors conditioned on an electrochemical basis (Jennings, 1979; Harold and Harold, 1980; for a review, see Stewart and Rogers, 1983).

9. REPRODUCTION OF ADIASPORES

The question whether adiaspores are able to reproduce without temperature manipulation was studied in the adiaspores of *C. parvum* var. *crescens* developing in experimentally infected animals and on cultivation media. There exist the following four views: (1) Adiaspores do not show any signs of proliferation or multiplication under the given conditions (Emmons *et al.*, 1971; Rippon, 1974; Chandler *et al.*, 1980). (2) Adiaspores are able to endosporulate, i.e., differentiate their protoplasm into spherical endospores, 2–5 μm in diameter (Hamáček and Semecký, 1972; Kodousek and Hejtmánek, 1972b). (3) Smaller secondary adiaspores can be formed inside the adiaspore (Hamáček and Semecký, 1972; Kodousek and Hejtmánek, 1972b; Šlais, 1976). (4) Adiaspores are able to multiply by budding (Hamáček and Semecký, 1972; Hejtmánek and Kodousek, 1971, 1972b; Štěrba *et al.*, 1973; Šlais, 1976). The characteristics of the respective morphological findings were summed up by Hamáček *et al.* (1972). They distinguish between exo- and endosporulation in adiaspores of *C. parvum* var. *crescens.* Exosporulation is expressed by budding and formation of "nipple-like prominences with exospores forming semilunar forms of secondary adiaspores." Endosporulation is morphologically expressed by small endospores in the adiaspore, by groups of internal bodies in the adiaspore, by a solitary internal body in the adiaspore, and by a secondary spherule in the adiaspore. In the authors' opinion, exosporulation (budding) appears to be quantitatively more important than endosporulation.

Šlais (1976) discovered nodules with necrotic centers in mice experimentally infected with *C. parvum* var. *crescens.* The zone bordering the nodule center harbored numerous spherules of different sizes in the superficial layer of the granulation tissue of the nodule. Spherules range from small, 3- to 4-μm forms to a large number of spherules averaging 20–40 μm with budding external bodies. Šlais suggests that these late-developing, budding spherical formations produce minute atypical spherules that are almost uniform in size and that gradually occupy the space of the necrotic center. Unfortunately, neither the inner structure nor the chemical composition of the external bodies is known. It is not clear whether they might correspond to Spendore–Hoeppli's material (Liber and Choi, 1973), which Chandler *et al.* (1980) think forms focal aggregates on the adiaspore surface interpreted as buds (Fingerland, 1972a; Fingerland and Vortel, 1972). However, there are probably physical and chemical conditions locally changed by the effect of the necrotic center in the nodule that inhibit the development of the conidia deposited from the inoculum. This explains the occurrence of conidia at the nodule center, transitional forms of various sizes in the pericentral part, and the largest and fully differentiated adiaspores at the periphery.

The ability of adiaspores developing in a constant temperature of 37°C to reproduce is open to question for the following reasons: (1) Signs of endo- and exosporulation in adiaspores are rare both in the cultivated material and in histological preparations of adiaspiromycotic granulomas. These changes can thus pass unnoticed. (2) Any conclusion about adiaspore reproduction by endospores must be regarded as provisional, since germination tests yielded both positive (Hamáček and Semecký, 1972) and negative results (Kodousek and Hejtmánek, 1972b). The endosporelike structures isolated from adiaspores by means of a micromanipulator and stained by the Feulgen fluorescence method did not contain any nuclei (Hejtmánek, unpublished observations). (3) Some of the findings of budding adiaspores (trophocytes) in animals can be interpreted in terms of thallic development. This means that the budding trophocytes found by Hejtmánek and Kodousek (1972a,b) in mice 4–12 days after inoculation with the mycelial stage of *C. parvum* var. *crescens* can, in fact, be short hyphal fragments with one, two, or more swollen places converting in a thallic manner into adiaspores. (4) Viability of the adiaspore buds rarely seen in some histological preparations could not be proved biologically. Neither has it been found whether such "buds" contain a nucleus and other cell structures indispensable for the autonomous cell cycle and for the processes of adiasporogenesis. On the other hand, a strikingly regular dissemination seen only in hematogenous dissemination of miliary tuberculosis and a great number (about 5–6 million) of adiaspiromycotic granulomas in the lung of a Czech boy could bring a

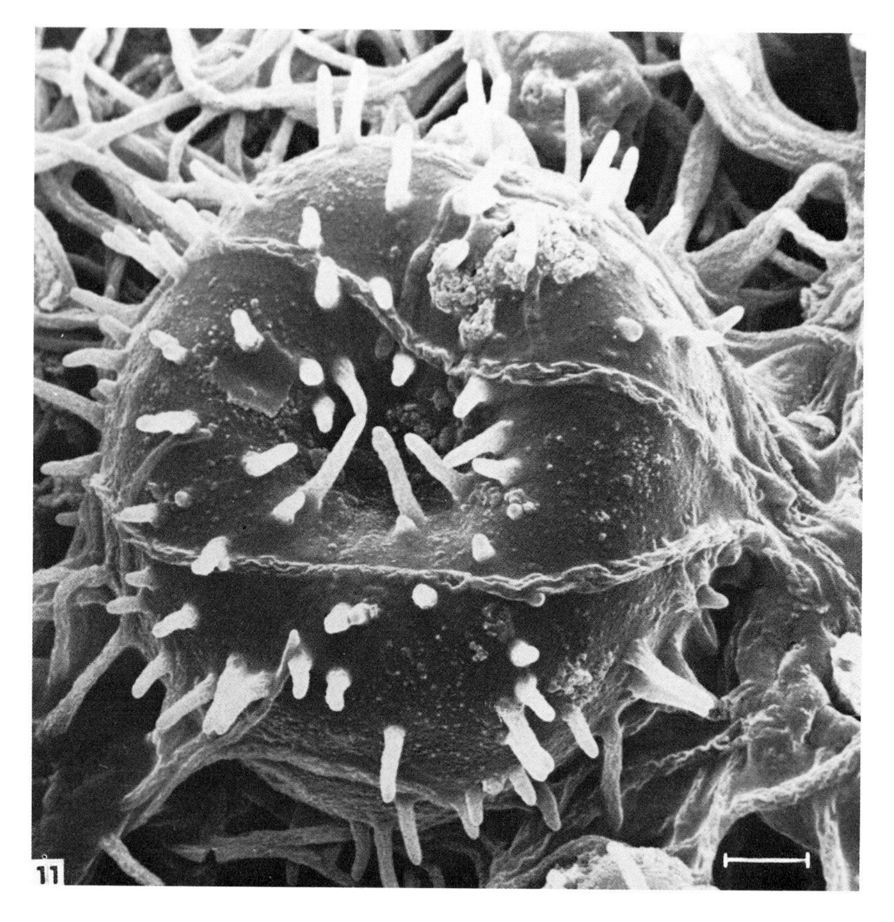

Figure 11. Multilocularly germinating *C. parvum* var. *crescens* adiaspore. Scanning electron micrograph. Scale bar: 10 μm.

pathologist to the conclusion that the causative agent can—under certain conditions in the host—still multiply (Fingerland, 1972b; Fingerland, personal communication, 1982).

No evidence for the reproduction of mature adiaspores of *C. parvum* var. *crescens* growing at a constant temperature of 37°C has been published that would stand methodological criticism. Conversely, it has repeatedly been confirmed that exposure of adiaspores to lower temperature (below 30°C) for several hours means initiation of the germination processes morphologically expressed by the growth of germ hyphae during cultivation at laboratory temperature (Figure 11) or by the growth of spherical cells ("buds") when cultivated at 37°C. Generally, trophocytes and immature adiaspores are induced to initiate these developmental processes more easily than are mature, thick-walled adiaspores (Hejtmánek, unpublished observations).

10. GENETIC CONTROL

Both adiaspores and conidia of *C. parvum* are the result of the expression of genetic information for specific sporogenesis under certain environmental conditions. Each sporogenesis has its genetic level that provides a sporogenic competence to the fungal cells and an ability to respond to environmental factors mediated through primary and then secondary metabolic pathways. The pathways are further subjected to positive and negative regulations (Turian, 1974). As in other fungi, sporogenesis in *C. parvum* var. *crescens* can be influenced by mutations.

Of 12 mutant strains of *C. parvum* var. *crescens* derived by ultraviolet irradiation, 9 demonstrated growth rates in their mycelial stage (31.2–89.6%) lower than the wild-type strain and differed in colony morphology. Four of the mutants did not produce thick-walled adiaspores at 37°C, but instead formed small, spherical, thin-walled trophocytes (Hejtmánek and Lenhart, 1976). A positive correlation for some of the mutants was found between adiaspore size *in vivo* and the growth rate of the mycelial stage *in vitro* and was also manifested by the smaller size of the adiasporic stage in granulomas (Hejtmánek and Bártek, 1976). The mutants of *C. parvum* var. *crescens* that were unable to differentiate typical adiaspores showed decreased virulence or were avirulent in mice. The loss or decrease in virulence is thought to be due to a pleiotropic effect of the mutations controlling adiaspore differentiation (Hejtmánek and Křivanec, 1977). Avirulent mutants have their antigenic and immunogenic activity preserved (Tomšíková *et al.*, 1979, 1982).

Evidence suggests that the virulence expressed during development of adiaspiromycotic granulomas in mice is not dependent solely on the ability of the fungus to form morphologically fully differentiated adiaspores on agar medium (Vacková-Janečková and Hejtmánek, 1983). The mutant M-2 of *C. parvum* var. *crescens* forms adiaspores on agar medium, but not in mice, and thus appears avirulent. Two other mutants (M-9 and M-12) produce thin-walled spherical cells (trophocytes) instead of adiaspores on agar medium and provoke adiaspiromycosis in mice. Normal adiaspores are formed in the granulomas. These results indicate that mutations expressed by inhibition of adiasporogenesis in the trophocyte phase need not provoke avirulence. Adiasporogenesis inhibited in the trophocyte phase on agar medium can in some mutants continue to a fully differentiated adiaspore in the host.

11. ENVIRONMENTAL CONTROL

Adiaspores of *C. parvum* var. *crescens* are produced at 37°C on various agar and liquid media, during surface and submerged cultivation, and in the bodies of various warm-blooded animals. A mycelium with conidia forms at temperatures below 30°C on the same media, but conidiation is inhibited by submerged cultivation. Adiaspores contained in the host's tissue can develop into the mycelial stage by germination, when tissue samples are kept refrigerated at 4°C for some time (Dvořák *et al.*, 1973).

Adiaspores are also differentiated (at 37°C) under decreased CO_2 tension and O_2 reduction (Dvořák *et al.*, 1973). Differentiation also takes place in liquid media with various sources of inorganic or organic nitrogen and in distilled water with 1% glucose; however, in water free of any admixture, it is inhibited (Hejtmánek, unpublished observation). The development of adiaspores from the mycelial stage is likewise inhibited in peptone solutions containing 0.5 M or more glucose (Weigl and Hejtmánek, 1973).

Adiasporogenesis is inhibited in the trophocyte phase on Sabouraud's agar medium enriched with glucose and glycerol at a final concentration above 0.5 M. The inhibition is attributed to the increased osmotic pressure of the medium. Adiaspores can develop in a medium of 10^{-4} M glucose (Hejtmánek *et al.*, 1971).

Elevated temperature (37°C) can be regarded as the determining factor controlling the conversion of mycelium to adiasporic stages in *C. parvum* var. *crescens.* Other external factors, such as medium components, have no effect on the processes of swelling (i.e., development of trophocytes and adiaspores) as long as the factors remain within physiological limits and allow growth.

The development of adiaspores of *C. parvum* var. *crescens* in experimentally infected mice is inhibited by amphotericin B. When determining the minimal inhibitory concentration (MIC) for the adiasporic stage using a mycelial inoculum, a conversion to the adiasporic stage was observed in the medium containing amphotericin B. The MIC of this antibiotic for the adiasporic stage is about twice that for the mycelial stage (Dvořák *et al.*, 1973).

Flavoprotein I inhibitor, 5-ethyl-5-isoamylbarbituric acid (Amobarbital SPOFA), added to Sabouraud's glucose medium in concentrations of 5×10^{-3} to 5×10^{-4} M blocks the differentiation of *C. parvum* var. *crescens* adiaspores in trophocyte phase at 37°C. During cultivation at 26°C, the inhibitor decreases the growth rate of the mycelial stage to 38 and 80% of control growth rate. Conidiation is inhibited as well. Other respiratory inhibitors, such as sodium azide or cyanide, do not show this action (Weigl, unpublished data).

No factor is known that alone or in combination with others replaces increased temperature in its adiasporogenic effect. It is generally agreed that in thermic-controlled sporogenesis, the spherical cells do not germinate, since the processes of apical growth are inhibited by increased temperature. Growth is not stopped, however, but occurs by isotropic wall deposition resulting in spherical cells of a definite size and wall thickness (Smith and Berry, 1978; for a review, see Bemmann, 1981).

The controlling mechanism of temperature in fungal morphogenesis is not clear, but by using imagination and the principles of regulation at the molecular level, it can be hypothetically deduced from present models of fungal-cell morphogenesis. The key role of temperature in the regulation of fungal-cell morphogenesis could be the rate of inactivation of the nascent plasmalemma-located polysaccharides of the cell wall due to specific inhibitor proteins located outside the plasmalemma (Farkaš, 1978, 1979).

12. CONCLUSION

Findings on the development of the mycelial and adiasporic stages and their morphology, ultrastructure, and cytochemistry and on the genetic and environmental control of sporogenesis can be the basis for further research making use of methods of biochemical analysis and genetics only infrequently applied to this organism.

Chrysosporium parvum var. *crescens* is especially suited for the study of dimorphism and morphogenesis of the cell wall because isotropic growth and enlargement under controlled conditions give rise to giant adiaspores with a wall several tens of micrometers thick, differentiating from both conidia and hyphal cells.

REFERENCES

Bartnicki-García, S., 1973, Fundamental aspects of hyphal morphogenesis, in: *Microbial Differentiation* (J. M. Ainsworth and J. E. Smith, eds.), Cambridge University Press, Cambridge, pp. 245–267.

Bemmann, W., 1981, Pilzdimorphismus—eine Literaturübersicht, *Zentralbl. Bakteriol. Parasitenkd. Infektionskr. Hyg. Abt. 2* **136:**369–416.
Blank, F., 1957, Note on chemical composition of cell wall of *Haplosporangium parvum, J. Histochem Cytochem* **5:**500–502.
Boisseau-Lebreuil, M. T., 1970, Particularités biologiques de l'infestation adiaspiromycosique par *Emmonsia crescens,* Emmons et Jellison, 1960 chez *Pitymys subterraneus* (DeSelys-Longchamps, 1936) et *Mustella nivalis nivalis* L. 1766, *Mycopathologia* **40:**183–191.
Boisseau-Lebreuil, M. T., 1975a, Sensibilité comparée de divers animaux de laboratoire a l'infection par instillations nasales de la phase saprophytique d'*Emmonsia crescens* Emmons et Jellison, 1960: Frequence et intensité du parasitism, réactions histopathologiques, *Mycopathologia* **56:**143–168.
Boisseau-Lebreuil, M. T., 1975b, Croissance et differentiation morphologique comparées à diverses temperatures de vingt-deux souches d'*Emmonsia* Ciferri et Montemartini 1959, agent d'adiaspiromycose, *Mycopathologia* **57:**63–72.
Boisseau-Lebreuil, M. T., 1981, *Emmonsia parva* (Emmons et Ashburn, 1942) Ciferri et Montemartini, 1959 = *Chrysosporium parvum* (Emmons et Ashburn) comb. nov.; *Emmonsia crescens* Emmons et Jellison, 1960 = *Chrysosporium parvum* var. *crescens:* Critères de differentiation des deux variétés, *Mycopathologia* **73:**135–141.
Carmichael, J. W., 1962, Chrysosporium and some other aleuriosporic hyphomycetes, *Can. J. Bot.* **40:**1137–1173.
Chandler, F. W., Kaplan, W., and Ajello, L., 1980, *A Colour Atlas and Textbook of the Histopathology of Mycotic Diseases,* Wolfe Medical, London.
Ciferri, R., and Montemartini, A., 1959, Taxonomy of *Haplosporangium parvum, Mycopathol. Mycol. Appl.* **10:**303–316.
Cole, G. T., and Samson, R. A., 1979, *Patterns of Development in Conidial Fungi,* Pitman, London, San Francisco, Melbourne.
Doby-Dubois, M., Chevrel, M. L., Doby, J. M., and Louvet, M., 1964, Premier cas humain d'adiaspiromycose par *Emmonsia crescens,* Emmons et Jellison 1960, *Bull. Soc. Pathol. Exot.* **57:**240–244.
Dowding, E. S., 1947, The pulmonary fungus, *Haplosporangium parvum* and its relationship with some human pathogens, *Can. J. Res.* **25:**195–206.
Dvořák, J., Otčenášek, M., and Rosický, B., 1973, *Adiaspiromycosis Caused by Emmonsia crescens,* Emmons et Jellison 1960, Academia, Prague, pp. 1–120.
Emmons, C. W., 1964, Budding in *Emmonsia crescens, Mycologia* **56:**415–419.
Emmons, C. W., and Ashburn, L. L., 1942, The isolation of *Haplosporangium parvum* n. sp. and *Coccidioides immitis* from wild rodents, *Public Health Rep.* **57:**1715–1727.
Emmons, C. W., and Jellison, W. L., 1960, *Emmonsia crescens* sp. n. and adiaspiromycosis (haplomycosis) in mammals, *Ann. N.Y. Acad. Sci.* **89:**91–101.
Emmons, C. W., Binford, C. H., and Utz, J. P., 1971, *Medical Mycology,* Lea and Febiger, Philadelphia, pp. 1–508.
Farkaš, V., 1978, The regulation of morphogenesis in fungi, *Biol. Listy* **43:**269–277 (in Czech with English summary).
Farkaš, V., 1979, Biosynthesis of cell walls of fungi, *Microbiol. Rev.* **43:**117–144.
Fingerland, A., 1972a, Some histological similarities and differences between adiaspiromycosis, rhinosporidiosis and other related mycoses, *Acta Univ. Palacki. Olomuc. Fac. Med.* **63:**59–66.
Fingerland, A., 1972b, Two cases of human adiaspiromycosis, in: *Advances in Antimicrobial and Antineoplastic Chemotherapy* (M. Hejzlar, M. Semonský, and S. Masák, eds.), Urban and Schwarzenberg, Munich, pp. 227–231.

Fingerland, A., and Vortel, V., 1972, The accidental finding of adiaspiromycosis caused by *Emmonsia crescens* in a case of lung tuberculosis, *Acta Univ. Palacki. Olomuc. Fac. Med.* **63:**19–22.

Hamáček, F., and Semecký, V., 1972, Conception of life cycle of *Emmonsia crescens* adiaspores and pathogenesis of experimental adiaspiromycosis in mice, *Acta Univ. Palacki. Olomuc. Fac. Med.* **63:**67–72.

Hamáček, F., Kyntera, F., Dvořák, J., and Otčenášek, M., 1971, Influence of some factors on the growth and development of adiaspores of the fungus *Emmonsia crescens*, Emmons et Jellison 1960, *Mycopathologia* **43:**201–209.

Hamáček, F., Dvořák, J., Otčenášek, M., and Semecký, V., 1972, The morphological manifestation of the adiaspores of *Emmonsia crescens in vitro* and *in vivo, Folia Parasitol. (Prague)* **19:**341–347.

Harold, R. L., and Harold, F. M., 1980, Oriented growth of *Blastocladiella emersonii* in gradients of ionophores and inhibitors, *J. Bacteriol.* **144:**1159–1167.

Hejtmánek, M., 1973, Can *Emmonsia crescens* Emmons et Jellison 1960—the causative agent of adiaspiromycosis—be distributed by the excrements of mice?, *Folia Parasitol. (Prague)* **20:**369–373.

Hejtmánek, M., 1976a, Conversion of adiasporic and mycelial stages of *Emmonsia crescens* examined in the scanning electron microscope, *Folia Parasitol. (Prague)* **23:**165–167.

Hejtmánek, M., 1976b, Raster-Elektronenmikroskopie des Adiaspiromykoseregers, *Mykosen* **19:**77–83.

Hejtmánek, M., 1976c, Scanning electron microscopy of experimental adiaspiromycosis, *Mycopathologia* **58:**91–95.

Hejtmánek, M., and Bártek, J., 1976, Mutants of *Emmonsia crescens*—their pathogenicity and size of adiaspores *in vivo, Folia Microbiol. (Prague)* **21:**297–300.

Hejtmánek, M., and Hejtmánková, N., 1976, Fluorescence microscopy of hyphal nuclei, *Ceska Mykol.* **30:**20–23.

Hejtmánek, M., and Kodousek, R., 1971, Zur Vermehrung von *Emmonsia crescens in vitro* and *in vivo, Mykosen* **14:**269–274.

Hejtmánek, M., and Kodousek, R., 1972a, Morphologie der Adiaspiromykose im Versuch an genetischen Mäusestämmen, *Mykosen* **15:**249–253.

Hejtmánek, M., and Kodousek, R., 1972b, The contribution to the experimental adiaspiromycosis, *Acta Univ. Palacki. Olomuc. Fac. Med.* **63:**81–85.

Hejtmánek, M., and Kodousek, R., 1985, Granulomas caused by devitalized adiaspores and cell wall fragments of *Chrysosporium parvum* var. *crescens*—the etiological agent of adiaspiromycosis, *Acta Univ. Palacki. Olomuc. Fac. Med.* (in press).

Hejtmánek, M., and Křivanec, K., 1977, Avirulence and decreased virulence in mutants of *Emmonsia crescens*, a causative agent of adiaspiromycosis, *Folia Parasitol. (Prague)* **24:**173–177.

Hejtmánek, M., and Lenhart, K., 1976, Morphological mutants of *Emmonsia crescens* Emmons et Jellison 1960—the causative agent of adiaspiromycosis, *Acta Univ. Palacki. Olomuc. Fac. Med.* **76:**25–31.

Hejtmánek, M., Hejtmánková-Uhrová, N., and Dvořák, J., 1968, Die Kerne der Adiasporen und Hyphenzellen von *Emmonsia crescens, Mykosen* **11:**353–358.

Hejtmánek, M., Lenhart, K., and Kodousek, R., 1971, Manifestations of morphological modifications and mutations of the fungus *Emmonsia crescens, Scr. Med. Fac. Med. (Brno)* **44:**219–220 (in Czech).

Hejtmánek, M., Nečas, O., and Havelková, M., 1974, The ultrastructure of the spherules of *Emmonsia crescens* studied by the technique of freeze–etching, *Mycopathologia* **54:**79–83.

Ingold, C. T., 1981, The validity of the concept of conidia as either blastic or thallic, *Trans Br. Mycol. Soc.* **77**:194–196.
Jellison, W. L., 1969, *Adiaspiromycosis (= Haplomycosis),* Mountain Press, Missoula, Montana, pp. 1–99.
Jennings, D. M., 1979, Membrane transport and hyphal growth, in: *Fungal Walls and Hyphal Growth* (J. H. Burnett and A. P. J. Trinci, eds.), Cambridge University Press, Cambridge, pp. 279–294.
Kashkin, K. P., 1980, Dimorphism and antigens, in: *Medical Mycology* (H. J. Preusser, ed.) *Zentralbl. Bakteriol. Parasitenkd. Infektionskr. Hyg. Abt. IA* (Suppl. 8) **15**:3–15.
Kendrick, W. E. (ed.), 1971, *Taxonomy of Fungi Imperfecti,* University of Toronto Press, Toronto.
Kirschenblatt, J. D., 1939, A new parasite in the lung of rodents, *Dokl. Akad. Nauk SSSR* **23**:406–408 (in Russian).
Kodousek, R., 1974, Adiaspiromycosis, *Acta Univ. Palacki Olomuc. Fac. Med.* **70**:1–68.
Kodousek, R., and Hejtmánek, M., 1971, Zur enzymatischen Aktivität der Sphaerulae vom Adiaspiromykose-Erreger *Emmonsia crescens* (Emmons et Jellison 1960), *Acta Histochem.* **41**:349–352.
Kodousek, R., and Hejtmánek, M., 1972a, Enzymatic activity of spherules of *Emmonsia crescens* Emmons et Jellison, *Ceska Mykol.* **26**:23–24.
Kodousek, R., and Hejtmánek, M., 1972b, Some morphological observations concerning problems of endosporulation in *Emmonsia crescens*—etiological agent in adiaspiromycosis, *Mycopathologia* **47**:343–384.
Kodousek, R., and Hejtmánek, M., 1975, The passage of *Emmonsia crescens* through gastrointestinal tract in experimental mice, *Acta Univ. Palacki. Olomuc. Fac. Med.* **73**:199–203.
Kodousek, R., Vortel, V., and Fingerland, A., 1970a, Pathology of human adiaspiromycosis due to fungus *Emmonsia crescens,* Emmons et Jellison 1960, *Stud. Pneumol. Phtiseol. Cech.* **30**:320–336 (in Czech with English abstract).
Kodousek, R., Vortel, V., Fingerland, A., Hájek, V., and Kučera, K., 1970b, Disseminated adiaspiromycosis of lungs due to *Emmonsia crescens*—a new nosological entity in man, *Cas. Lek. Cesk.* **109**:923–924 (in Czech).
Kodousek, R., Vortel, V., Fingerland, A., Vojtek, V., Šerý, Z., Hájek, V., and Kučera, K., 1971, Pulmonary adiaspiromycosis in man caused by *Emmonsia crescens, Am. J. Clin. Pathol.* **56**:394–399.
Kodousek, R., Hejtmánek, M., Havelková, M., and Štrachová, Z., 1972a, Enzyme cytochemistry of *Emmonsia crescens*—an etiological agent in adiaspiromycosis, *Acta Univ. Palacki. Olomuc. Fac. Med.* **63**:93–98.
Kodousek, R., Hejtmánek, M., Havelková, M., and Štrachová, Z., 1972b, A survey of the ultrastructural organization of spherules of fungus *Emmonsia crescens* Emmons et Jellison 1960, *Acta Univ. Palacki. Olomuc. Fac. Med.* **63**:87–98.
Kodousek, R., Hejtmánek, M., Havelková, M., and Štrachová, Z., 1972c, The ultrastructure of spherules of fungus *Emmonsia crescens*—a causative agent of adiaspiromycosis, *Beitr. Pathol.* **145**:83–88.
Liber, A. R., and Choi, H.-S. H., 1973, Spendore–Hoeppli phenomenon about silk sutures, *Arch. Pathol.* **95**:217–220.
Malínský, J., Hejtmánek, M., and Kodousek, R., 1972, Electron microscopy of experimental adiaspiromycosis, *Acta Univ. Palacki. Olomuc. Fac. Med.* **63**:99–104.
McGinnis, M. R., 1980, *Laboratory Handbook of Medical Mycology,* Academic Press, New York, London, Toronto, Sydney, San Francisco.

Otčenášek, M., and Zlatanov, Z., 1975, Natural variability in mycelial form of *Emmonsia crescens*, *Mycopathologia* **55**:97–104.

Otčenášek, M., Prokopič, K., and Hamáček, F., 1982, Adiaspiromykose—eine wenig bekannte Lungenerkrankung, *Z. Erkr. Atmungsorgane* **159**:131–145.

Padhye, A. A., and Carmichael, J. W., 1968, *Emmonsia brasiliensis* and *Emmonsia ciferrina* are *Chrysosporium pruinosum*, *Mycologia* **60**:445–447.

Rippon, W. J., *Medical Mycology: The Pathogenic Fungi and the Pathogenic Actinomycetes*, W. B. Saunders, Philadelphia, London, Toronto.

Šlais, J., 1976, Histopathological changes and the genesis of adiaspiromycomas in mice infected intraperitoneally with *Emmonsia crescens*, Emmons et Jellison, 1960, *Folia Parasitol. (Prague)* **23**:373–381.

Smith, J. E., and Berry, D. R., 1978, *Developmental Mycology, The Filamentous Fungi*, Vol. 3, Edward Arnold, London.

Štěrba, J., Hamáček, F., Tomšíková, A., and Nováčková, D., 1973, The pattern of experimental infection with the fungus *Emmonsia crescens* in mice, *Folia Parasitol. (Prague)* **20**:361–366.

Stewart, P. R., and Rogers, P. J., 1983, Fungal dimorphism, in: *Fungal Differentiation—A Contemporary Synthesis* (J. E. Smith, ed.), Marcel Dekker, New York, pp. 267–314.

Tomšíková, A., Hejtmánek, M., and Nováčková, D., 1979, Antigenic activity of *Emmonsia crescens* mutants, *Mycopathologia* **66**:83–90.

Tomšíková, A., Šlais, J., Štěrba, J., Hejtmánek, M., and Nováčková, D., 1982, Beitrag zur aktiven und passiven Immunisierung bei Organmykosen: *Chrysosporium parvum* var. *crescens* als Modell, *Mykosen* **25**:393–403.

Turian, G., 1974, Sporogenesis in fungi, *Annu. Rev. Phytopathol.* **12**:129–137.

Vacková-Janečková, I., and Hejtmánek, M., 1983, Mutants of *Chrysosporium parvum* var. *crescens*—a causative agent of adiaspiromycosis, *Acta Univ. Palacki. Olomuc. Fac. Med.* **105**:27–37.

Vanbreuseghem, R., De Vroey, C., and Takashio, M., 1978, *Practical Guide to Medical and Veterinary Mycology*, Masson, New York.

Watts, J. C., Callaway, C. S., Chandler, F. W., and Kaplan, W., 1975, Human Pulmonary adiaspiromycosis, *Arch. Pathol.*, **99**:11–15.

Weigl, E., and Hejtmánek, M., 1973, Growth of the spherules of *Emmonsia crescens*, Emmons et Jellison—a causative agent of adiaspiromycosis, *Acta Univ. Palacki. Olomuc. Fac. Med.* **65**:51–57 (in Russian with English summary).

Ždárská, Z., and Šlais, J., 1972, Morphology and histochemistry of the differentiated adiaspore of *Emmonsia crescens*, *Acta Univ. Palacki. Olomuc. Fac. Med.* **63**:73–79.

Zíková, Z., Štěrba, J., Šlais, J., Kůdová, H., and Tošovská, A., 1973, Ultrasture of the mycelium of *Emmonsia crescens*, *Plzen. Lek. Sb.* **39**:257–258 (in Czech).

Chapter 11

Phialophora verrucosa and Other Chromoblastomycotic Fungi

Billy H. Cooper

1. INTRODUCTION

The tissue form of the agents of chromoblastomycosis is quite unique among human pathogenic fungi. The yeast cells, hyphae, pseudohyphae, or spherules that are typical of other human pathogenic fungi are not customarily observed. Instead, richly pigmented brown cells (Figure 1) that form transverse septations are seen by microscopic observation of the lesions of chromoblastomycosis. In some instances, multicellular bodies that form both longitudinal and transverse septa as they divide (muriform cells) are observed. Early investigators of chromoblastomycosis (Medlar, 1915), thinking that these muriform cells represented the development of a sclerotium, named these cells "sclerotic cells" or "sclerotic bodies." The cells have also been called "Medlar bodies," "chromobodies," "fumagoid bodies," and even "copper pennies" by various observers (McGinnis, 1983). For convenience, they will be referred to herein as *sclerotic cells,* even though it is recognized that the term may be somewhat misleading, since the multicellular form seen in tissue is not a sclerotium, nor does it represent a stage in the development of a sclerotium.

Sclerotic cells are similar to chlamydospores in many respects, as pointed out by early investigators (Medlar, 1915; Lane, 1915). The exact

Billy H. Cooper • Department of Pathology, Baylor University Medical Center, Dallas, Texas 75246.

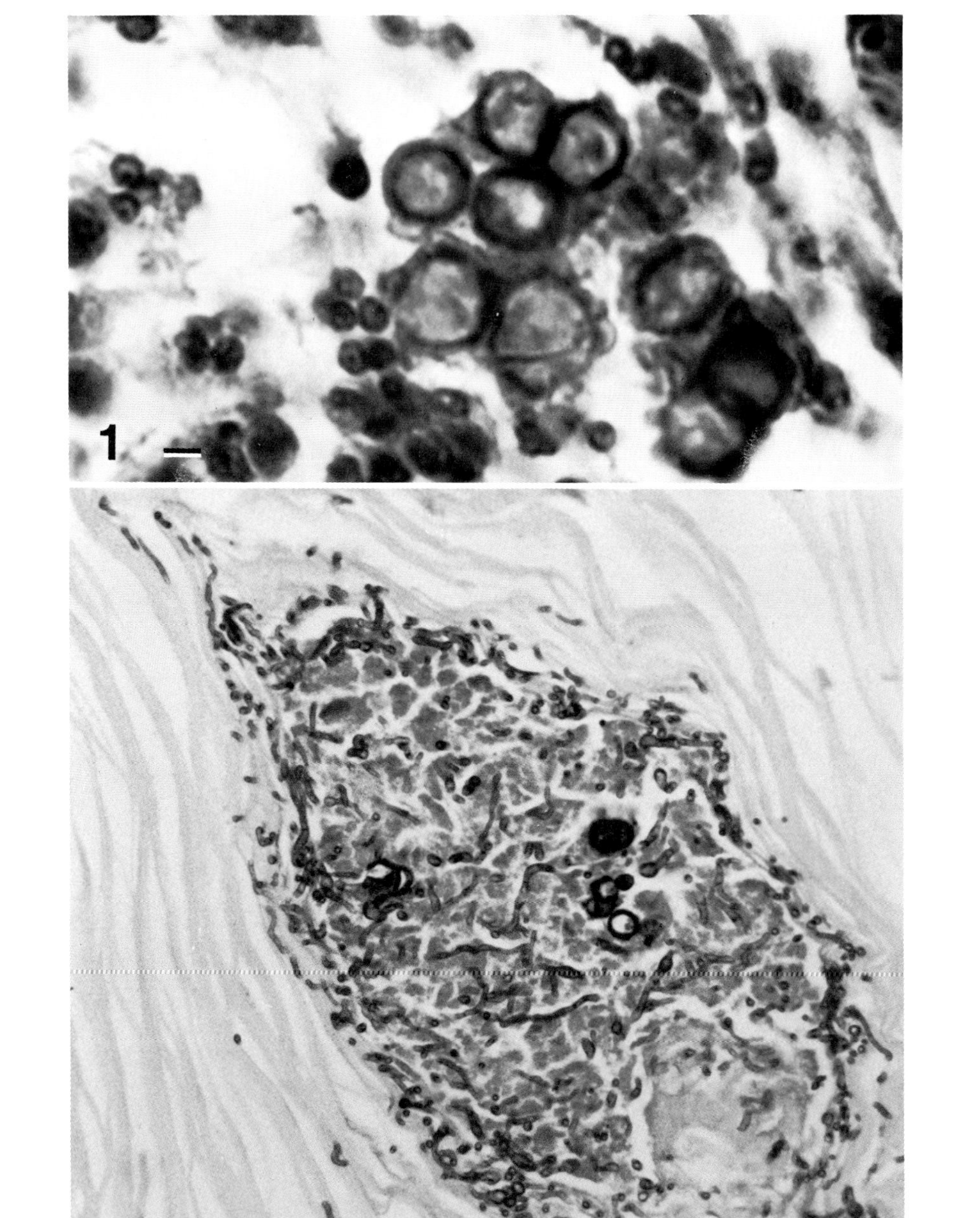
1
2

mechanism by which hyphae of dematiaceous fungi are induced to form into sclerotic cells is not known at present. Even less well understood is the mechanism that causes continued replication of sclerotic cells deep within infected tissues. As sclerotic cells are forced to the outer crusts of the epidermis by transepithelial elimination (Batres *et al.*, 1978), they can be seen to germinate into hyphae (Figure 2) (Al-Doory, 1972; Zais, 1978). It appears from this observation that whatever controls the host's tissue exerts on the morphology of the infecting fungus are reversed or eliminated as the sclerotic cells are forced to the outer crusts of lesions.

Chromoblastomycosis is thought to be initiated by traumatic implantation of a hypha or conidium into skin. The disease progresses slowly, and any hyphae or conidia inoculated deeply within the skin of a patient disappear, so that only sclerotic cells are observed within the dermis when tissue sections are microscopically examined. Sclerotic cells may, in fact, simply be resistant forms that survive in tissue. However, the disease is a chronic, but dynamic, process with new satellite lesions arising close to older lesions. Reaction of the skin is disproportionately exuberant in light of the relatively few sclerotic cells observed deep within the dermis. Large, verrucous lesions result from the pseudoepitheliomatous hyperplasia, microabscesses, and granulomatous tissue reaction that are characteristic of the disease. The dynamic reaction of the skin to the infecting fungus and the occurrence of new lesions suggest that sclerotic cells are not just inactive resistant foreign bodies, but are instead actively growing, dividing, viable fungi.

It has been suggested that sclerotic cells result when polar cell growth (bud or hyphal development) is retarded but isotropic cell enlargement and division continue (Szaniszlo *et al.*, 1976, 1983). *In vitro* experiments have shown that manganese deprivation (Reiss and Nickerson, 1974) and low pH (approximately 2.5–3.0) (Szaniszlo *et al.*, 1976) can induce hyphae to convert to sclerotic cells. The mechanism by which the absence of manganese or an acid pH might inhibit polar growth while permitting cell enlargement and division to continue is not known at present, but these observations probably provide important clues

←

Figure 1. Sclerotic cells of *Fonsecaea pedrosoi* in tissue from a chromoblastomycosis patient. Hematoxylin and eosin stain. Scale bar: 1.0 μm.

Figure 2. Sclerotic cells and hyphae in outer crust of skin from a chromoblastomycosis lesion. Same patient as in Figure 1. Periodic acid–schiff stain. Scale bar: 5.0 μm.

to the nature of the mechanisms that control sclerotic-cell morphogenesis.

2. CLINICAL FEATURES OF CHROMOBLASTOMYCOSIS

The disease chromoblastomycosis is caused by at least four species of fungi that belong, taxonomically, to the form-family Dematiaceae. The species that cause the disease include *Phialophora verrucosa, Fonsecaea pedrosoi, F. compacta* (possibly a variant of *F. pedrosoi*), and *Cladosporium carrionii* (Carrion and Silva-Hutner, 1971; Al-Doory, 1972; McGinnis, 1983). The clinical features of the diseases caused by these fungi are essentially the same regardless of the infecting species. The four species can be identified (albeit sometimes not easily) by careful microscopic examination of their conidia as produced in slide culture mounts. To date, no biochemical tests have been devised that aid in distinguishing one species from another. In like manner, the tissue form produced by all four species is essentially identical. It is not possible, even for trained observers, to differentiate the four species in tissue by microscopic examination of fungal elements.

Other species of dematiaceous fungi, which are similar in morphology and metabolism to the agents of chromoblastomycosis, can cause diseases characterized by subcutaneous abscesses, subcutaneous cysts, lesions of joints, or lesions of the central nervous system. The clinical features of these diseases are different from the verrucous lesions of classic chromoblastomycosis. Brown yeast cells, short muriform hyphae, and occasionally sclerotic cells can be seen by microscopic examination of stained sections of such lesions (Figure 3). These other types of infection are customarily lumped together under the name "phaeohyphomycosis" to dramatize their differences from chromoblastomycosis (Ajello, 1975). In actual fact, the distinction between chromoblastomycosis and phaeohyphomycosis may not be that dramatic. However, the factors that cause the agents of chromoblastomycosis to form sclerotic cells deep within infected tissues, whereas the agents of phaeohyphomycosis produce a mixture of hyphae, yeast cells, and sclerotic cells, are not known.

Figure 3. Yeast cells, moniliform hyphae, and sclerotic cells of *Exophiala jeanselmei* in tissue from a patient with phaeohyphomycosis. Gomori methenamine silver stain. Scale bar: 5.0 μm.

Figure 4. Sclerotic cells and hyphae of *F. pedrosoi* strain SA-9 incubated at 37°C in glucose yeast nitrogen base broth adjusted to pH 3.0. Unstained. Scale bar: 5.0 μm.

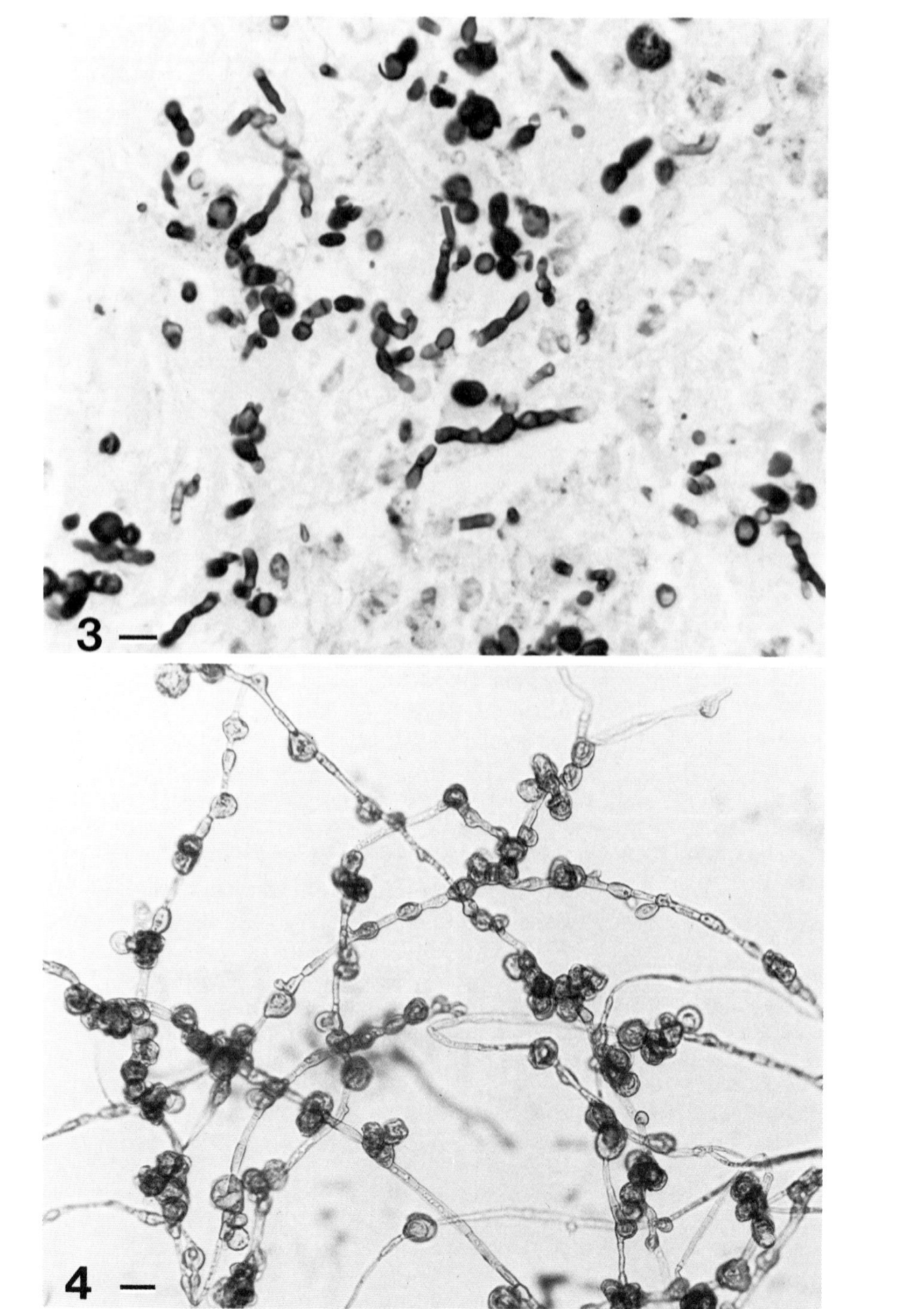
3
4

3. MICROSCOPIC OBSERVATIONS OF INFECTED TISSUE

3.1. Light Microscopy

When observed under the light microscope, sclerotic cells are yellow-brown to dark chestnut brown in color in hematoxylin-and-eosin-stained tissue sections. The average diameter of a sclerotic cell is approximately 10 μm. The cells may be arranged singly, in pairs, in clusters, or in short chains. Most of the cells observed at the magnification provided by a light microscope ($\times$400–1000) appear to be viable, intact, and quite resistant to the inflammatory response of the host.

3.2. Scanning Electron Microscopy

Techniques for processing tissues infected with fungi for observation with scanning electron microscopy (SEM) have not yet been perfected. For this reason, very few such observations have been reported. However, it has been possible to process scrapings of skin for SEM. One such effort by Hanada and Kusunoki (1983) describes observations made with scrapings from the outer crusts of a lesion on the hand of a woman infected with *F. pedrosoi.* Those investigators observed spherical cells, sclerotic cells, and hyphae in scrapings that were digested with 1% sodium hydroxide prior to processing for SEM.

In addition to sclerotic cells in clusters and hyphae, Hanada and Kusunoki (1983) illustrate in their report sclerotic cells that appear to be dividing. Dividing cells are shown to be splitting into two hemisperical cells that remain attached on one side. Subsequent cell division occurs in the same fashion with the cells remaining attached. As the cells enlarge, they assume a spherical shape so that a cluster of round cells is formed. These observations verify that sclerotic cells continue to divide and clarify the process by which this takes place. Sclerotic cells that produced germ tubes are also described, suggesting that transition from the sclerotic cell form into hyphae occurs by means of germ-tube development.

3.3. Transmission Electron Microscopy

Examination of sclerotic cells with transmission electron microscopy (TEM) reveals considerable variation in ultrastructure as a consequence of the dynamic interaction between host tissues and the invading fungus. In addition to cells that appear to have normal internal organelles, cells with extensive lipid and glycogen vacuoles and cells with complete internal disintegration can be observed (Nishimoto, 1970; Rosen *et al.,* 1980).

Frequently, the sclerotic cells are seen to be surrounded by a multilayered, electron-dense outer wall. The electron density of the outer wall is thought to be due to melanin pigment; however, the number of layers seen in the cell wall is greater than the number of layers observed by TEM of vegetative hyphae (Cooper *et al.*, 1973). Occasional sclerotic cells appear to be splitting apart in that the layers of the cell wall of some are more widely separated and are more distinct than in others. Even so, the internal ultrastructure appears to be quite normal in these cells. In other sclerotic cells, the outer wall appears to be intact, but the internal organelles have been totally replaced by myelin figures (Rosen *et al.*, 1980). Still other sclerotic cells are observed to have a very thin outer wall and to be surrounded by an electron-lucent halo. While this halo may be just a fixation artifact, it has been interpreted as representing antibody complexed with the fungal wall (Nishimoto, 1970; Rosen *et al.*, 1980). All these forms observed in infected tissues appear to represent various stages in the complex interaction between a patient's tissues and the invading fungus.

4. EXPERIMENTAL AND NATURAL INFECTIONS OF ANIMALS

Natural infections with chromoblastomycotic fungi have been observed in frogs and toads, and these poikilothermic animals have been utilized to study experimental chromoblastomycosis (Velasquez and Restrepo, 1975; Beneke, 1978). The majority of the fungal cells observed in infected tissues of these amphibians have been sclerotic cells, although some short hyphae have also been noted.

5. *IN VITRO* CULTIVATION OF SCLEROTIC CELLS

5.1. Early Cultural Methods

Attempts to cultivate the tissue form of the agents of chromoblastomycosis *in vitro* have, to date, met with only partial success. Medlar (1915) and Lane (1915) described the formation of sclerotic cells by *P. verrucosa* grown on hydrocele agar and Loeffler's serum agar. On these media, sclerotic cells were observed to arise as gradual enlargements of hyphal cells (usually near the hyphal tip) and develop into round to oval cells, 8–15 μm in diameter. When this kind of development took place in a nonterminal cell, the enlargement was usually toward one side. The

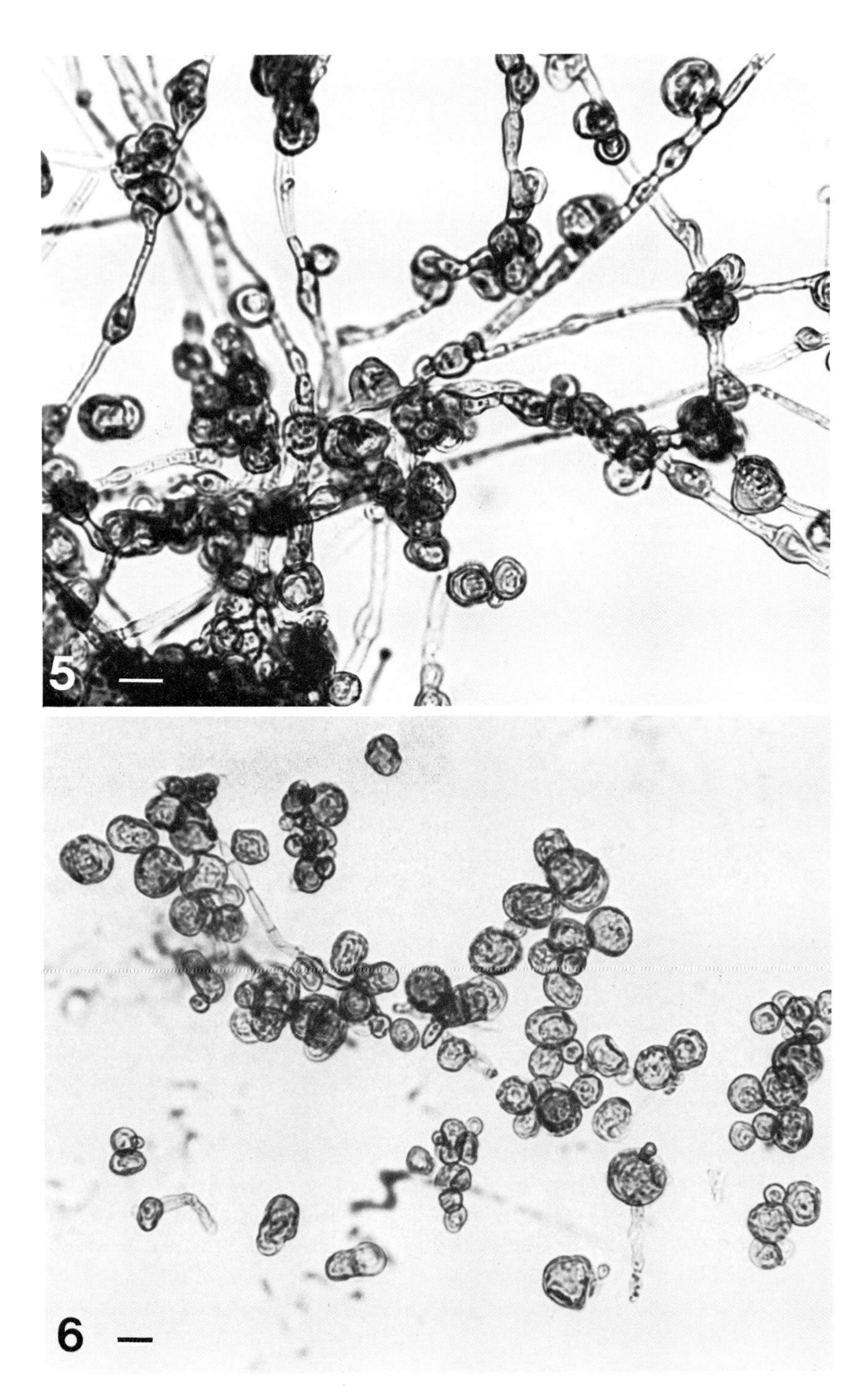
5
6

enlarged cells then divided into several cells by forming septa in more than one plane. While the original swollen cells described by Medlar and Lane are similar to chlamydospores, the subsequent development of multicellular forms by septation is not typical of chlamydospores that are produced by other fungi. I have verified that the formation of these chlamydosporelike cells is essentially the same as described by Medlar and Lane (Figures 4–7), as have other investigators (Silva, 1957; Reiss and Nickerson, 1974; Szaniszlo *et al.*, 1983). It is interesting to note that a recently described (de Vries *et al.*, 1984) *Phialophora* species produces aggregates of chlamydosporelike cells that resemble the sclerotic cells seen in chromoblastomycosis when cultivated on 2% malt extract agar and incubated at 20°C. This fungus has not been reported to be a cause of chromoblastomycosis, but was isolated from a human case of mycetoma.

Silva (1957, 1958, 1960) studied the nutritional requirements of both the saprophytic and parasitic growth phases of chromoblastomycotic fungi. She attempted to produce large quantities of sclerotic cells by injecting 19 different isolates of dematiaceous fungi into the chorioallantoic membrane of embryonated eggs, into mice, and into silkworm pupae. She also utilized *in vitro* culture with (1) a "synthetic lymph" consisting of a glucose–urea–minimal salts medium supplemented with human blood plasma and bits of skin, (2) the triple peptone medium devised by Salvin (1947), and (3) Francis's cystine–blood–glucose medium. The rate of success for converting chromoblastomycotic fungi to sclerotic cells achieved by Silva was highly variable and depended on the culture system and the fungal strain utilized for individual experiments. A maximum of 85% conversion to sclerotic cells was achieved in the most successful experiments, and Francis's medium was found to produce a high yield of sclerotic cells. The sclerotic cells developed in Silva's experiments (Figures 8 and 9) resembled the chlamydosporelike cells described by Medlar and Lane.

5.2. Chick-Embryo and Tissue-Culture Methods

In addition to Medlar and Lane, Howles *et al.* (1954) succeeded in growing the tissue form of a chromoblastomycotic fungus by directly

←

Figure 5. Sclerotic cells and hyphae of *F. pedrosoi* strain SA-9 incubated at 37°C in yeast nitrogen base glucose broth adjusted to pH 3.0. Unstained. Scale bar: 2.0 μm.

Figure 6. Disarticulated sclerotic cells of *F. pedrosoi* strain 9311 incubated at 37°C in glucose yeast nitrogen base broth adjusted to pH 3.0. Unstained. Scale bar: 2.0 μm.

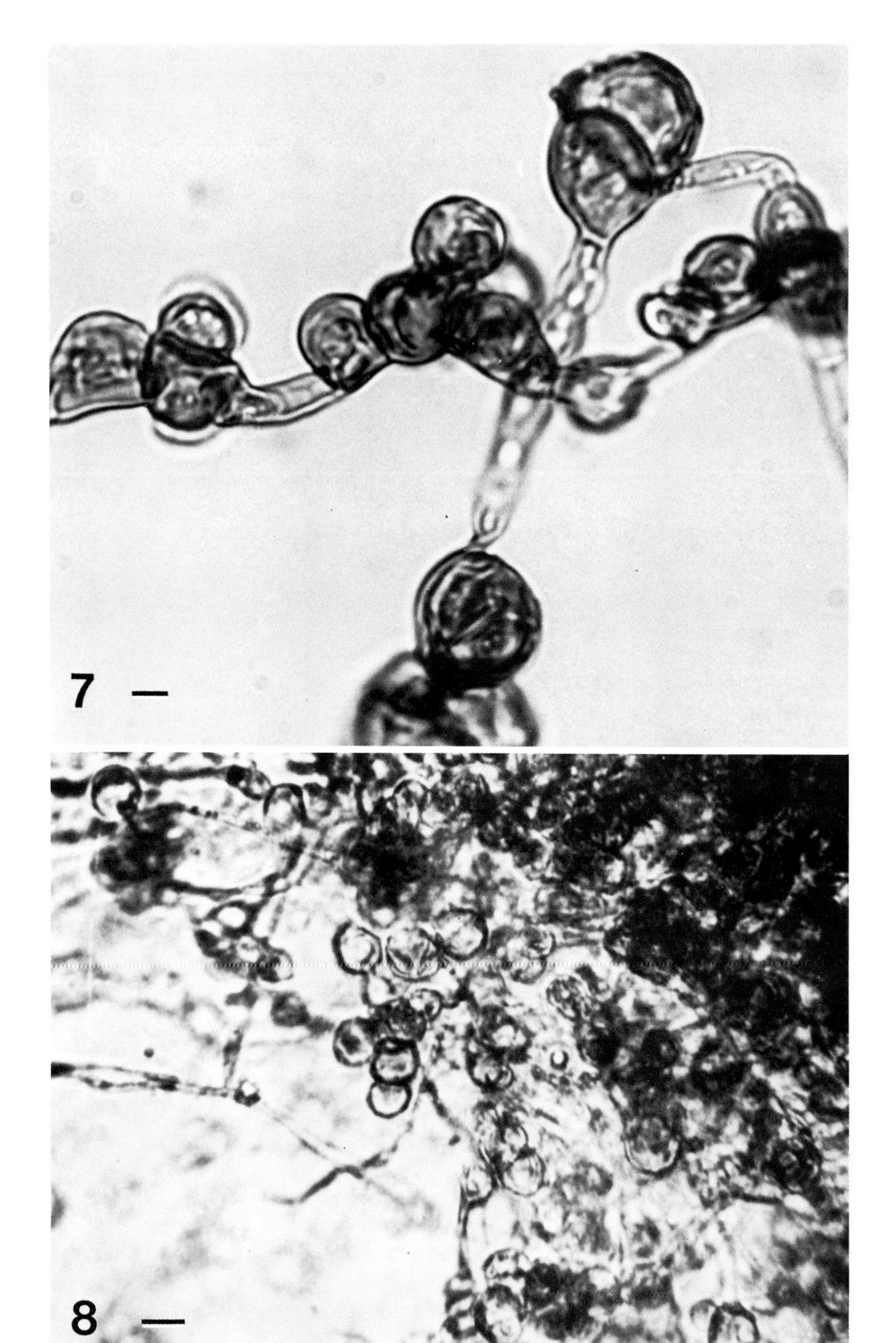
7
8

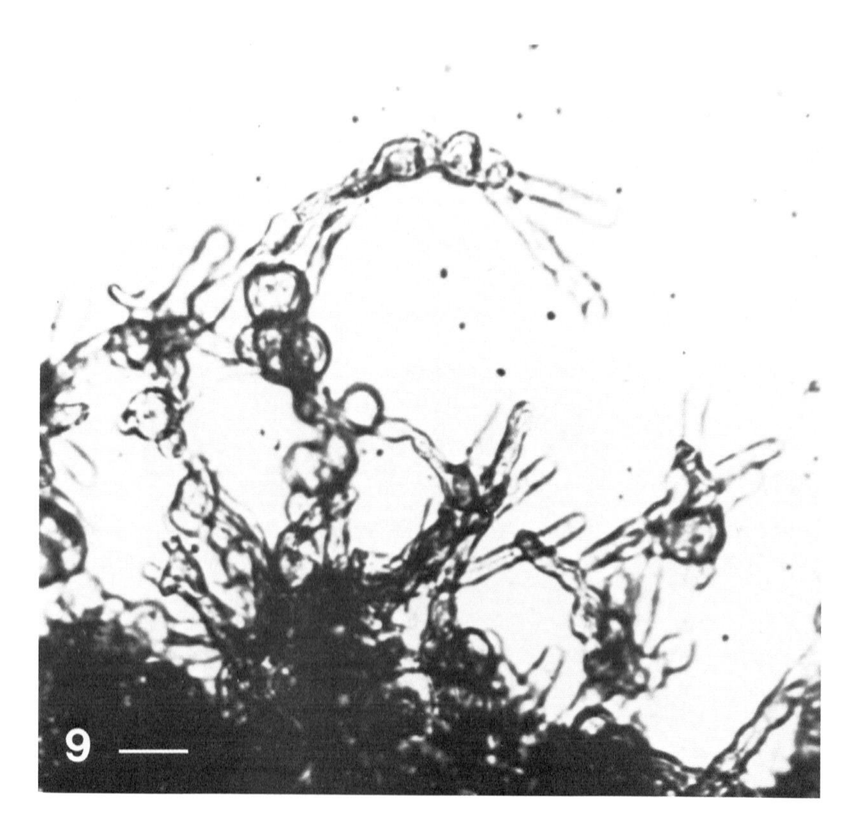

Figure 9. Sclerotic cells of *P. verrucosa* grown on Francis's glucose cystine blood agar at 37°C. Unstained. Scale bar: 5.0 μm. (From Silva, 1957. Used with the author's permission.)

injecting tissue from a chromoblastomycosis patient into the yolk sacs of embryonated hen's eggs. According to their description, the fungus continued to multiply in the sclerotic cell form without producing hyphae. Moore (1941) had previously reported a similar finding based on experiments using *P. verrucosa* inoculated into the chorioallantoic membrane of embryonated eggs. We (B. H. Cooper, unpublished observations) have

←

Figure 7. Sclerotic cells (intercalary chlamydospores) and hyphae of *F. pedrosoi* strain SA-9 incubated at 37°C in glucose yeast nitrogen base broth adjusted to pH 3.0. Unstained. Scale bar: 1.0 μm.

Figure 8. Sclerotic cells of *P. verrucosa* developed in chick embryo chorioallantois. Unstained. Scale bar: 5.0 μm. (From Silva, 1957. Used with the author's permission.)

attempted to cultivate sclerotic cells of *F. pedrosoi, P. verrucosa,* and *C. carrionii* using modern tissue-culture techniques. Incubation of several isolates with WI38 or Vero cells in Eagle's medium at 37°C yielded only vegetative hyphae and no sclerotic cells. These observations, along with the experiments with poikilothermic animals, suggest that neither a temperature of 37°C nor contact with mammalian cells is essential for growth of sclerotic cells.

5.3. Nutritional Studies in Chemically Defined Media

West (1967) studied the nutritional requirements of a single isolate of *P. verrucosa* in the hope of inducing the peritheciumlike structure reported earlier by Ajello and Runyon (1953). He succeeded in producing sclerotic cells, but no perithecia, in a medium containing sucrose, glutamic acid, and mineral salts and in a medium consisting of glucose, ammonium chloride, and mineral salts. Lesser numbers of sclerotic cells were also produced when either proline or guanine was substituted for ammonium chloride in the latter medium.

The definitive study of Reiss and Nickerson (1974) suggests that manganese plays a pivotal role in controlling sclerotic-cell formation by *P. verrucosa.* With a number of isolates of that species, these investigators studied the effects of divalent cations on growth, sporulation, and sclerotic-cell formation. Using a chemically defined medium that had been made deficient in Zn^{2+}, Cu^{2+}, Fe^{3+}, and Mn^{2+} by extraction with 8-hydroxyquinoline, they investigated the effects on growth that were produced by supplementation of the basal medium with one or more of these cations. Cultures were incubated at 25°C, and when all four cations were added to the medium, normal filamentous growth ensued. By contrast, only short hyphae with terminal swollen cells were produced when Mn^{2+} was omitted from the medium. These terminal cells lacked septations, but were otherwise identical to the cells seen in tissues infected with *P. verrucosa.* When the basal medium was supplemented with yeast extract, another organic nitrogen source, or ammonium phosphate, identical structures were produced whether Mn^{2+} was excluded or not. Curiously, *F. pedrosoi* and *P. richardsiae* could not be induced to form sclerotic cells under the same conditions as those that regularly caused their formation by *P. verrucosa.*

When ammonium sulfate was substituted for potassium nitrate, a striking difference in the results was noted. Sclerotic cells were formed whether Mn^{2+} was added to or excluded from the medium. The effect was attributed solely to the pH of the medium, which decreased to 2.6 during incubation. When ammonium phosphate was used, the pH remained neutral and no sclerotic cells were produced. Conversion to sclerotic-cell morphology was independent of the temperature of incubation, indicating that the control of morphogenesis in *P. verrucosa* is not related to temperature.

Fractionation of cells that had been labeled with radioactive ^{54}Mn revealed that the Mn^{2+} concentrated mostly in the cytoplasm, but appreciable amounts also localized in the cell walls and in phialoconidia. The ^{54}Mn in the cytoplasm appeared to be associated with a low-molecular-weight organometallic compound. From these observations, Reiss and Nickerson hypothesized that Mn^{2+} is stored in the cytoplasm in the form of an organometallic chelate and ultimately functions as a cofactor in cell-wall biosynthesis.

The effect of acid pH on morphogenesis in chromoblastomycotic fungi was illustrated by Szaniszlo *et al.* (1976, 1983). Using Czapek-Dox medium supplemented with amino acids and thiamine, conversion of hyphae of *P. verrucosa, F. pedrosoi,* and *C. carrionii* to sclerotic cells could regularly be demonstrated when the pH was adjusted to 2.5. The percentage conversion to sclerotic cells was low with the three chormoblastomycosis species named above, whereas almost 100% conversion of yeast cells of the phaeohyphomycotic fungus *Wangiella dermatitidis* was achieved. Other species tested included *C. trichoides, Exophiala jeanselmei,* and *E. spinifera.* However, these species failed to convert to sclerotic cells under any of the conditions tested. Another species, *Aureobasidium pullulans,* has also been reported (Park, 1984) to produce large, chlamydosporelike cells when cultivated at pH 3.0 or lower.

Ultrastructural examination of sclerotic cells produced in acidified medium reveals them to have characteristics that are similar to those of hyphae (Figure 10). The cell wall is thicker than the hyphal wall and is multilayered. The rounded form of the sclerotic cell contains internal organelles (e.g., ribosomes, mitochondria) and lipid bodies that are quite typical of those seen in hyphae (Cooper *et al.,* 1973) and of sclerotic cells observed in tissues (Nishimoto, 1970; Rosen *et al.,* 1980). Septa with Woronin bodies are occasionally observed that are typical of those seen in hyphae (Szaniszlo *et al.,* 1983). The cytoplasm of young sclerotic cells is typical of actively growing cells. In older sclerotic cells, the cytoplasm contain numerous lipid bodies and glycogen deposits and resembles the cytoplasm of a resistant spore.

It has recently been possible to verify the results obtained with acidified, modified Czapek-Dox broth (Szaniszlo *et al.,* 1976, 1983) by using Yeast Nitrogen Base (YNB, Difco) broth supplemented with glucose. When isolates of *P. verrucosa, F. pedrosoi,* and *C. carrionii* were incubated in this chemically defined medium adjusted to pH 3.0, abundant sclerotic cells in the form of terminal and intercalary chlamydospores were produced (see Figures 4–7). Cultures were incubated at 37°C

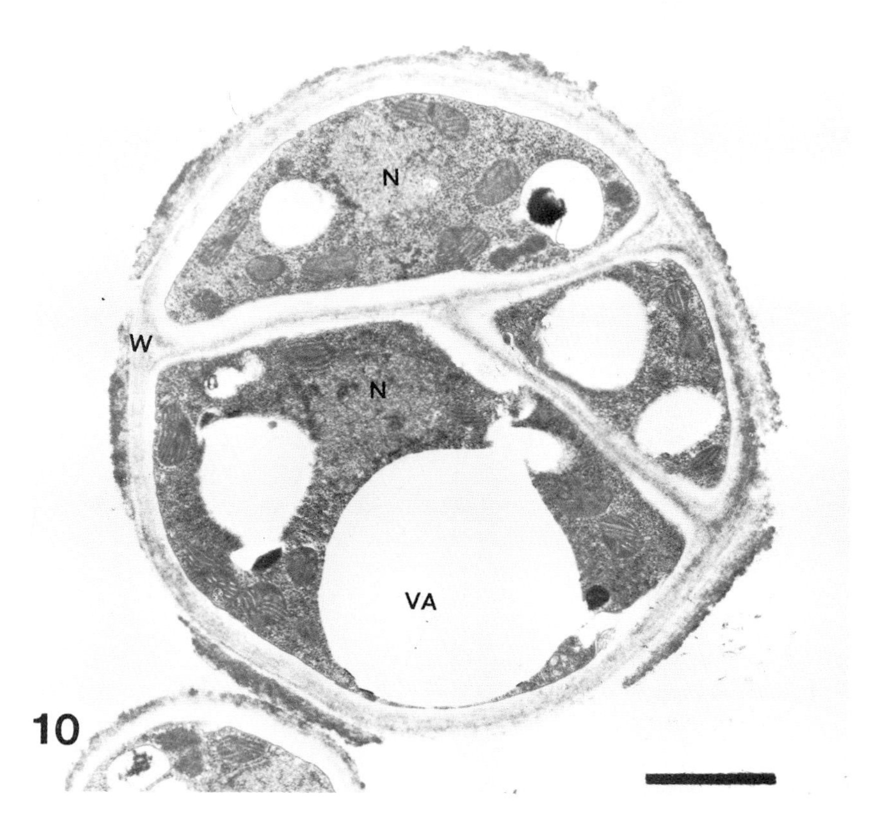

Figure 10. Transmission electron micrograph of sclerotic cell of *F. pedrosoi,* in a modified Czapek–Dox broth adjusted to pH 2.5 (Szaniszlo *et al.*, 1976). (W) Cell wall; (N) nuclei; (VA) vacuole. Scale bar: 1 μm. (Unpublished micrograph courtesy of P. J. Szaniszlo and J. D. Marlowe.)

and were not aerated. The overall percentage of conversion to sclerotic-cell morphology was not calculated, but it was relatively small. The septate sclerotic cells remained attached to normal-appearing hyphae.

6. CONTROL OF MORPHOGENESIS IN CHROMOBLASTOMYCOTIC FUNGI

The results of *in vitro* experiments with synthetic culture media suggest methods that can be used for cultivating large numbers of sclerotic cells. Previous studies of metabolism, pathogenicity, and antigenicity with chromoblastomycotic fungi have been handicapped because it was impossible to easily produce large numbers of the tissue forms of these fungi. Sclerotic cells produced in synthetic media appear to be identical to those observed in the lesions of chromoblastomycosis. However, it remains to be proved that the conditions that induce sclerotic cells in synthetic media also induce conversion to the sclerotic-cell morphology in human tissues, in the yolk sac or choroallantois of chicken embryos, in silkworm pupae, or in the tissues of frogs and toads. It seems very unlikely that the pH of human skin could drop as low as 2.5 for even a few hours without some tissue necrosis and some pain. Necrosis is not a common feature of chromoblastomycosis, and patients describe the lesions to be only slightly irritating and not painful. However, the possibility that such a low pH could persist within well-circumscribed microabcesses like those observed in lesions of chromoblastomycosis cannot be ruled out by available evidence.

The effect of extreme acid pH may simply be to inhibit transport of Mn^{2+} into hyphae. This was suggested by Reiss and Nickerson (1974), who demonstrated that sclerotic cells were formed by *P. verrucosa* in the presence of Mn^{2+} concentrations that were adequate to maintain the hyphal morphology when the pH of the growth medium was 2.6. There is at present no evidence that transport of Mn^{2+} is restricted in infected tissue, although this could be one of the effects of the host's inflammatory response. Human serum may also bind Mn^{2+} and sequester it from invading fungi. Binding by transferrin, conalbumin, and lactoferrin deprives infecting microorganisms of iron and is regarded as a natural defense mechanism (Weinberg, 1984). A similar mechanism for withholding Mn^{2+} from infectious agents has not, to my knowledge, been demonstrated. It seems reasonable that iron is not unique in this regard and that other metal ions including Mn^{2+} are bound to serum proteins for transport within the human blood vascular system. Manganese bound to serum protein would thus be sequestered from utilization by an infectious agent. Proof that a Mn^{2+}-binding protein exists in human tissue and functions in this fashion must await further experimentation.

Reiss and Nickerson (1974) suggested that melanin in the cell walls of chromoblastomycotic fungi may serve as protection against intracellular destruction by phagocytes. Sclerotic cells in infected tissues appear to be more intensely pigmented than vegetative hyphae of the same fungi. The walls of sclerotic cells also appear to be thicker than the walls of hyphae. It may be that such changes in cell-wall structure inhibit transport of Mn^{2+} into the cell just as they render the sclerotic cell impermeable to phagocytic cells. However, the opposite hypothesis seems to be more likely on the basis of available evidence, i.e., that inhibition of Mn^{2+} transport, by whatever mechanism, leads to the formation of a cell wall that is thicker and more intensely pigmented.

Sclerotic cells resemble spores in some respects, and it is tempting to assert that Mn^{2+} deprivation may cause effects in chromoblastomycotic fungi that are analogous to those demonstrated in bacterial spores (Szaniszlo *et al.*, 1983). Manganese is known to be a cofactor for a large number of enzymes and to affect the synthesis of cell walls, DNA, RNA, and fatty acids. It also influences the transport of other ions across cell membranes. In most metabolic processes, Mg^{2+} is an effective substitute for Mn^{2+}. However, the DNA-dependent RNA polymerases involved in sporulation in *Bacillus subtilis* have an absolute requirement for Mn^{2+}. As the intracellular Mg^{2+}/Mn^{2+} ratio changes, differences in polymerase specificity are thought to occur that lead to the production of "sporulation-specific" messenger RNA and synthesis of proteins that are essential for sporulation (Fukuda *et al.*, 1975). Sclerotic cells are resistant forms that may or may not be spores. An attractive, but speculative, hypothesis is that sclerotic cells are spores and that regulatory processes similar to those operative in *B. subtilis* control the morphogenesis of sclerotic cells in chromoblastomycotic fungi.

Obviously, more questions remain to be answered than are clearly understood regarding morphogenesis in chromoblastomycotic fungi. An intriguing question concerns the reasons for the differences *in vivo* of the fungi that cause chromoblastomycosis and those that cause phaeohyphomycosis. Isolates of *C. trichoides, E. jeanselmei,* and *E. spinifera* could not be induced to form sclerotic cells when cultured at pH 2.5. These agents of phaeohyphomycosis appear to be very similar to those that cause chromoblastomycosis. However, the failure of these three phaeohyphomycotic agents to form sclerotic cells *in vivo* or when cultured *in vitro* at pH 2.5 may reflect a fundamental difference between them and *P. verrucosa, F. pedrosoi, F. compacta,* and *C. carrionii.*

REFERENCES

Ajello, L., 1975, Phaeohyphomycosis: Definition and etiology, in: *Proceedings of the Third International Conference on the Mycoses,* Scientific Publication No. 304, Pan American Health Organization, Washington, D.C., pp. 126–130.

Ajello, L., and Runyon, L., 1953, Abortive "perithecial" production by *Phialophora verrucosa, Mycologia* **45**:947–950.

Al-Doory, Y., 1972, *Chromomycosis,* Mountain Press, Missoula, Montana.

Batres, E., Wolf, J. E., Jr., Rudolph, A. H., and Knox, J. M., 1978, Transepithelial elimination of cutaneous chromomycosis, *Arch. Dermatol.* **114**:1231–1232.

Beneke, E. S., 1978, Dematiaceous fungi in laboratory-housed frogs, in: *the Black and White Yeasts,* Proceedings of the Fourth International Conference on the Mycoses, Scientific Publication No. 356, Pan American Health Organization, Washington, D.C., pp. 107–108.

Carrion, A. L., and Silva-Hutner, M., 1971, Taxonomic criteria for the fungi of chromoblastomycosis with reference to *Fonsecaea pedrosoi, Int. J. Dermatol.* **10**:35–43.

Cooper, B. H., Grove, S., Mims, S., and Szaniszlo, P. J., 1973, Septal ultrastructure in *Phialophora pedrosoi, Phialophora verrucosa* and *Cladosporium carrionii, Sabouraudia* **11**:127–130.

De Vries, J. A., de Hoog, J. S., and de Bruyn, H. P., 1984, *Phialophora cyanescens* sp. nov. with *Phaeosclera*-like synanomorph, causing white-grain mycetoma in man, *Antonie van Leeuwenhoek J. Microbiol. Serol.* **50**:149–153.

Fukuda, R., Keilman, J., McVey, E., and Doi, R. H., 1975, Ribonucleic acid polymerase pattern of sporulating *Bacillus subtilis* cells, in: *Spores IV* (P. Gerhardt, R. N. Costilon, and H. L. Sadoff, eds.) American Society for Microbiology, Washington, D.C., pp. 213–220.

Hanada, S., and Kusunoki, T., 1983, Scanning electron microscopic observation of the parasitic forms of *Fonsecaea pedrosoi* in a human skin lesion, *Mycopathologia* **82**:33–37.

Howles, J. K., Kennedy, C. B., Jarvin, W. H., Brueck, J. S., and Buddingh, G. S., 1954, Chromoblastomycosis: Report of nine cases from a single area in Louisiana, *Arch. Dermatol. Syphilol.* **69**:83–90.

Lane, C. G., 1915, A cutaneous lesion caused by a new fungus *(Phialophora verrucosa), J. Cutan. Dis.* **33**:840–846.

McGinnis, M. R., 1983, Chromoblastomycosis and phaeohyphomycosis: New concepts, diagnosis, and mycology, *J. Am. Acad. Dermatol.* **8**:1–16.

Medlar, E. M., 1915, A cutaneous infection caused by a new fungus, *Phialophora verrucosa,* with a study of the fungus, *J. Med. Res.* **32**:507–521.

Moore, M., 1941, The virulence of strains of *Phialophora verrucosa* determined by inoculating chorioallantoic membranes of chick embryos, *J. Invest. Dermatol.* **5**:411–422.

Nishimoto, K., 1970, Electron microscopic findings of lymph nodes affected by chromomycosis, *Jpn. J. Dermatol. Ser. A* **80**:181–195.

Park, D., 1984, Low pH and the development of large cells in *Aureobasidium pullulans, Trans. Br. Mycol. Soc.* **82**:717–720.

Reiss, E., and Nickerson, W. J., 1974, Control of dimorphism in *Phialophora verrucosa, Sabouraudia* **12**:202–213.

Rosen, T., Gyorkey, F., Joseph, L. M., and Batres, E., 1980, Ultrastructural features of chromoblastomycosis, *Int. J. Dermatol.* **19**:461–468.

Salvin, S. B., 1947, Cultural studies of the yeast-like phase of *Histoplasma capsulatum* Darling, *J. Bacteriol.* **54**:655–660.

Silva, M., 1957, The parasitic phase of the fungi of chromoblastomycosis: Development of sclerotic cells *in vitro* and *in vivo, Mycologia* **49**:318–331.

Silva, M., 1958, The saprophytic phase of the fungi of chromoblastomycosis: Effect of nutrients and temperature upon growth and morphology, *Trans. N. Y. Acad. Sci.* **21**:46–57.

Silva, M., 1960, Growth characteristics of the fungi of chromoblastomycosis, *Ann. N. Y. Acad. Sci.* **89**:17–29.

Szaniszlo, P. J., Hsieh, P. H., and Marlowe, J. D., 1976, Induction and ultrastructure of the multicellular (sclerotic) morphology in *Phialophora dermatitidis, Mycologia* **68**:117–130.

Szaniszlo, P. J., Jacobs, C. W., and Geis, P. A., 1983, Dimorphism: Morphological and biochemical aspects, in: *Fungi Pathogenic for Humans and Animals,* Part A, *Biology* (D. H. Howard, Ed.), Marcel Dekker, New York, pp. 323–426.

Velasquez, L. F., and Restrepo, A. M., 1975, Naturally acquired chromomycosis in the toad *Bufo marinus:* Comparison of the etiologic agent with fungi causing human chromomycosis, *Sabouraudia* **13**:1–9.

Weinberg, E. D., 1984, Iron withholding: A defense against infection and neoplasia, *Physiol. Rev.* **64**:65–102.

West, B., 1967, Nutrition of *Phialophora verrucosa* A126, *Mycopathololologia* **31**:12–16.
Zais, N., 1978, Chromoblastomycosis: A superficial minimycetoma, in: *The Black and White Yeasts,* Proceedings of the Fourth International Conference on the Mycoses, Scientific Publication No. 356, Pan American Health Organization. Washington, D.C., pp. 17–18.

Chapter 12

Arthroconidium–Spherule–Endospore Transformation in *Coccidioides immitis*

Garry T. Cole and S. H. Sun

1. INTRODUCTION

Coccidioides immitis is a peculiar pathogen that remains a taxonomic enigma. Its natural habitat is soil, geographically limited with rare exceptions to the arid and semiarid regions of the western hemisphere, where it grows as a mold, producing dry arthroconidia. The conidia are dispersed as aerosols when soil is disturbed and serve as infectious propagules for humans and other animals. Infection is associated with morphological transformation of the conidium into a multinucleate spherule, the contents of which subsequently differentiate into a myriad of tiny, uninucleate endospores. The latter are released from the parent spherule, and each endospore is potentially capable of initiating a second generation of spherules within the host. Thus, *C. immitis* is a diphasic microorganism, characterized by distinct saprobic and parasitic cycles (Figure 1). The saprobic phase of *C. immitis* differs little from that of other soil fungi that produce arthroconidia (Sigler and Carmichael, 1976; Carmichael *et al.*, 1980) and reveals morphological features that suggest an ascomycetous relationship, e.g., septate hyphae, simple septal pores, and Woronin

Garry T. Cole • Department of Botany, The University of Texas at Austin, Austin, Texas 78712. **S. H. Sun** • Mycology Research Laboratory, Veterans Administration Hospital, San Antonio, Texas 78284. This chapter is dedicated to the memory of Milton Huppert (1920–1984), a pioneer in studies of the biology of *Coccidioides immitis*, a highly respected immunologist, and, most important, a dear friend.

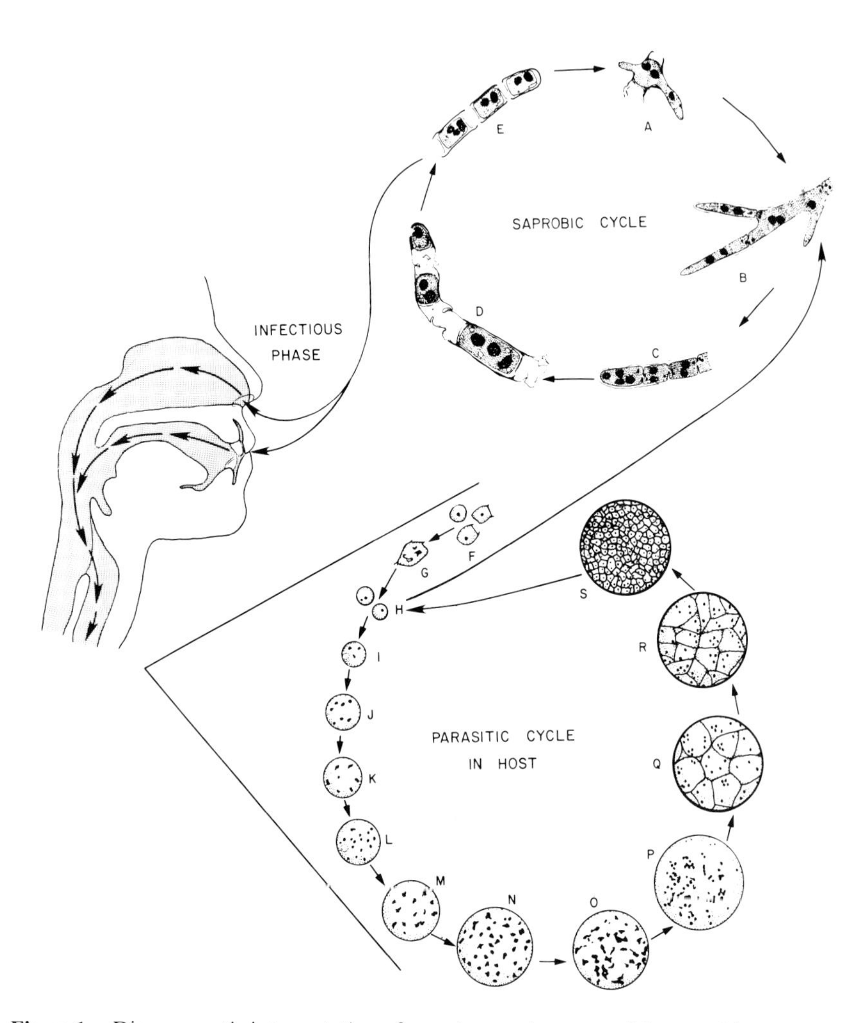

Figure 1. Diagrammatic interpretation of morphogenetic events of the saprobic (A–E) and parasitic (F–S) cycles of *C. immitis.* Nuclei in (A–E) are indicated by darkly stippled cell inclusions. The arthroconidia (E) are infectious propagules that invade the host via the respiratory tract. Arthroconidia convert to spherules (F–H), which become multinucleate (I–P) and then undergo segmentation (Q, R) and endosporulation (S–H) within host tissue. The endospores may convert back to the saprobic phase if they are released from the host (H-B). Nuclei in (F–S) are also represented by darkly stippled regions. (After Sun and Huppert, 1976; Cole *et al.,* 1983.)

bodies. On the other hand, it is the only species of arthroconidial fungus known to produce a primary infection in humans and to be capable of undergoing transformation from conidium to spherule to disseminating endospores within the host. Hence, *C. immitis* is unique among fungi that cause human mycoses, being distinguished from morphogenetically similar saprobes by its pathogenicity and from other pathogenic fungi by its unusual parasitic cycle. *Coccidioides* remains a monospecific form-genus.

The disease coccidioidomycosis was first described in 1892 by Posadas and Wernicke in Argentina and a short time later by Rixford, Thorne, and Gilchrist in the United States (Posadas, 1892; Wernicke, 1892; Rixford, 1894; Thorne, 1894; Rixford and Gilchrist, 1896). All believed the causative agent to be a protozoan because *in vivo* it resembled *Coccidium*. Fiese (1958) and Deresinski (1980) presented informative accounts of the early history of this disease, and the latter author reproduced some of the drawings of Rixford and Gilchrist (1896) of the alleged protozoan. It is evident that these early workers recognized features that were atypical of the coccidial protozoans, many representatives of which are parasitic in the digestive epithelium of vertebrates. In fact, it was these same authors in 1896 who named the etiological agent *Coccidioides* ("like *Coccidium*") *immitis* ("not mild"), because the few cases described were severe, disseminated disease. Four years later, Ophüls and Moffitt (1900) confirmed earlier suspicions that the causative agent of coccidioidomycosis was a fungus. The authors reported the third recognized American patient with coccidioial disease, who, like the first two, was a Portuguese farm laborer from the Azores and had worked in the San Joaquin Valley of southern California. In this case, however, it was possible to examine the entire course of the disease from primary pulmonary infection to death with miliary dissemination three months later. Pathological sections revealed the protozoanlike microbe described by Rixford and Gilchrist, but cultures of infected tissue, obtained both from the patient and from inoculated guinea pigs, consistently gave rise to a mold. Although the organism was at first suspected to be a contaminant, the authors were soon convinced on the basis of satisfaction of Koch's postulates that the fungus was the elusive pathogen. Ophüls later presented detailed reports of the pathology and histology of the disease (Ophüls, 1905a) and published the first fairly accurate account of the saprobic and parasitic phases of *C. immitis* (Ophüls, 1905b). Subsequent studies established that soil is the natural habitat of the fungus (Stewart and Meyer, 1932), that inhalation of arthroconidia is the principal route of infection (Dickson, 1937; Dickson and Gifford, 1938), and that coccidioidomycosis occurs in a multiplicity of clinical forms, including asymptomatic or symptomatic primary respiratory disease usually with uncomplicated recovery, chronic residual pulmonary disease, and the classic but rare disseminated disease that can be either acute or chronic and is often fatal (Salkin, 1961). Early studies revealed that recovery from infection is accompanied by strong resistance to reinfection, apparently determined by cell-mediated immunity (C. E. Smith, 1942, 1943; C. E. Smith *et al.*, 1946). Cases of coccidioidomycosis acquired by direct percutaneous inoculation are rare (Pappagianis, 1973, 1980), and person-to-person transmission has not been confirmed (Drutz and Catanzaro, 1978; Brewer *et al.*, 1982). However, a possible example of the latter is maternal–fetal transmission. Several cases of coccidioidomycosis in neonates have been reported, and the maternal uterus or birth canal was the likely source of infection (Bernstein *et al.*, 1981). Although endospores and spherules are excreted by the host, no direct evidence is yet available that these cells are capable of spreading the disease among humans. However, contaminated materials must be considered potentially dangerous fomites because cells of the parasitic cycle under proper conditions can revert to the infectious, sporulating mycelial phase (Lones *et al.*, 1971). The small size of arthroconidia (typically 3–6 × 2–4 μm) allows them to penetrate even the lowermost reaches of the respiratory tract (Austwick, 1966). Endemic areas of *C. immitis* in North America include northern Mexico and southwest regions of the United States, incorporating parts of Texas, New Mexico, Arizona, and California (Maddy, 1958; Rao *et al.*, 1972). Several areas of South and Central America have also been identified as endemic, these areas including regions of Argentina, Paraguay, Venezuela, Guatemala, Honduras, and possibly Colombia (Pappagianis, 1980). Skin reactivity tests using mixtures of antigens prepared from *C. immitis* mycelia by a variety of methods (Huppert and Bailey, 1963), and collectively referred to as *coccidioidin,* have been employed for about 60 years in immunological investigations aimed at surveying populations for exposure to the airborne arthroconidia (Catanzaro, 1979). Arid climatic and edaphic conditions are adequate for growth and sporulation of the saprobic phase of *C. immitis* and are particularly well suited for wind dissemination of the infectious propagule (Flynn *et al.*, 1979).

2. SAPROBIC CYCLE

2.1. Mycelial Growth

The fungus grows as a mycelial culture on virtually all laboratory media at most temperatures (optimum approximately 30°C). Although vegetative hyphal growth still occurs at 37°C, sporulation of certain strains is inhibited at this elevated temperature (Walch, 1982). Good mycelial growth is usually obtained on glucose–yeast extract (GYE) medium consisting of 1% glucose, 0.5% yeast extract, and 1.5% agar, as well as Sabouraud's dextrose agar and potato dextrose charcoal agar (Keuhn *et al.*, 1961). Most strains of *Coccidioides* grown on agar plates demonstrate small, gray, membranous colonies in about 3–5 days and develop white to gray aerial hyphae that form a loose, cobwebby to cottony texture during the next 1–2 weeks. Some strains develop a light brown pigment in the aerial mycelium at about 2 weeks that may intensify to dark brown with aging. The nature of this pigment is unknown (see Section 4.1). When a large number of isolates are examined, strain variablity is clearly apparent in size, conformation, rate of growth, and pigmentation of the colonies (Huppert *et al.*, 1967). Liquid GYE medium is also commonly used for production of mycelia in shake culture. Roessler *et al.* (1946) experimented with different synthetic media for growth of the saprobic phase and found that a basal medium of K_2HPO_4, KH_2PO_4, $MgSO_4$, $NH_4C_2H_3O_2$, and glucose supported development of septate mycelia and "spores" that "arose from the swollen and rounded contents of the" hyphal cells. "As the spores became more mature, the longer fragments broke up and short chains of spores appeared. After 10 days incubation, numerous single spores having thick capsules were observed." Our studies of strain C634 (Cole *et al.*, 1983) have demonstrated that mycelia grown in liquid GYE media at 24°C for 9–16 days give rise to similar rounded hyphal compartments, or moniliform hyphae (Figures 2 and 3). After prolonged incubation, the chains of thick-walled cells (chlamydospores?) disarticulate. These cells, however, should not be confused with the dry arthroconidia that differentiate from aerial hyphae. Further comparison of such cell types requires ultrastructural examination of the morphogenetic events that occur in submerged culture. Levine *et al.* (1960) determined that if the basal medium used by Roessler *et al.* (1946) was modified by addition of 2% mannitol and omission of glucose, vegetative mycelia free of "spores" could be harvested within 48 hr. No moniliform hyphae of strain C634 appeared in GYE shake culture during the initial 120-hr incubation period (Figure 2). Of possible significance is another observation presented by Roessler *et al.* (1946) that addition of low levels of zinc to their basal medium (2–4 ppm as $ZnSO_4$) greatly enhanced mycelial growth and disarticulation of the chains of rounded cells. The importance of zinc in the morphogenesis of *Candida albicans* is well documented (Bedell and Soll, 1979), and its apparent association with development of the saprobic phase of *C. immitis* deserves further investigation.

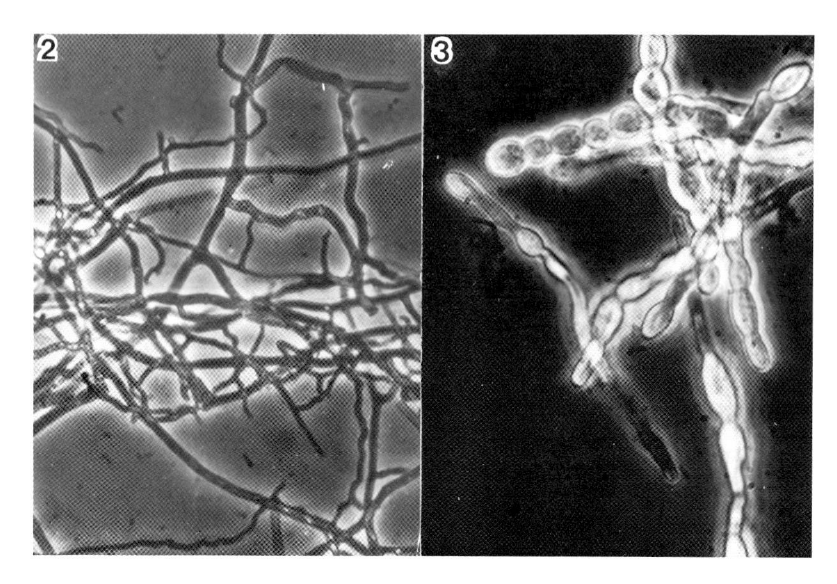

Figures 2 and 3. Vegetative (2) and moniliform hyphae (3) produced in GYE liquid media at 24°C after 5 and 9 days, respectively. Note the chain of rounded cells (chlamydospores?) in (3). ×240.

2.2. Conidiogenesis

Arthroconidia are multinucleate, thick-walled and barrel-shaped cells that show considerable variation in length-to-width ratios. Conidiogenesis occurs by differentiation of propagules within the fertile hyphae, a process that has been termed *enteroarthric* development (Cole and Samson, 1979, 1983). Initially, the hypha ceases apical extension and undergoes septation (Figure 4). Certain compartments delimited by these septa are soon distinguished by their thickened lateral walls and apparently condensed cytoplasm, which contrasts with adjacent, nonrefractile compartments (Figure 5). Both the lateral and cross walls of the former continue to thicken and the endogenously formed arthroconidia become clearly visible (Figures 6 and 7). The nonrefractile compartments do not develop further, but instead appear to undergo autolysis. As the conidia

Figures 4–9. Time-lapse photomicrographic sequence of enteroarthric conidium formation in *C. immitis*. The fungus was grown on GYE agar in a thin glass culture chamber (Cole and Kendrick, 1968). Arrowheads in (4) locate cross walls. Time: (4) 0 hr; (5) 4 hr; (6) 15 hr; (7) 27 hr; (8) 44 hr; (9) 68 hr. Magnification: (4–7) ×1700; (8, 9) ×1300.

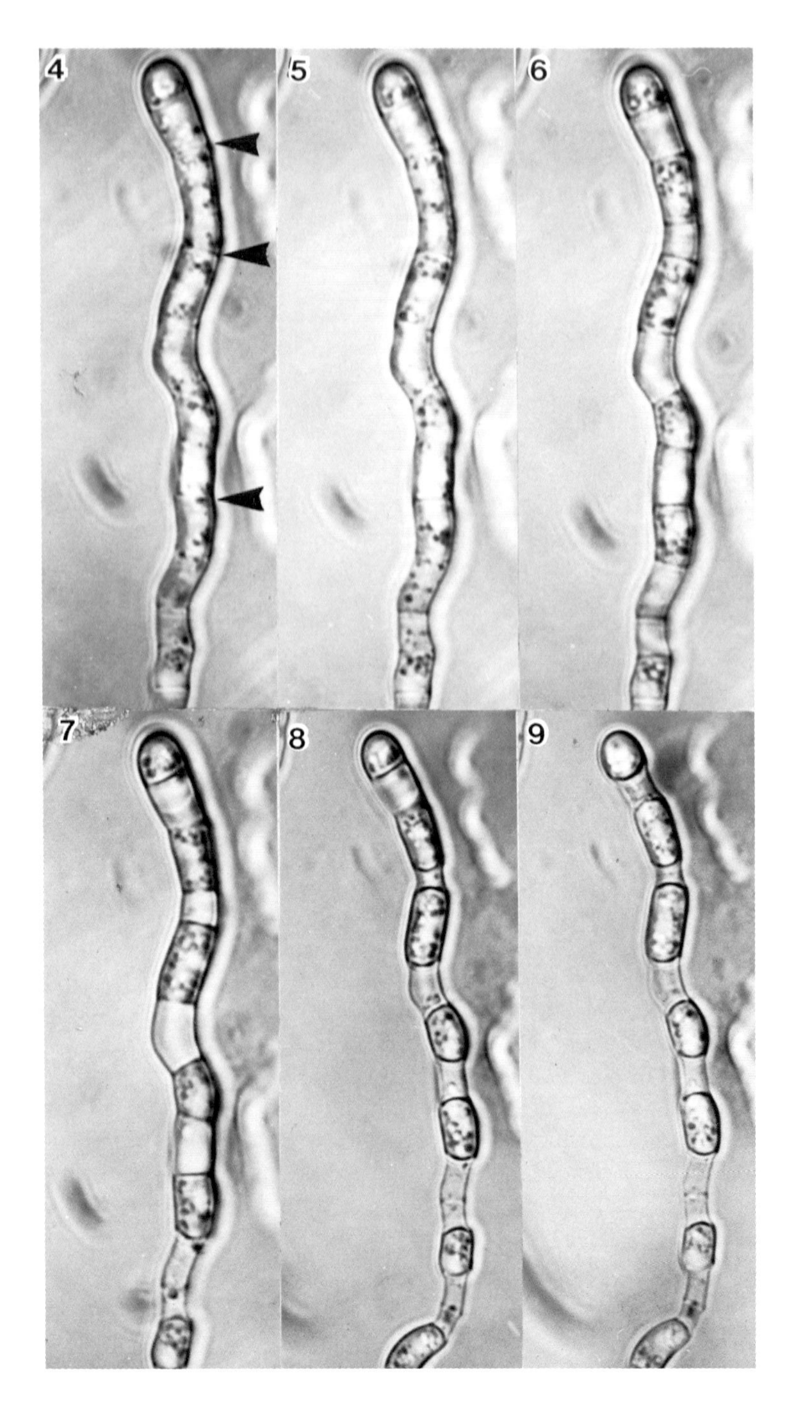
4
5
6
7
8
9

continue to enlarge and their end walls become convex (Figure 8), the lateral walls of the intervening cells become thin and fragile (Figure 9) and eventually fracture, resulting in disarticulation of the arthroconidial chain. This mechanism of conidial secession has been termed *rhexolytic* (Hughes, 1971a,b), and may occur as a result of mechanical stress, lytic enzyme activity, or both (Cole and Samson, 1979). Conidia are commonly dispersed with the original sleeve of the fertile hyphal wall still intact.

These same features of conidium ontogeny, which are diagramatically summarized in Figure 10, are demonstrated by a number of other imperfect fungi including strains of *Sporendonema* and *Malbranchea* (Cole and Samson, 1979; Sigler and Carmichael, 1976), *Coremiella* (Emmons, 1967; Cole, 1975), and *Ovadendron* (Carmichael *et al.*, 1980). Ultrastructural and karyological examinations, discussed below, have further illustrated developmental relationships between these soil fungi. Since *C. immitis* was originally described solely on the basis of endosporulating spherules in tissue (Rixford and Gilchrist, 1896), and because the mycelial form shows particularly striking morphological similarities to *Malbranchea,* Sigler and Carmichael (1976) have referred to the saprobic form of the pathogen as the *Malbranchea* state of *C. immitis.* These same authors have suggested that *Coccidioides* is a member of the Gymnoascaceae. Nevertheless, the taxonomic position of *C. immitis* remains uncertain (McGinnis, 1980) and awaits further developmental, biochemical, and genetic studies to clarify the affinities of this fungus to other fungi. At present, identification of *C. immitis* cannot be based exclusively on the morphology of the saprobic phase, but necessitates *in vivo* or *in vitro* tests for transformation of conidia into endosporulating spherules (Sun *et al.,* 1976; Huppert and Sun, 1980b). Despite its morphogenetic similarity to the saprobic phase of *C. immitis,* attempts to transform conidia of *M. dendritica* into spherules by intraperitoneal inoculation of mice have failed (Orr, 1972).

The identification of *C. immitis* has also been performed successfully using an immunological procedure developed by Standard and Kaufman (1977). Mycelial broth cultures were placed on a shaking incubator at 25°C for 3–6 days and then killed with thimerosal. The supernatant (exoantigen) was concentrated (10 to 25-fold) and tested for the presence of antigens in an agar gel double-diffusion system against a reference antigen–antibody complex that produced three distinct precipitin lines. Culture extracts from common saprobic fungal contaminants such as *Penicillium* and *Aspergillus* apparently do not interfere with the exoantigen test (DiSalvo *et al.,* 1981). In an extensive evaluation of this diagnostic technique, Huppert and Sun (1980b) concluded that if the exoantigen of

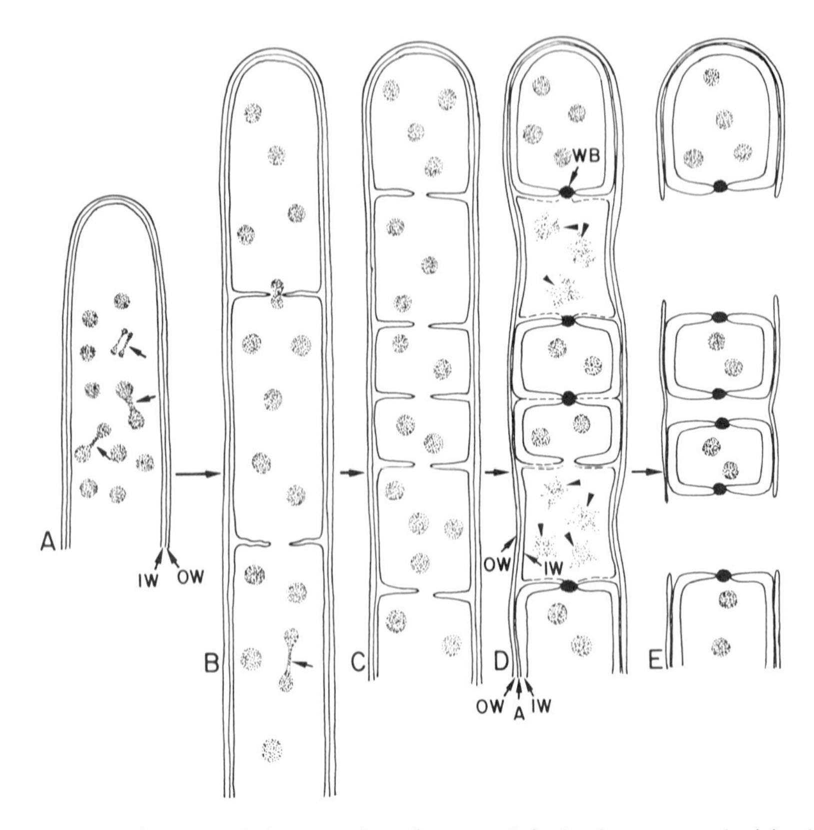

Figure 10. Diagrammatic interpretation of enteroarthric development emphasizing karyological events and aspects of wall differentiation. Arrows in (A, B) indicate dividing nuclei. Arrowheads in (D) point to degenerating nuclei. (A) Amorphous wall layer of fertile hypha; (IW) inner wall layer; (OW) outer wall layer; (WB) Woronin body. (After Cole and Samson, 1979.)

an unknown isolate developed one or more lines of identity with the reference system, this was sufficient evidence for concluding that the fungus was *C. immitis.*

2.3. Ultrastructure

Thin sections of successive stages of conidial development are shown in Figures 11 and 12. The rough surface of the outer hyphal wall (OW) that encloses the conidia (Figure 11), and the contrasting smooth-surfaced outer-wall layer (Figure 12), correlate with the variation in conidial surface texture demonstrated by the scanning electron microscope. Inside

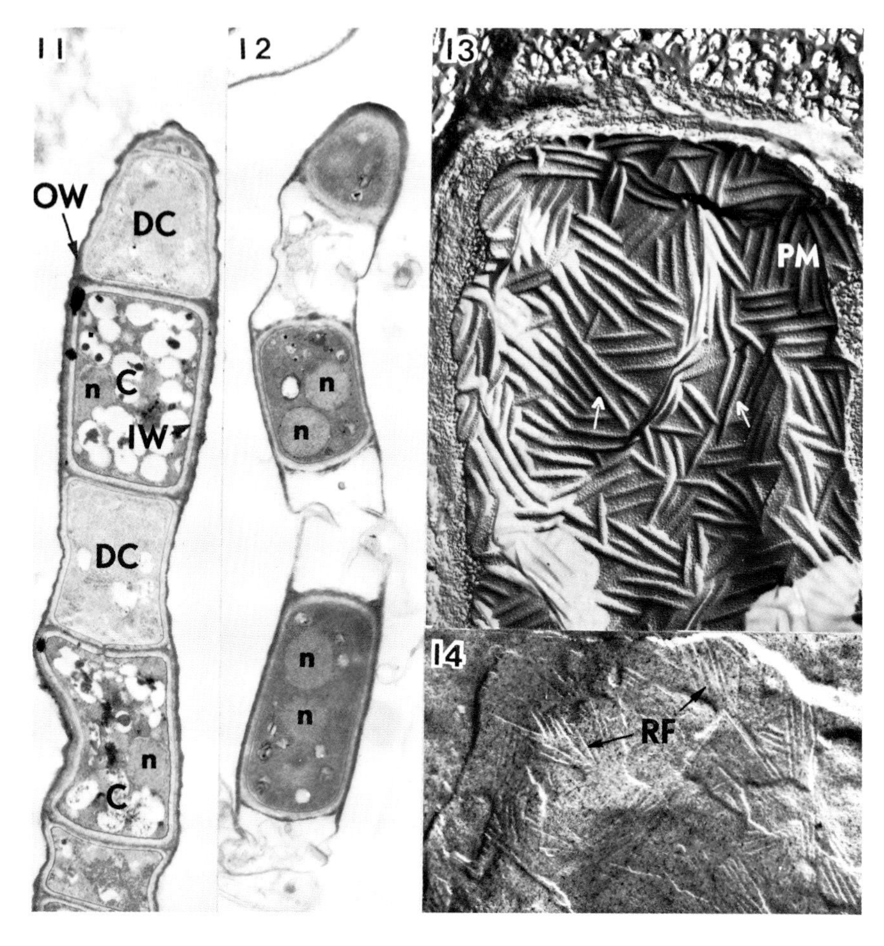

Figures 11 and 12. Thin sections of successive stages of arthroconidium formation showing differentiated outer-wall layer of original fertile hypha (OW) and newly formed inner wall (IW). (DC) Degenerate cell; (C) arthroconidium; (n) nucleus. Magnification: (11) ×3000; (12) ×2500.

Figures 13 and 14. Freeze–fractures of "dormant" conidia showing plasmalemma [PM in (13)] and surface-fractured wall (14). Arrows in (13) locate plasmalemma invaginations. (RF) Rodlet fascicles. Magnification: (13) ×19,000; (14) ×72,600.

this sleeve of the original outer wall of the fertile hypha is an electron-translucent layer (IW in Figure 11) that delineates two cell types: the vacuolate conidia (C) and intervening cells destined to undergo autolysis (DC). The cytoplasm of the latter is not vacuolate and is less dense than that of the conidia. Thin sections of arthroconidial chains of *Sporendo-*

nema purpurascens at comparable developmental stages have revealed that cells located between differentiating conidia contain hypertrophied mitochondria and nuclei with structural irregularities in their membranous envelope (Cole, 1975). Such organelle deformations are suggested to indicate the onset of autolysis. From a comparison of adjacent cells (Figure 11), it is evident that some difference exists in thickness of their respective inner-wall layer (IW). By the time the conidia are mature (Figure 12), the inner wall of autolysing cells is no longer visible. At this stage, only the outer electron-dense wall layer holds the conidia together in a chain and encloses small amounts of incompletely digested, cytoplasmic deposits within the intervening cells (Figure 12). The thin remnant of the fertile hyphal wall eventually ruptures, allowing individual propagules to be dispersed. Such conidia are capable of surviving extremes of desiccation and temperature variation (0–40°C; possibly higher temperatures). In our laboratory, arthroconidia of *C. immitis* are grown on GYE agar at 24°C and then stored on dry culture plates for 60–90 days. Viability of these "dormant" conidia has been estimated at 85–90% (Cole *et al.*, 1983). Freeze–fractured conidia reveal large numbers of plasmalemma invaginations (Figure 13) that are characteristic of mature conidia produced by other imperfect fungi (Cole, 1975). Hess (1973) has shown that when conidia germinate, the portion of the cell membrane surrounding the germ tube is smooth except for faint scars that represent previously invaginated regions. Such observations suggest that the invaginations simply increase the surface area of the cell membrane in preparation for the initial rapid expansion of the plasmalemma during germ-tube emergence and before synthesis of new membrane becomes synchronized with tube growth. No attempts have yet been made to determine whether comparable ultrastructural changes in the cell membrane occur during arthroconidium-to-spherule transformation. Freeze–fractures of the conidial wall surface (Figure 14) demonstrate small clusters or fascicles of fibrous wall components identified as "rodlets" (Cole, 1973). The fracture plane that exposes these wall components seems to pass between the persistent outer hyphal wall and newly formed conidial wall. Shadow replicas of intact conidia show only an amorphous layer, indicating that rodlets of *C. immitis* are not exposed on the cell surface. A similar distribution of rodlet fascicles has been reported for arthroconidia of *S. purpurascens* (Cole and Samson, 1979). In each case, the native conidia are extremely hydrophobic, but if the outer wall components are removed by sonication, the cells readily suspend in water and swell, presumably as a result of hydration of the residual cell envelope (Cole *et al.*, 1983). In a recent investigation of rodlet function, conidia produced by a hydrophilic mutant strain of *Neurospora crassa,* easily wettable or *eas* (Selitrennikoff,

1976), were shown to lack rodlet fascicles, while hydrophobic conidia of the wild-type *Neurospora* strain has an intact rodlet layer (Beever and Dempsey, 1978). The latter authors concluded that rodlet fascicles contribute to cell hydrophobicity and to the efficiency of air dissemination of conidia. Drutz and Huppert (1983) have suggested that the outer conidial wall layer of *C. immitis* has an antiphagocytic function and demonstrated that its removal by mechanical means, such as sonication, prompts phagocytosis (>25%) by human polymorphonuclear neutrophils (PMNs). On the other hand, Pesanti (1979) reported that conidia of the *eas* mutant of *N. crassa* were much less readily ingested by macrophage than were the hydrophobic conidia produced by the wild-type strain. The author pointed out that reduced ability to ingest certain bacteria has also been correlated with diminished hydrophobic forces to the cell surface (Van Oss, 1978). No explanation is available for these apparently contradictory results obtained from phagocytic studies of *C. immitis* and *N. crassa.* In any case, both native arthroconidia and those stripped of their outer-wall layer are capable of surviving the attack of PMNs. The cell wall undoubtedly contributes to the survival capacity of conidia within the host.

2.4. Karyology: Mycelium–Arthroconidium Transformation

Details of the nuclear cycle in *C. immitis* are still unresolved, and these represent important gaps in our knowledge of the biology of this respiratory pathogen. The most pressing issue in this regard is whether or not the fungus produces meiospores at some stage of the saprobic or parasitic cycle. The dénouement would contribute significantly to *in vitro* studies of cell synchrony as well as considerations of the taxonomic status of the pathogen. Information available on the saprobic cycle suggests that nuclear events are typical of members of the Fungi Imperfecti that give rise to arthroconidia (Cole 1975)(see Figure 10). Kwon-Chung (1969) described the nucleus in vegetative mycelia of *C. immitis* as a round, dense chromatin mass that develops into a ring with apparently three chromatinic bodies. During nuclear division, the ring opens and becomes rodlike, stretching into a thin filament. The degree of resolution of chromatin in these and subsequent studies, however, is insufficient to determine the karyotype, and controversy persists over the number of chromosomes in each nucleus of the different cell types (Sun and Huppert, 1976). Nevertheless, the light-microscopic observations of Kwon-Chung (1969) are comparable to those reported by Robinow (1981) in his exquisitely illustrated description of mitosis in conidial fungi. His technique, which is a modification of the methodology of Clutterbuck and Roper

(1966), may be particularly useful for further studies of *C. immitis*. Once septation and conidial differentiation begin, the nuclei appear to be distributed within the fertile hypha so that each compartment contains 2–4 nuclei (Figure 15). Such distribution of organelles is probably not entirely random, but involves interaction of signals during septation, nuclear division, and nuclear migration (Raudaskoski, 1970, 1972). On the other hand, a large percentage of the total cytoplasmic and wall material synthesized by the organism during early stages of enteroarthric development is apparently wasted during subsequent events of selected cell autolysis. The chromatin in those cells in Figure 15 that were destined to autolyse appears somewhat diffuse in contrast to that of the adjacent arthroconidia. Once the conidial chain is mature and has begun to disarticulate, chromatin is no longer detected in the degenerate cells (Figures 16 and 17). Comparision of the average number of nuclei in mature conidia (e.g., 60 days, Figure 17) to that of young propagules (e.g., 5-day slide culture, Figure 15) indicates that a reduction in total chromatin has also occurred in these cells, perhaps by a process of selected nuclear abortion. Such an event may have important genetic implications, but to our knowledge has not been examined in this pathogen.

3. PARASITIC CYCLE

3.1. Karyology: Arthroconidium–Spherule–Endospore Transformation

An important milestone in morphogenetic studies of *C. immitis* was reached when Converse (1955, 1956, 1957) defined the physical and chemical conditions for *in vitro* growth of endosporulating spherules (Gilardi, 1965). Although several earlier workers had reported *in vitro* generation of cells of the parasitic cycle (MacNeal and Taylor, 1914; Ciferri and Redaelli, 1936; Lack, 1938, E. E. Baker and Mrak, 1941; E. E. Baker *et al.,* 1943), their results were less consistent than those of Converse. His medium, which was partly based on that of Roessler *et al.* (1946) and later modified slightly by Levine and co-workers (Levine, 1961; Levine *et al.,* 1960), contains basal salts with dextrose and ammonium acetate as the sole sources of organic carbon and nitrogen. With the simple addition of refined agar to modified Converse medium, Brosbe (1967) provided the recipe for a substrate that could be used for rapid conversion of cell types and identification of *C. immitis in vitro* which is still used extensively today (Sun *et al.,* 1976). Initiation of morphogenesis of cell types of the parasitic cycle is witnessed by swelling of the arthroconidia that occurs when these cells are incubated on modified Converse

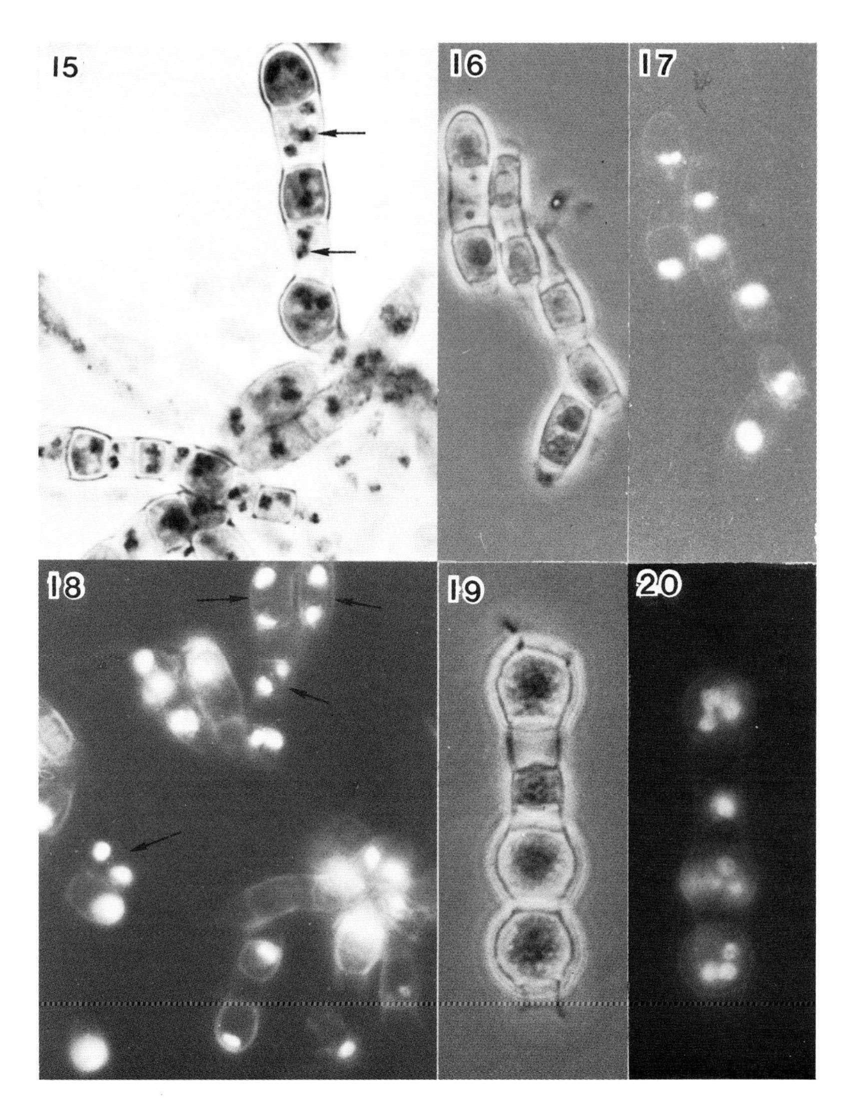

Figures 15–17. Nuclear-stained preparations (15, 17) and phase-contrast micrograph (16) of saprobic phase cells. (15) 5-Day slide culture stained with acetoorcein showing multinucleate cells. Arrows indicate diffuse chromatin in degenerate cells. (16, 17) Matching micrographs of the same cells. The cells in (17), stained with mithramycin (Slater, 1978), are uni- and binucleate. The degenerate cells are enucleate. Magnification: (15) ×1900; (16, 17) × 1800.

Figures 18–20. Nuclear-stained preparations of parasitic-phase cells obtained from modified Converse agar at 12 hr (18) and 24 hr (19, 20) after inoculation with arthroconidia. Arrows in (18) locate binucleate cells. (19, 20) Matching phase-contrast/fluoresence micrographs of the same cells. (18, 20) Mithramycin fluorescent stain. ×1800.

agar at 39–40°C in the presence of 20% CO_2–80% air. Further discussion of the possible significance of CO_2 in cell transformation is presented in Section 3.4. The karyological events associated with the parasitic cycle were examined by Sun and Huppert (1976), and their interpretation is summarized in Figure 1 F–S. The authors suggested that the swollen arthroconidium contains a single nucleus and that this uninucleate condition persists for only a short time (8–24 hr on Converse agar; less in liquid medium). In fact, the duration also varies considerably among strains grown *in vitro.* These same authors reported that the size of the single nucleus in the round cell is approximately 2–3 times greater than each nucleus of the multinucleate conidium. The uninucleate cell continues to round up and soon becomes binucleate (Figure 18). Relatively rapid and apparently synchronous nuclear divisions follow (Figures 19 and 20) to give rise to large, multinucleate spherules (Figures 21 and 22). When mitotic figures are present in the developing spherule, virtually all nuclei are involved in division (Figure 21). Karyokinesis then apparently ceases simultaneously among all nuclei (Figure 22) because mitotic figures are not present during stages of spherule–endospore differentiation. Cessation of mitosis is followed shortly by initiation of spherule septation. This latter process first involves differentiation of multinucleate compartments (Figure 23), but culminates in the formation of uninucleate endospores (arrows in Figure 24) that are clustered in packets surrounded by a thin, membranous layer. The endospores may grow and their nuclei divide while still within the packet or even within the unruptured spherule. These events initiate reproduction of a new generation of endosporulating spherules (see Figure 1H–S). A fundamental difference exists in the nuclear cycle between the first generation beginning with arthroconidia and successive generations initiated with endospores. The mature arthroconidum is multinucleate, but becomes uninucleate early in transformation (i.e., early growth phase). The pivotal but still unresolved problem is whether this change in nuclear content is the result of karyogamy or degeneration of all but one nucleus. In contrast, uninucleate endospores are derived from progressive segmentation of the multinucleate protoplasm in the maturing spherule. The possibility of karyogamy occurring at some stage of spherule maturation cannot be excluded, but careful study of successive preparations shows only an interval of rapid nuclear division followed by a stage in which all nuclei appear in interphase while segmentation proceeds. Thus, although each spherule–endospore cycle begins with a uninucleate cell, the first generation originates from a multinucleate cell in which all but one nucleus have disappeared, while succeeding generations originate from primary uninucleate cells.

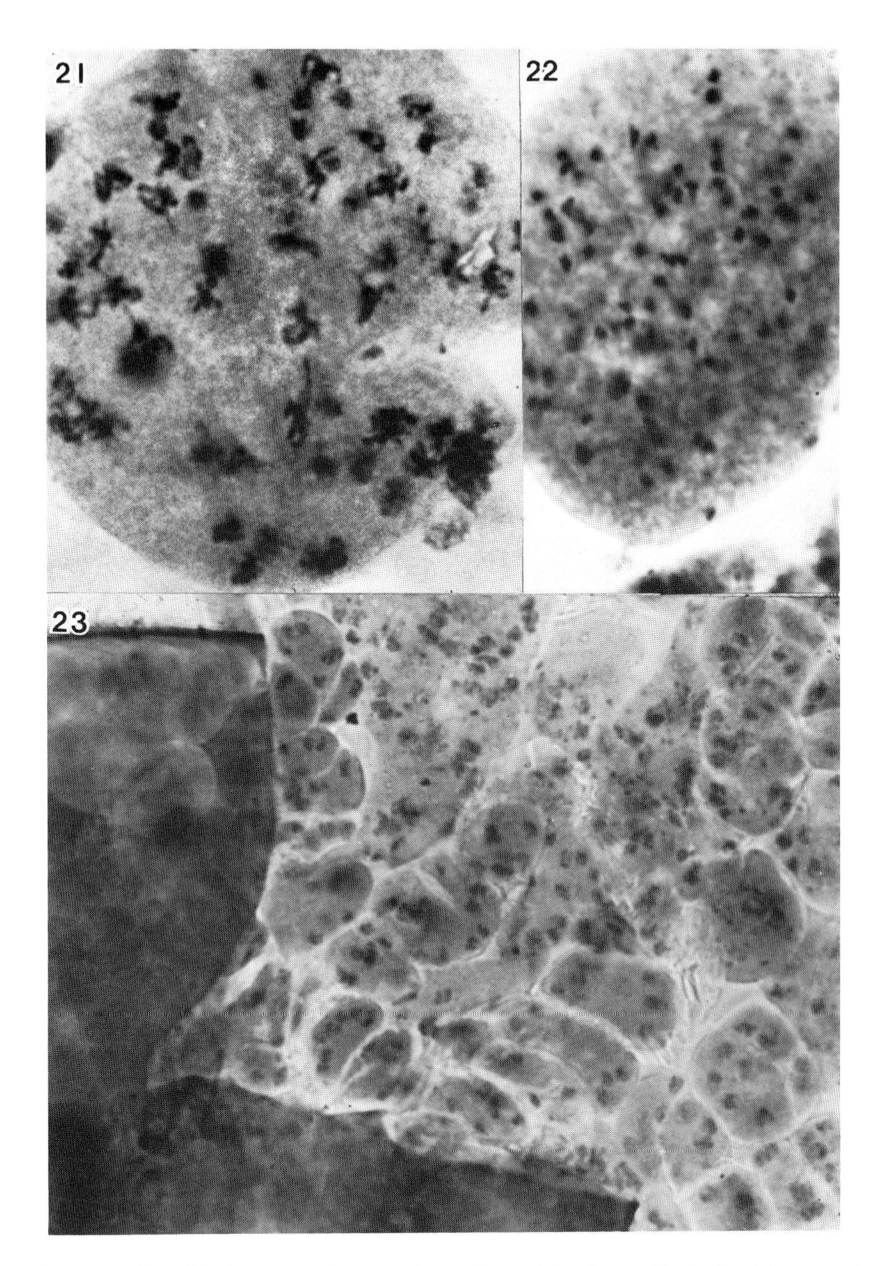

Figures 21–23. Nuclear-stained preparations of parasitic-phase cells obtained from modified Converse agar at approximately 36 hr (21), 48 hr (22), and 72 hr (23) after inoculation with arthroconidia. Note that all nuclei in (21) are in a stage of division, contrasting with the nondividing nuclei in (22). The spherule in (23) was crushed to release multinucleate segments (i.e., still undifferentiated endospore packets). Acetoorcein stain. ×1500.

Current investigations in our laboratories involve use of specific DNA fluorescent stains, such as mithramycin, combined with light-microscopic spectrophotometric analyses to examine the DNA content of individual nuclei in cell types obtained from different stages of the saprobic and parasitic cycles. The aim of these studies is to determine whether a change in ploidy occurs during arthroconidium–spherule or spherule–endospore transformation or both. Because of our inability to isolate uninucleate cells (rounded arthroconidia and endospores) in sufficiently large numbers, application of conventional microfluorimetry and flow cytometry (Roberts and Szaniszlo, 1980) for examining the cell cycle of *C. immitis* has been so far unsuccessful.

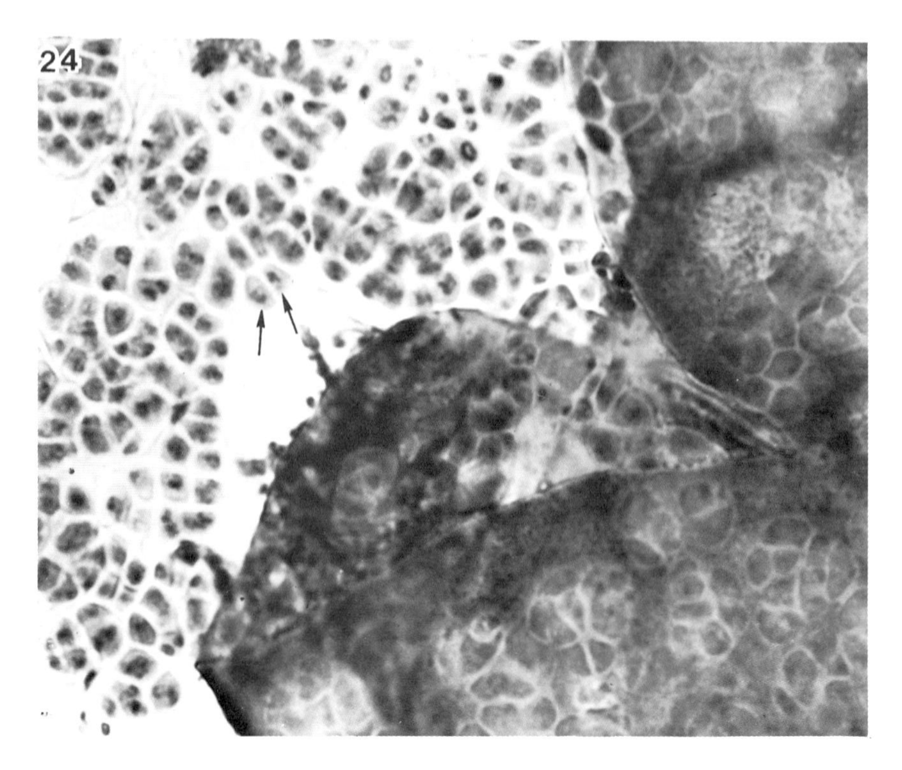

Figure 24. Nuclear-stained preparation of endosporulating spherule 96 hr after inoculation and incubation on Converse agar. Individual, uninucleate endospores (arrows) are enclosed by hyaline, packet membrane. Acetoorcein stain. ×1500.

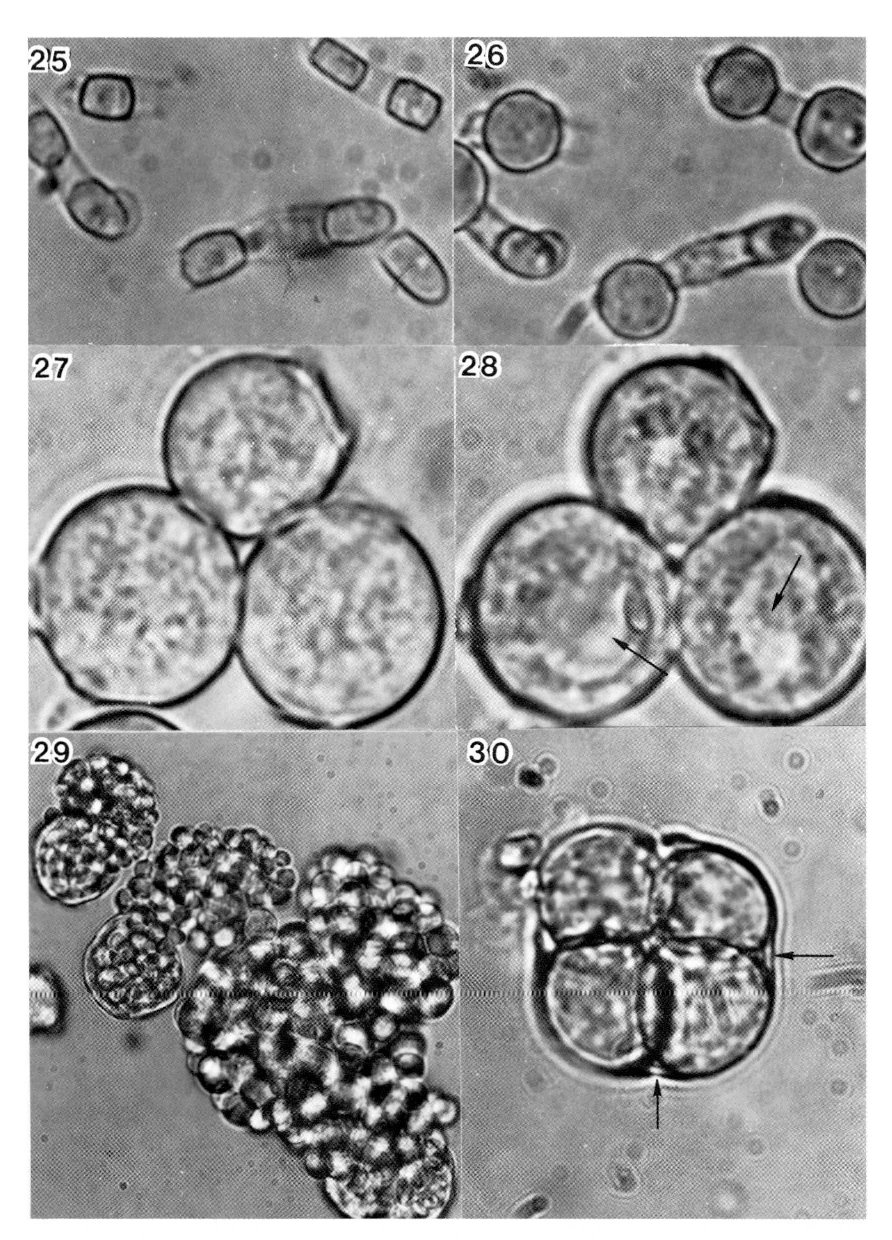

Figures 25–28. Time-lapse photomicrographic sequences of arthroconidial growth phase (25, 26) and spherule segmentation (27, 28) during parasitic cycle *in vitro.* Arrows in (28) locate the central cavity (cf. Figure 31). Time after inoculation of Converse agar: (25) 12 hr; (26) 24 hr; (27) 48 hr; (28) 72 hr. ×1800.

Figures 29 and 30. Endosporulating spherules (29) and released endospore "packet" (30). The latter is a cluster of endospores enclosed by a thin, membranous layer (arrows). Note the difference in the size of endospores (29). The lower spherule in (29) was the first to release endospores that had doubled in size, initiating the second generation of spherules.

3.2. Spherule Segmentation and Endospore Formation

Using a simple slide culture inoculated with arthroconidia and incubated under proper conditions, it is possible to observe stages of spherule and endospore development with the light microscope (Figures 25–28). A diagrammatic interpretation of cell differentiation during this first generation of the parasitic cycle is presented in Figure 31. The conidia in Figure 25 are slightly swollen 12 hr after inoculation of modified Converse agar (Brosbe, 1967), but show an approximate 2-fold increase in volume during the next 12 hr (Figure 26). Over the following 48-hr period (Figures 27 and 28), progressive septation of the spherules occurs. A faint outline of the segmented protoplasm is visible in Figure 27, whereas certain spherules in Figure 28 show a central, vacuolate region (arrows). The latter is suggested to be an optical section of the unsegmented spherule protoplasm. It appears that this central region persists as a cavity throughout endospore differentiation. Each peripheral compartment of the segmented spherule, on the other hand, gives rise to multiple, uninucleate endospores, some of which are released into the central cavity. The endospores continue to grow *in situ* and eventually cause the outer spherule wall to rupture (Figures 29 and 31). Closer examination of the products released from the ruptured spherules reveals that endospores are initially in packets, enclosed by a thin, membranous layer (arrows in Figure 30). However, the latter soon ruptures as a result of endospore growth, and remnants of the packet membrane can subsequently be found on the surface of the endospore wall (see Section 3.3). The endospore packets are about 10 μm in diameter, whereas individual endospores measure only 2–4 μm in diameter and can thus be easily disseminated hematogenously within the host. The remarkable simplicity of the requirements for cell differentiation in *C. immitis* attests further to its uniqueness among microorganisms pathogenic for humans.

3.3. Ultrastructure

Thin sections of different stages of spherule and endospore formation have contributed especially to our understanding of wall differentiation during endosporulation (Sun *et al.*, 1979). The swollen arthroconidium, or round cell, in Figure 32 was formed 24 hr after inoculation of the growth medium. Similar electron-dense and -translucent wall layers are visible as demonstrated by the mature conidia in Figure 12, and the relative thickness of these layers has not significantly changed. Despite an obvious increase in cell volume, no apparent wall synthesis has taken place. Closer examination of the wall ultrastructure, however, reveals a thin, newly formed layer (arrows in the Figure 32 inset) adjacent to the

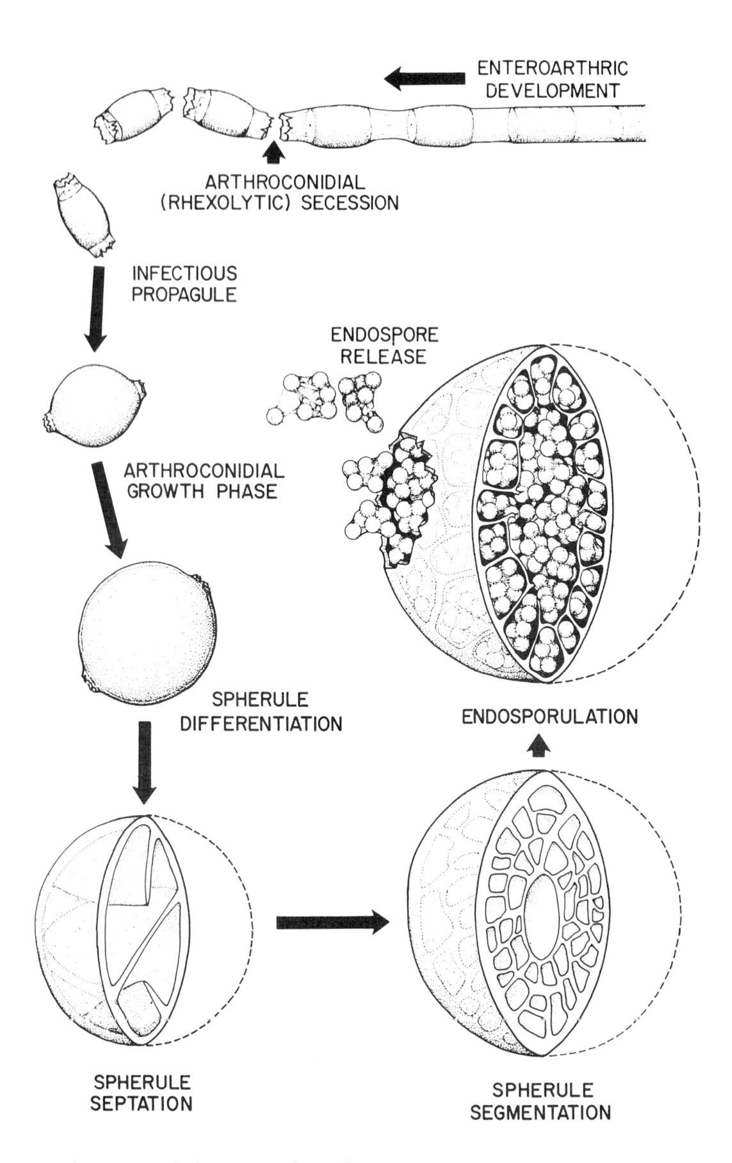

Figure 31. Diagrammatic interpretation of morphogenesis during first-generation arthroconidium–spherule–endospore transformation.

→

Figures 32 and 33. Thin sections of arthroconidial growth phase (32) and initial stage of septation (33). Arrows in the (32) inset locate thin, inner wall layer. The arrow in (33) points to invaginated inner wall. Arrows in the (33) inset locate the newly formed innermost wall layer that corresponds to the thin inner wall in (32). (n) Nucleus; (PM) plasmalemma. Magnification: (32, 33) ×12,000; (insets) ×25,000.

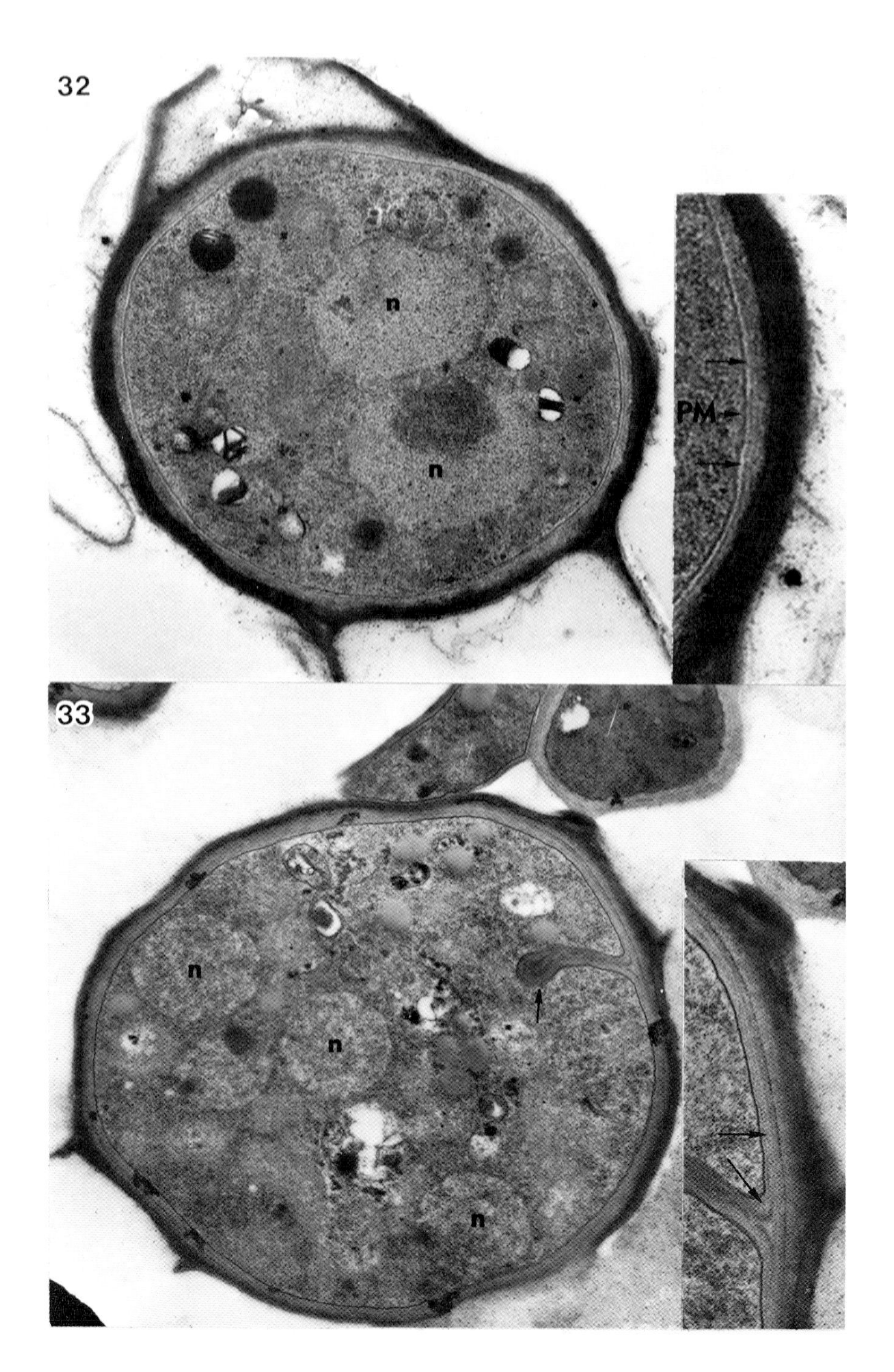
32
n
n
PM
33
n
n
n

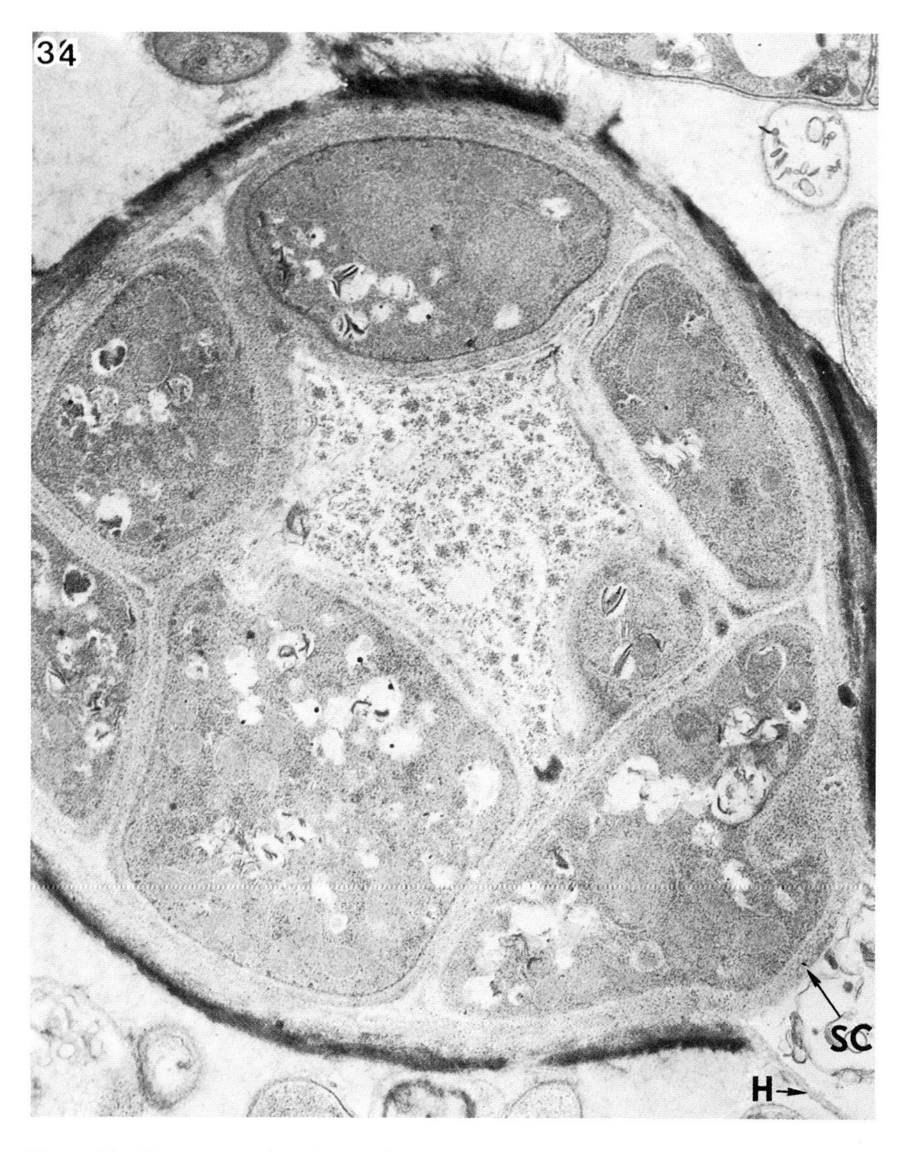

Figure 34. Segmented spherule, showing remnants of fertile hypha (H) and secession scar (SC). Note that the wall enclosing cytoplasmic material is differentiated from the inner and outer wall layers that encompass the spherule. Note also the central cavity, which appears to contain cytoplasmic debris. ×12,000.

plasmalemma (PM). This inner wall layer is more clearly visible in Figure 33. The multinucleate spherule, which was formed after 48 hr incubation, had initiated septation. Note that only the innermost wall layer is continuous with the invaginated wall (arrows in the Figure 33 inset). This same process of wall ingrowth continues and results first in the formation of multinucleate compartments (Figure 34) and ultimately in differentiation of uninucleate endospores. Huppert and Sun (1980a) have referred to the invaginated walls that originate from the inner circumference of the spherule as the primary cleavage planes (see Figure 31). They suggested that these initially fuse, separating the protoplasm into relatively large, multinucleate compartments, and then give rise to secondary cleavage planes that further subdivide the cytoplasmic contents into endospores. In Figure 34, the wall comprising each spherule compartment appears separate from both the outer and inner circumferential layers. The central region appears to be a cavity (cf. Figures 28 and 31) occupied by degenerated cytoplasmic material. It is not yet clear how this central cavity is formed during segmentation. It is also not clear how the endospores differentiate from the primary multinucleate chambers of the segmented spherule. Resolution of these problems will necessitate application of serial-section and freeze–fracture techniques. The compartmentalized interior of the spherule is referred to as a segmentation apparatus to distinguish it from the cleavage apparatus of multispored sporangia produced by certain zygomycetous fungi. In *C. immitis,* endospores are delimited by invagination, growth, and branching of the inner wall of the spherule. In contrast, the thin-section examinations by Bracker (1966, 1968) of sporangial development in *Gilbertella persicaria* have revealed that sporangiospores are formed by coalescence of vesicles to form a tubular cleavage apparatus that subdivides the cytoplasm into spore initials. Thus, resemblance of endosporulating spherules of *C. immitis* to sporangia is only superficial. As endospores emerge from the spherule, almost all are in packets bound by the smooth membranous, outer layer (Figure 35). When the endospores grow and begin to separate, the membrane is reduced to a fibrillar network covering endospores and is stretched or twisted into fibrils that bridge between adjacent spores (Figure 36). Eventually, the fibrils break, leaving freed endospores with the potential to reproduce a new generation of endosporulating spherules. If transferred to conditions that promote saprobic growth, the endospores give rise to one or more germ tubes (Figure 37), and thereby reestablish the mycelial phase.

3.4. *In Vivo* Morphogenesis and Fungus–Host Interaction

The question of whether *in vivo* and *in vitro* development are identical cannot be answered completely as yet. Morphological and ultrastruc-

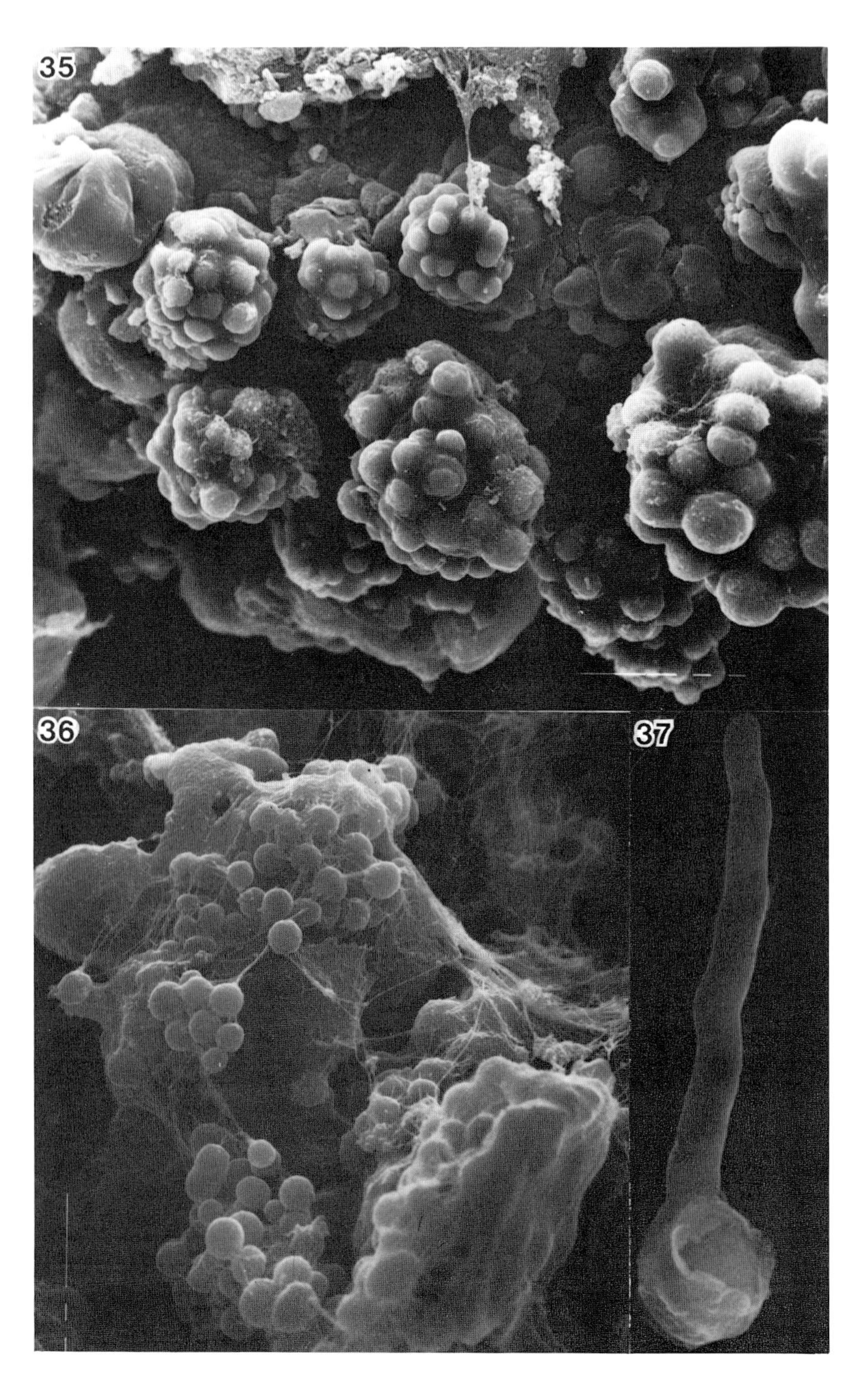
35
36
37

tural details appear the same (Huppert *et al.*, 1983), but comparability of biochemical and antigenic composition has not been ascertained. With respect to this last point, however, we can say that at least some of the antigens produced by the *in vitro*-grown fungus must also be produced by *in vivo* forms, since patients develop immunological responses to apparently specific antigens prepared from the cultured pathogen (Gifford and Catanzaro, 1981; Weiner, 1983). Huppert *et al.* (1983) studied *in vivo* morphogenesis by examining mice infected intranasally with conidia. Transformation into the parasitic cycle was followed by pulmonary lavage at successive intervals. Lavage materials were collected on membranes and processed for electron microscopy. Infected animal lung tissue was also frozen in liquid nitrogen, cryofractured, and subsequently processed for the scanning electron microscope (SEM). As previously discussed, the outer wall of arthroconidia may contain an antiphagocytic factor that provides some protection against host defense. Even if the conidium is phagocytosed, it often remains intact and survives within the host cell (Figure 38). Beaman and Holmberg (1980) determined that alveolar macrophages obtained from rhesus monkeys by bronchial lavage were unable to kill arthroconidia *in vitro,* nor was killing induced by addition of immune serum, complement, or lung lining material extracted from the bronchial lavage fluid. The authors suggested that such inability to kill was at least partly attributable to the failure of phagolysosomal fusion. Using the same *in vitro* assay, the authors also showed that phagocytosed endospores were able to survive and develop into endosporulating spherules while still within alveolar macrophages. On the other hand, Beaman *et al.* (1981) demonstrated that in the presence of lymphocytes from *C. immitis*-immune mice, murine macrophages were capable of killing the pathogen *in vitro.* Such observations attest to the major role of cell-mediated immunity in host defense against *C. immitis* (Drutz and Huppert, 1983).

There is some evidence to suggest that viable leukocytes may actually induce conversion of arthroconidia to spherules and concomitantly inhibit reversion of spherules to the mycelial phase (O. Baker and Braude, 1956; Galgiani *et al.*, 1982). This concept, which was based on *in vitro* studies, has recently been tested using an *in vivo* model (Klotz *et al.*, 1984). A polyallomer chamber inoculated with arthroconidia was implanted subcutaneously into mice. The contents of the chamber and body fluids were separated by a dialysis membrane that allowed the accu-

←

Figures 35–37. Scanning electron micrographs of endospore packets (35) and individual endospores (36) showing fibrous network. (37) An endospore that has germinated on Converse agar. Magnification: (35, 36) ×1100; (37) ×8000.

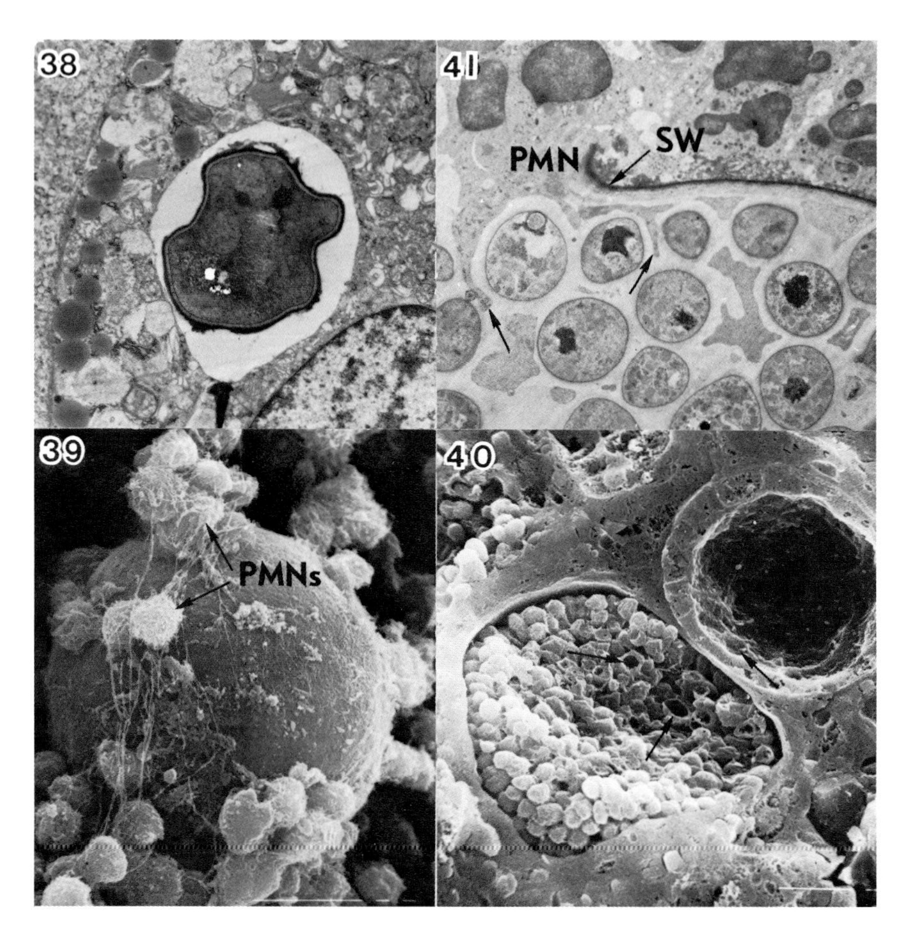

Figures 38–41. Thin sections (38, 41) and SEM preparations (39, 40) showing *in vivo* morphology of pathogen and nature of host interaction. An apparently intact arthroconidium has been engulfed by an alveolar macrophage in (38). Numerous PMNs are attached to the surface of the spherule in (39), the wall of which appears partially digested. Cryofracture of mouse lung tissue (40) reveals two adjacent spherules that contain endospores. Arrows in (40) locate empty chambers of segmentation apparatus. In (41), numerous PMNs adjacent to the opening of the endosporulated spherule were in the process of phagocytosis of endospores (arrows). (SW) Ruptured spherule wall. Magnification: (38) $\times 4000$; (39) $\times 1900$; (40) $\times 2200$; (41) $\times 3500$.

mulation of a sterile dialysate of tissue fluid within the chamber while preventing exchange of cellular elements. The chamber was also equipped with a rubber diaphragm that permitted arthroconidia or exogenous phagocytic cells to be introduced, or cell-free dialysate to be removed for studies *in vitro*. The authors concluded that leukocytes are neither necessary nor beneficial to the process of spherule conversion in their chamber, but rather CO_2 concentration is the pivotal factor affecting morphogenesis. Their results support the conclusions of earlier workers that CO_2 is an essential factor for consistent *in vitro* production of endosporulating spherules (Converse, 1955; Lones and Peacock, 1960). The exact role of CO_2 in regulating development of *C. immitis* is still unresolved.

In experiments involving nonimmune, intranasally challenged mice, Drutz and Huppert (1983) obtained spherules from pulmonary lavages that frequently showed numerous PMNs associated with their surfaces (Figure 39). Most histological studies of coccidioidomycosis indicate, however, that both immature and endosporulating spherules generate a granulomatous, macrophage response in the host (Chandler *et al.*, 1980). Nevertheless, indirect evidence is available that PMNs are capable of digesting at least the surface-wall components of spherules, probably by release of lysozyme, and thereby may reduce the resistance of the pathogen to subsequent attack by macrophages (Collins and Pappagianis, 1973; Drutz and Huppert, 1983). The cryofracture of an infected mouse lung in Figure 40 shows two adjacent, thick-walled spherules, one still containing many endospores. Visible in both spherules are empty compartments (arrows) that represent remnants of the segmentation apparatus (see Figure 31). On the basis of ultrastructural studies, Drutz and Huppert (1983) have suggested that when endospores excape from a ruptured spherule, they generate a chemotactic response of PMNs (Figure 41). Despite this apparent mobilization of phagocytes, *in vitro* studies with human PMNs indicate that only 10–20% of ingested endospores are killed (Drutz and Huppert, 1983). In addition, young endospores are commonly released from spherules still within membrane-bound packets (cf. Figure 35), and at least some of these are consequently inaccessible to phagocytes. As the surviving endospores begin to transform into the next generation of spherules, a new wave of macrophages attack and engulf the cells. However, the pathogen has often firmly established residence in the host at this stage, since hundreds of endospores have been released from the first generation of spherules. Survival and sporulation of a few of these newly formed spherules provide for further dissemination of the fungus. Thus, *C. immitis* is a formidable pathogen and is apparently well equipped to survive in the hostile environment of the host.

4. CELL ENVELOPE

4.1. Wall Isolation and Chemical Composition

The majority of fungus–host interactions involve cell surfaces, as in phagocytosis; therefore, comprehension of the nature of both the microbial and host envelope and its respective role in host–parasite interactions is crucial to a proper understanding of microbial pathogenicity (H. Smith, 1977). The cell wall of *C. immitis* has been receiving particular attention as the primary site of interaction between host and fungal cells. Justification for this lies in evidence that spherule walls contain antigen(s) capable of protecting experimental animals against fatal disease challenge (Lecara *et al.,* 1983), that enzyme treatment of spherule walls releases clinically significant antigens (Collins *et al.,* 1977), that extracts of mycelial and spherule walls elicit cell-mediated immune responses among sensitized hosts (Huppert, 1983), and that arthroconidial walls possess an antiphagocytic factor and, even when phagocytosed after opsonization, may be responsible for protecting the fungus against intracellular killing by host phagocytes (Drutz and Huppert, 1983).

Several early investigations involved analysis of total carbohydrate and protein content of cell walls of *C. immitis* (Blank and Burke, 1954; Pappagianis and Kobayashi, 1958, 1960; McNall, 1962; Tarbet and Breslau, 1953; Goldschmidt and Taylor, 1958). More recently, the chemical composition of mycelial and arthroconidial walls has been reported by Wheat and co-workers (Wheat *et al.,* 1977, 1978; Wheat and Chung, 1977; Wheat and Scheer, 1977), who noted that protein and *N*-acetylglucosamine together constitute about 50% of the isolated mycelial wall, whereas other polysaccharides account for most of the remainder. Comparison of amino acid content of whole arthroconidial and mycelial walls revealed significant differences, while the carbohydrate composition showed basic similarities, with glucosamine, glucose, and mannose as the major components. A minor constituent of both the mycelial and the arthroconidial wall was 3-*O*-methylmannose (Porter *et al.,* 1971), originally characterized as an extracellular polysaccharide by Goldschmidt and Taylor (1958). While these earlier studies all involved examinations of whole cell walls obtained from homogenized mycelia, arthroconidia, and spherules, Cole *et al.* (1982, 1983, 1985a,b) have mechanically dissected the walls of different cell types into outer and inner fractions and compared their chemical composition. A crucial aspect of the latter investigations was the methodology for obtaining relatively pure suspensions of cells from selected stages of the saprobic and parasitic cycles. Sporulating mycelia were grown on GYE medium in petri dishes incubated for 60 days at 24°C in continuous darkness. The conidia were collected from plates using a vacuum harvesting apparatus (Cole *et al.*, 1983), and high yields ($\approx 1 \times 10^{10}$ conidia from 8–10 petri plates) were obtained with virtually no contaminating mycelia. *In vitro* production of spherules and endospores was achieved using the specially equipped

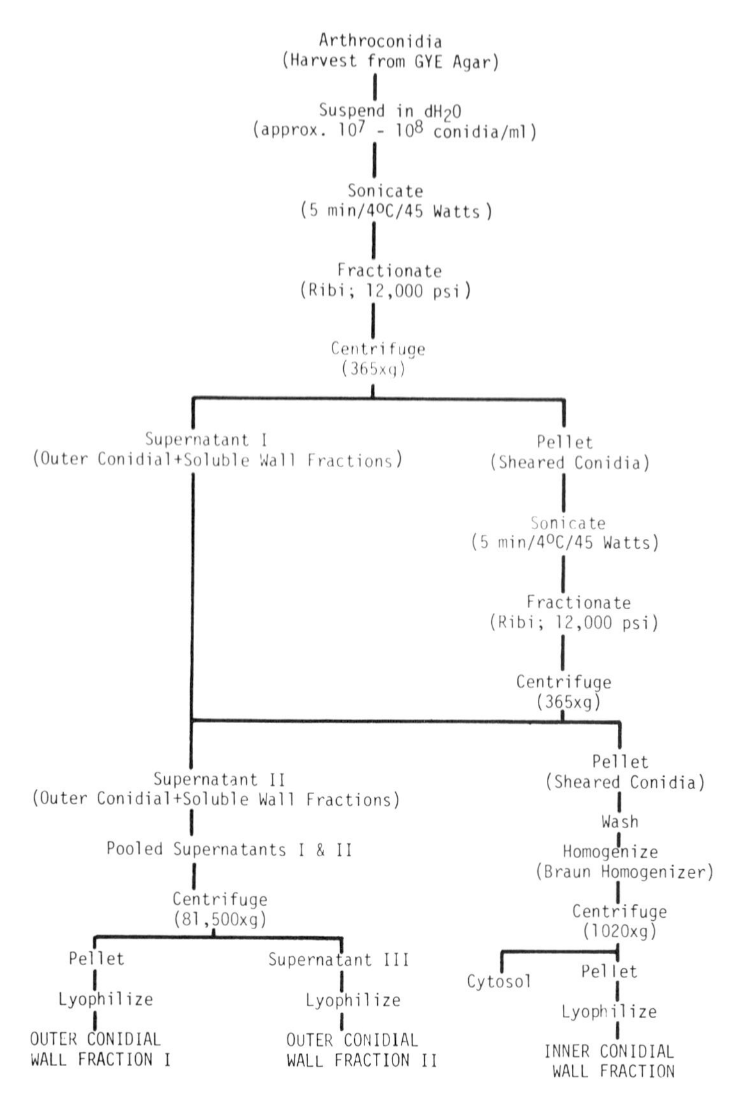

Figure 42. Outline of the procedure for isolation and purification of outer and inner arthroconidial wall fractions of *C. immitis*. (After Cole *et al.*, 1982.)

flasks (Cole *et al.*, 1985b). Either an 1800-ml or a 250-ml Erlenmeyer flask was used containing 800 or 100 ml, respectively, of modified Converse medium (Levine *et al.*, 1960). In each case, the inoculum contained a final concentration of 10^6 conidia/ml obtained from GYE agar plates. In the case of strain C634, presegmented, segmented, and endosporulating spherules were obtained after growth for 48, 72, and 96 hr, respectively. Cell morphogenesis was fairly synchronous, perhaps because 60- to 90-day ("dormant") conidia were used as the inoculum. Endospores of variable size were separated from ruptured and intact spherules by differential centrifugation. Individual endospores were further released from unruptured spherules and endospore packets (cf. Fig. 30) by sonication of the cell suspension (3 × 5 min, 4°C, 45W) using a Branson sonicator (Branson Sonic Power Co., Danbury, Connecticut).

Surface-wall components were separated from the inner-wall layer of different cell types by a succession of treatments using an ultrasonicator, a Ribi cell fractionator (Sorvall Model RF-1, refrigerated), and a Braun homogenizer (Model MSK, Bronwill Scientific, Inc., Rochester, New York). An outline of the procedure used for isolation and purification of outer and inner arthroconidial wall fractions is presented in Figure 42. Results of the sonication–Ribi fractionation treatment are shown in Figures 43 and 44. The stripped conidia are slightly swollen (Figure 43), probably as a result of hydration of their cell wall, but show the same viability (85–90%) as untreated conidia. The outer-wall components (Figure 44) were separated from stripped conidia by differential centrifugation, and the pooled supernatants were subsequently partitioned into an 81,500*g* pellet and supernatant. The latter are referred to as outer conidial wall fractions I (OCWI) and II (OCWII), respectively. OCWII contained any solubilized components released during the cell "shearing" procedure. The stripped but unruptured conidia were homogenized, and the inner conidial wall (ICW in Figure 45) was separated from the cytosol and washed several times. All fractions were examined by electron microscopy and lyophilized in preparation for chemical analysis.

A striking but not surprising feature of the inner conidial wall was the presence of a network of intertwined fibrils (Figure 46), which is characteristic of the arrangement of chitin microfibrils. No such layer was observed in the outer-wall fractions. Comparative analysis of the chemical composition of the conidial-wall fractions confirmed that ICW contained the highest percentage of amino sugars (Table I) and that glucosamine was the only amino sugar present. Spectrophotometric analysis of released *N*-acetylglucosamine using the method of Reissig *et al.* (1955) suggested that most hexosamine in ICW occurred as chitin. Comparison of the carbohydrate, protein, and lipid content also showed that differences exist between the conidial wall fractions. The higher protein and

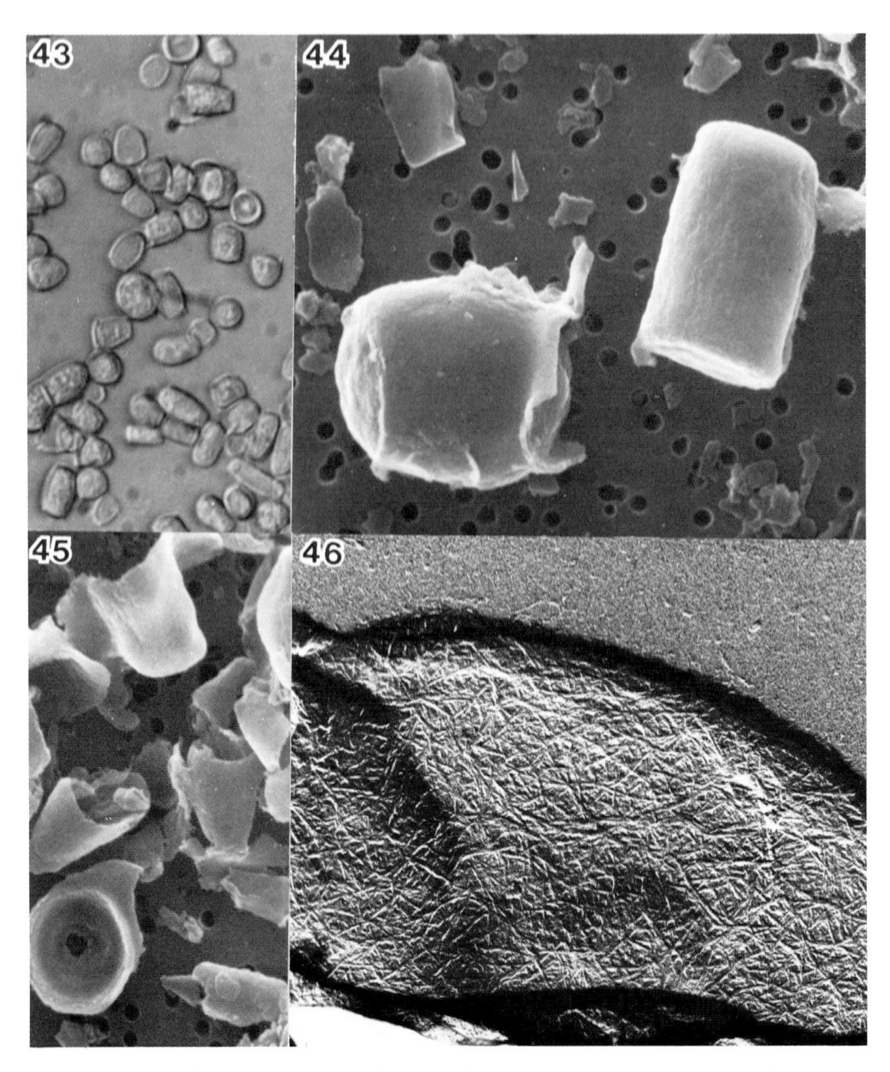

Figures 43–46. Sheared arthroconidia (43, 44) and isolated inner conidial wall (45, 46) obtained by the procedure outlined in Figure 42. Note that few cells are ruptured after the shearing process (43) and that conidia are effectively stripped of their outer wall layer (44). A shadow replica of the isolated inner conidial wall shows a network of microfibrils reminiscent of chitin. Sheared conidia and inner conidial wall were collected on a Nuclepore filter for SEM preparation. Magnification: (43) ×1500; (44, 45) ×5000; (46) ×45,000.

Table I
Summary of the Chemical Composition of Outer and Inner Conidial Wall Fractions and 48-Hour Whole Spherule Wall of *C. immitis* Strain 634[a]

	Conidial wall fractions			
	Outer			
	Fraction I (%)	Fraction II (%)	Inner (%)	Whole spherule wall (%)
Total neutral carbohydrate				
By GLC[b]	12.0	31.6	32.3	42.0
By anthrone[c]	(3.2)	(5.3)	(20.5)	(24.9)
Mannose[d]	(64.6)	(30.3)	(45.8)	(36.4)
Glucose[d]	(22.5)	(58.7)	(35.1)	(46.1)
Galactose[d]	(11.5)	(7.9)	(7.1)	(5.0)
3-*O*-Methylmannose[d]	(1.4)	(3.1)	(12.0)	(12.5)
Total hexosamine	1.7	0.6	21.9	26.6
Peptides	49.8[e]	28.5[e]	27.4[e]	17.1[e]
	(29.0)[f]	(21.5)[f]	(15.5)[f]	(10.5)[f]
	(21.8)[g]	(8.1)[g]	(12.9)[g]	(7.8)[g]
Lipids				
Readily extractable	15.4	7.4	4.5	4.0
Bound	9.7	5.2	12.9	6.5
Other	NM[i]	20.0[h]	NM	NM
Ash	NM	ND[j]	ND	NM
Phosphorus	0.1	ND	0.02	0.02
Recovery	88.7	93.3	99.0	96.2

[a]Values are expressed as percentages of total dry weight of each wall fraction.
[b]Determined by summation of monosaccharides identified by gas–liquid chromatographic (GLC) analysis.
[c]Percentage of total neutral carbohydrate based on the anthrone method. These values were not used to calculate recovery.
[d]Monosaccharide content is expressed as percentage of total neutral carboydrate. The content was determined by GLC analysis. These values were not used to calculate recovery.
[e]Determined by the Kjeldahl method (Kabat and Mayer, 1961; Campbell *et al.*, 1970).
[f]Determined by the Lowry method. These values were not used to calculate recovery.
[g]Determined by summation of amino acids. These values were not used to calculate recovery.
[h]Lyophilized pigment component obtained from methanol–H_2O layer during isolation of readily extractable lipids from outer conidial wall fraction II.
[i]Not measurable.
[j]Not determined.

lipid content of OCWI may reflect the presence of the rodlet layer (cf. Figure 14), which was largely removed during sonication and fractionation (Cole *et al.*, 1983). Reports concerning other fungi indicate that morphologically similar wall components are mainly proteinaceous (Beever *et al.*, 1979) or lipoproteinaceous in nature (Cole and Pope, 1981). A major component of OCWII is an amber-colored pigment that was isolated in the methanol–water layer during lipid extraction of the purified wall fraction. Although the chemical composition of this pigment is unknown, its infrared spectrum is not characteristic of melanin (Li, 1983). Whole-wall preparations of 48-hr, presegmented spherules were also obtained by homogenization, and the chemical composition of this fraction was compared to that of the conidial fractions (Table I). The spherule and inner conidial-wall fractions demonstrate the highest carbohydrate/protein ratios, and their most abundant monosaccharides are mannose, glucose, and 3-*O*-methylmannose. Further discussion of the distribution and earlier speculations on immunogenicity of the methylated polysaccharide in *C. immitis* is presented in Section 4.2. Using an alternative approach to compositional analysis, which involved enzymatic dissection of the spherule wall, Hector and Pappagianis (1982) have demonstrated that the inner wall is a matrix of chitin and β(1-3)-glucan. On the other hand, the outer portion of the spherule wall was determined to be largely α(1-3)-glucan. The authors suggested that a mannan–protein complex was interspersed throughout the wall and was effective in binding the layers together as well as anchoring the wall to the cell membrane.

Our recent attempts to mechanically dissect the cell wall (Cole *et al.*, 1985b) have permitted isolation and purification of inner- and outer-wall fractions of the principal cell types of both the saprobic and parasitic cycles (Figures 47 and 48). The aim of these studies is to critically analyze the chemical composition of each fraction. Our earlier investigations have demonstrated that clear quantitative and certain qualitative differences exist between wall fractions of selected cell types (Cole *et al.*, 1983). It seems logical that during initial contact and subsequent interaction of conidia, spherules, and endospores with host tissue, different spectra of chemical components may be presented to the host, which in turn may generate different host responses. The available information about immunoreactivity to cells of selected stages of the parasitic cycle indicates that differences in host response do occur (see Section 3.4). Analysis of the antigenic composition of solubilized wall fractions, using a coccidioidin/anticoccidioidin (CDN/anti-CDN) reference system (Huppert *et al.*, 1979), also reveals that immunological differences exist between cell types. Thus, *C. immitis* represents both a primary fungal pathogen with a morphogenetically unique parasitic cycle and an excellent model for evaluating the role of cell-wall antigens in host response.

4.2. Identification of Wall Antigens

Coccidioidin (CDN), which was prepared by the method of Huppert *et al.* (1978), was used as the source material in our analysis of the antigenic content of the wall fractions. The two-dimensional immuno-

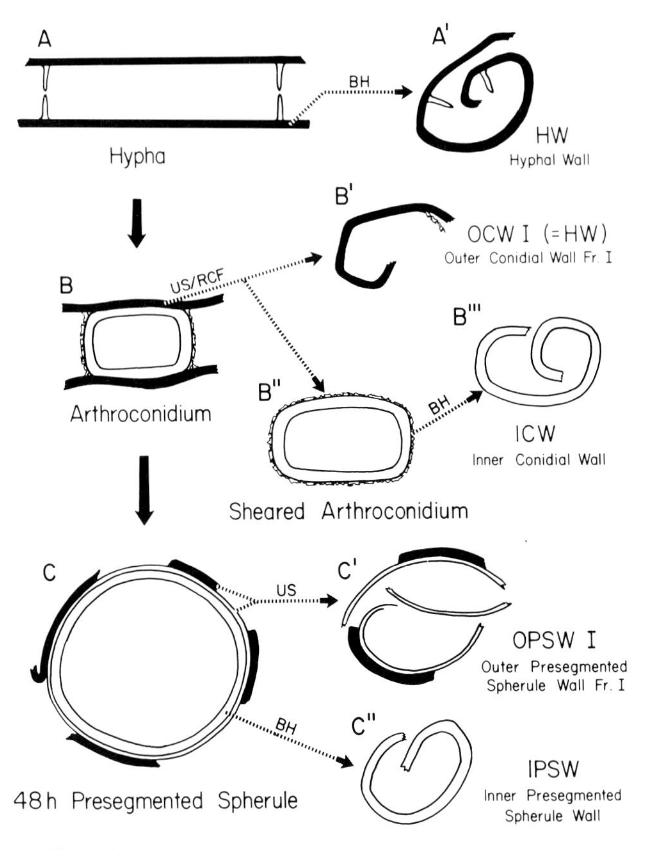

Figures 47 and 48. Diagrammatic representations of various cell types of the saprobic and parasitic cycles, and cell-wall fractions isolated from each cell type by Braun homogenization (BH), ultrasonication (US), and Ribi cell fractionation (RCF).

electrophoresis (2D-IEP) procedure employed for antigen detection has a sensitivity of 10–100 ng (Axelsen, 1971, 1973, 1975). Huppert *et al.* (1978, 1979) used anti-CDN serum of a hyperimmunized burro in the 2D-IEP technique to demonstrate at least 26 antigens (Ags) in CDN and thereby established a reference system for monitoring antigenic content of various soluble extracts (Figure 49). We extracted antigens from lyophilized wall fractions either with 1 N NaOH using a modification of the method of Cox and Larsh (1974) or with phosphate-buffered saline (PBS), (pH 7.4). In the former extraction procedure, the wall material was not pretreated with trypsin, but rather was suspended directly in 1 N NaOH (1 mg sample/ml), agitated for 3 hr at room temperature on a wrist-action

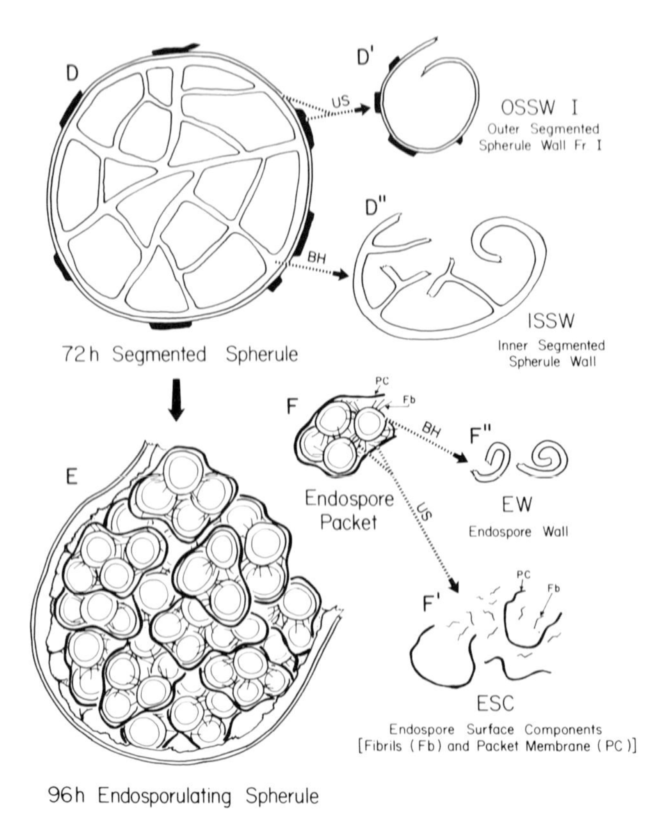

Figures 47 and 48. *(continued)*

shaker, centrifuged (27,000*g*), and the supernatant dialyzed (cutoff: mol. wt. 12,000–14,000) against distilled water (4 changes) at 4°C for 48 hr. The retentate was lyophilized and then resolubilized in PBS for analysis of Ag composition. The PBS or alkali-soluble water-soluble (ASWS) extracts were concentrated by ultrafiltration as required (Minicon B-15; Amicon Corp.). The cell-wall antigens were identified in gels both by the tandem 2D-IEP method (Figure 50) as modified by Cox *et al.* (1984) and by including an internal reference of bovine serum albumin (BSA) added to the antigen well and anti-BSA added to agarose in the second-dimension gel (Figure 51). Measurement of the peak of antigen–antibody precipitates in both dimensions from the well center, relative to that for BSA/anti-BSA, identified antigen–antibody reactions in the test plates (Figures 50 and 51) compared with those in the reference plate (Figure 49) (Cole *et al.,* 1983). The wall antigens were designated by numbers according to the CDN/anti-CDN reference system. The burro immuno-

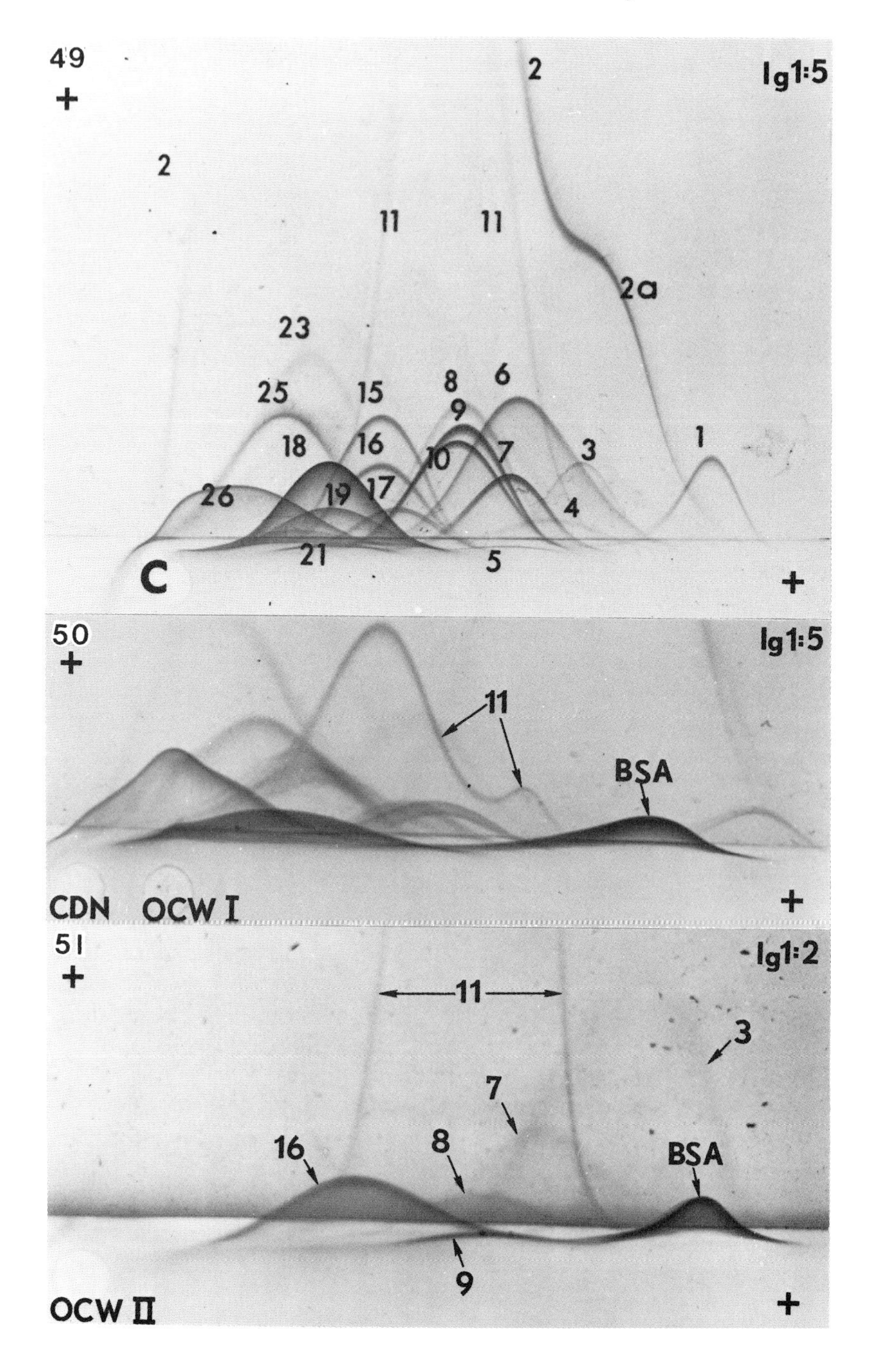
49
+
2
Ig1:5
2
11
11
2a
23
25
15
8
6
9
1
18
16
10
7
3
26
19
17
4
21
5
C
+
50
+
Ig1:5
11
BSA
CDN
OCW I
+
51
+
Ig1:2
11
3
7
16
8
BSA
9
OCW II
+

globulin concentrations were 1:2, 1:5, or 1:8 dilutions of precipitated immunoglobulin reconstituted to 5 mg protein/ml electrophoresis buffer. A summary of the antigenic composition of arthroconidial and 48-hr spherule wall fractions is presented in Table II. This may not represent the complete spectrum of wall antigens present, especially since all material in certain fractions was not solubilized by PBS or alkali treatment. Also, some antigens may have been lost from inner-wall fractions during repeated washing to remove cytoplasmic material. Collins *et al.* (1977) demonstrated that chitinase digestion of the cell wall yielded a supernatant rich in antigens, contrasting with the comparatively few antigens solubilized in buffer. Application of purified and immobilized enzyme extraction or other solubilizing procedures (e.g., Wheat *et al.*, 1983) may yield additional antigens from the isolated wall fractions. Use of an alternative antigen–antibody reference system, such as hyperimmunized goat antiserum against CDN derived from a large number of clinical isolates, is at present under investigation in our laboratories. Nevertheless, our results have revealed that antigenic differences between arthroconidial and spherule walls do exist, and these may be a reflection of the chemical differentiation reported in Table I. The relative ease of isolation and purification of wall fractions and the high degree of reproducibility of their chemical and antigenic composition provide the basis for further purification of clinically relevant antigens.

Our attention has recently focused on the distribution of a prominent antigen, identified as Ag 2, in the various wall fractions of *C. immitis.* Cox and co-workers have reported that this is the sole antigen in ASWS extracts of mycelial and spherule walls (Cox *et al.,* 1984). They have also demonstrated that the ASWS extract exhibits delayed-type hypersensitivity in *Coccidioides*-sensitized guinea pigs (Ward *et al.,*

←

Figure 49. Two-dimensional immunoelectrophoresis of CDN against burro immunoglobulin in the second dimension. The cathode is at the C-well end of the plate. The dilution of immunoglobulin (Ig) used was 1:5, which displays most of the 26 antigens of the CDN/anti-CDN reference system. (+) Indicates anodes and direction of migration in each dimension. (Procedure from Huppert *et al.,* 1979.)

Figures 50 and 51. Immunoelectrophoresis plates of outer conidial wall fraction I (50) and II (51). (50) Tandem 2D-IEP (PBS wall extract of OCWI, concentrated 10-fold, Ig 1:5) showing fusion between Ag 11 of the CDN reference antigen and Ag 11 in the wall extract. (51) 2D-IEP (PBS wall extract of OCWII, concentrated 10-fold, Ig 1:2) showing six antigen–antibody precipitins (numbered 3, 7, 8, 9, 11, and 16 according to the CDN/anti-CDN reference system). A BSA/anti-BSA system was added as a reference antigen–antibody precipitin. (+) Indicates anodes and direction of migration in each dimension. (From Cole *et al.,* 1983.)

Table II
Antigens Detected in Phosphate-Buffered Saline and Alkali-Soluble Water-Soluble Extracts of Arthroconidial and 48-Hour Spherule Wall Fractions[a]

Reference antigen number[b]	Extracts of wall fractions[c]											
	OCWI		OCWII		ICW		OSWI		OSWII		ISW	
	PBS	ASWS	PBS	ASWS	PBS	ASWS	PBS	ASWS	PBS	ASWS	PBS	ASWS
2	+	+	+	+	+	+	+	+	+	+	+	+
3	−	−	+	−	−	−	−	−	−	−	−	−
6	−	−	+	−	−	−	−	−	−	−	−	−
7	−	−	+	−	−	−	−	−	−	−	−	−
8	−	−	+	−	−	−	−	−	+	−	−	−
9	−	−	+	−	−	−	−	−	−	−	−	−
11	+	−	+	−	−	−	+	−	+	−	−	−
12a	−	−	−	−	−	−	−	−	+	−	−	−
16	−	−	+	−	−	−	−	−	−	−	−	−
25	−	−	−	−	−	−	−	−	?[d]	−	−	−
26	−	−	−	−	−	−	−	−	?[d]	−	−	−

[a](+)Identified by 2D-IEP using internal reference peak (BSA/anti-BSA) and confirmed by tandem 2D-IEP and advancing-line IEP with reference CDN/anti-CDN system. (−) Not detected.
[b]Based on the CDN/anti-CDN reference system (Huppert *et al.*, 1978, 1979).
[c](OCWI) Outer conidial wall fraction I; (OCWII) outer conidial wall fraction II; (ICW) inner conidial wall; (OSWI) outer 48-hr spherule wall fraction I; (OSWII) outer 48-hr spherule wall fraction II; (ISW) inner 48-hr spherule wall fraction; (PBS) phosphate-buffered saline; (ASWS) alkali-soluble/water-soluble.
[d]Not confirmed.

1975), confers immunoprotection to mice against intranasal challenge with viable arthroconidia (Lecara *et al.*, 1983), and is effective in detecting anti-*Coccidioides* IgE serum antibody (Cox and Arnold, 1979) and IgM tube precipitin antibody (Cox *et al.*, 1984). Of particular interest is that one of the monosaccharide components of the ASWS extract is 3-*O*-methylmannose (3-*O*-MM) (Olsberg and Cox, 1983), a sugar that has been suspected to be unique to *C. immitis* (San-Blas, 1982; Wheat *et al.*, 1983). Although 3-*O*-methylated heteromannans have been identified in prokaryotes (Nimmich, 1970; Maitra and Ballou, 1974), no reports of this sugar in other fungi have been published. The questions that we have raised are whether 3-*O*-MM is, in fact, unique to *C. immitis* and whether the occurrence of this sugar correlates with the presence of Ag 2. Gas chromatography and mass spectroscopy were used to characterize synthesized 3-*O*-MM (Figure 52), which was subsequently employed as a standard to determine the distribution of the methylated sugar in wall extracts of *C. immitis* as well as those of other pathogenic and nonpathogenic fungi (Cole *et al.*, 1985a). For example, in Figure 53, gas chromatographs and mass spectra of trimethylsilyl (TMS) methylglycosides of neutral sugars present in *Blastomyces dermatitidis* and *Malbranchea dendritica* cell walls are demonstrated. Comparison of retention times and mass spectra to those of the standard confirms the absence of 3-*O*-MM in *B. dermatitidis* but its presence in *M. dendritica.* The possible taxonomic relatedness of *C. immitis* and *M. dendritica* is further supported by the common presence of this unusual sugar. Similar analysis of the cell walls of *Aspergillus fumigatus, Histoplasma capsulatum,* and *Candida albicans* failed to detect 3-*O*-MM.

Because of the suspected correlation between occurrence of 3-*O*-MM and presence of Ag 2, the advancing-line IEP technique (Reiss *et al.*, 1985) was used to examine the antigenic content of solubilized wall extracts of these same fungi. The advancing-line IEP plate (e.g., Figure 54) is composed of three separately prepared agarose gels that are as follows: a lower gel with barbital buffer (pH 8.6), an upper gel with precipitated and resolubilized immunoglobulins from burro anti-CDN serum, and an intermediate gel with the CDN reference antigen at a dilution of 1:128 in barbital buffer. The antigen placed in the cathodal well is also CDN, but at a dilution of 1 : 8 in buffer. This dilution was optimal for development of a major antigen–antibody precipitate in the upper gel. The base of this peak is continuous with a precipitin line that has advanced from the intermediate gel. The antigen has been identified as Ag 2 on the basis of comparison to the reference system (Huppert *et al.*, 1979). Solubilized extracts of cell walls were added to the anodal wells and subjected to one-dimensional ("rocket") IEP. Distortion of the precipitin line of Ag 2 confirms the presence of this antigen in the anodal

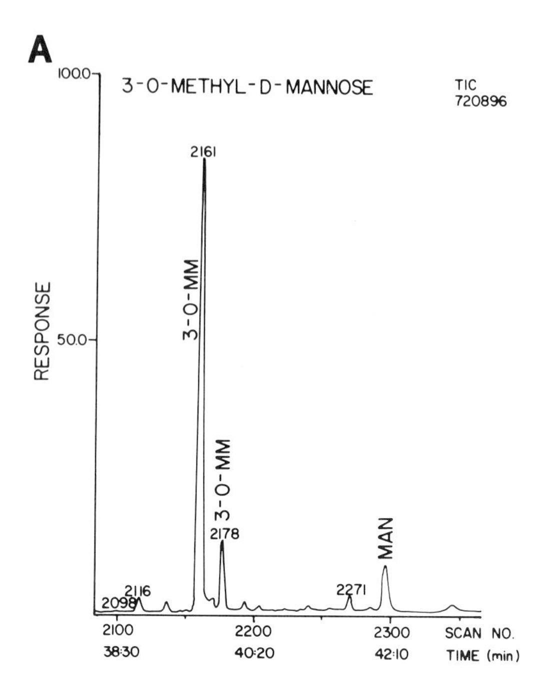

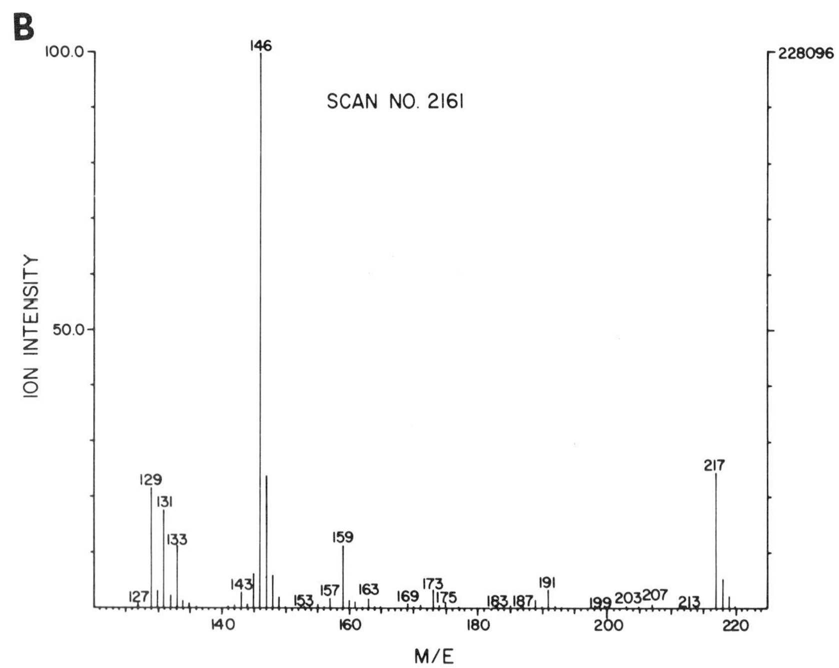

Figure 52. GLC spectrum of TMS derivative of synthesized 3-*O*-methyl-D-mannose (A, kindly supplied by R. W. Wheat) using a 50-m BP1 capillary column and temperature program [40°C (2 min) 5C°/min to 260°C]. Positive ion mass spectra of α- and β-isomers of

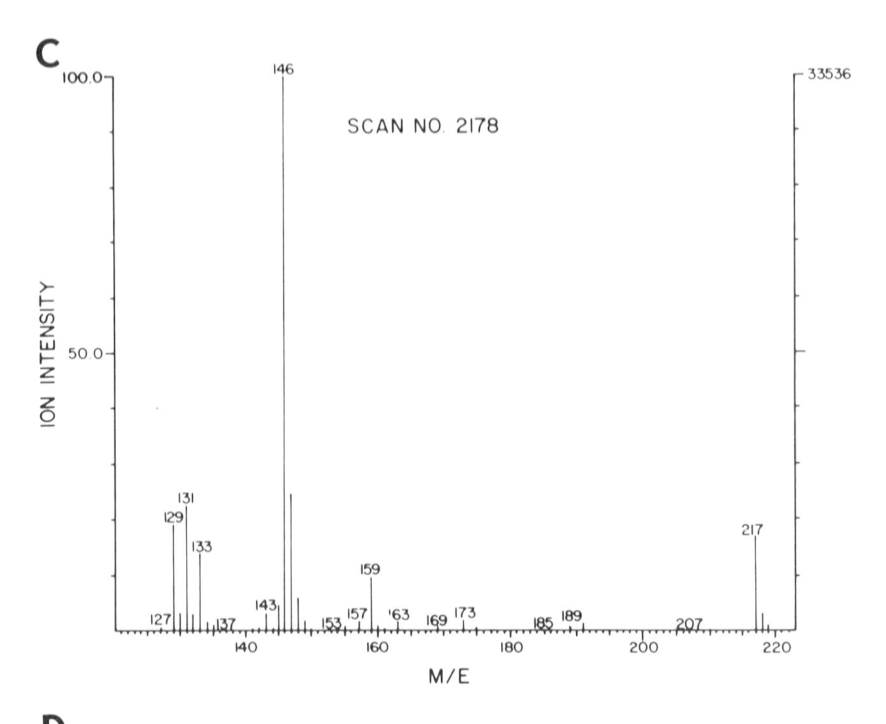

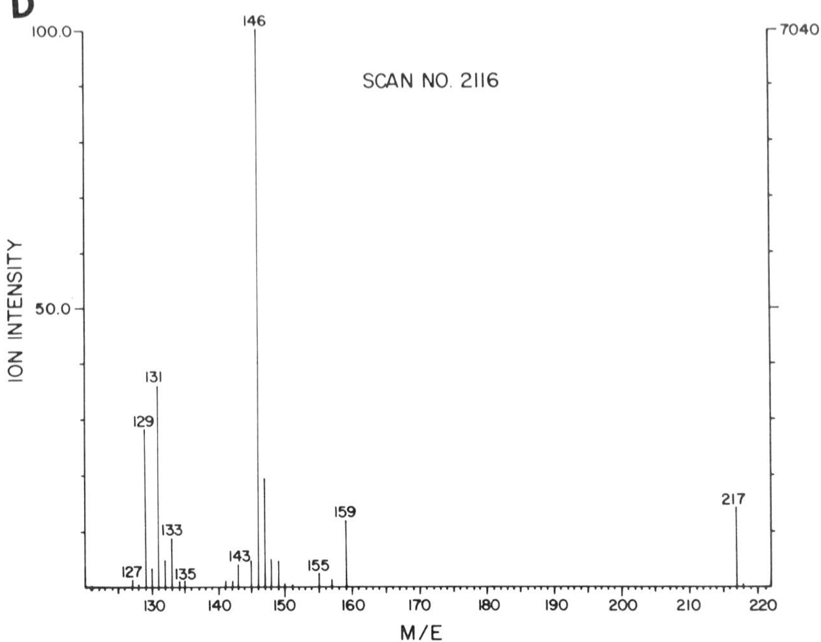

synthesized sugar (B and C, respectively) and compound designated by scan No. 2116 (D) suspected to be third isomer of same sugar. (3-*O*-MM) 3-*O*-Methylmannose; (MAN) mannose; (TIC) total ion count. (From Cole *et al.*, 1985a.)

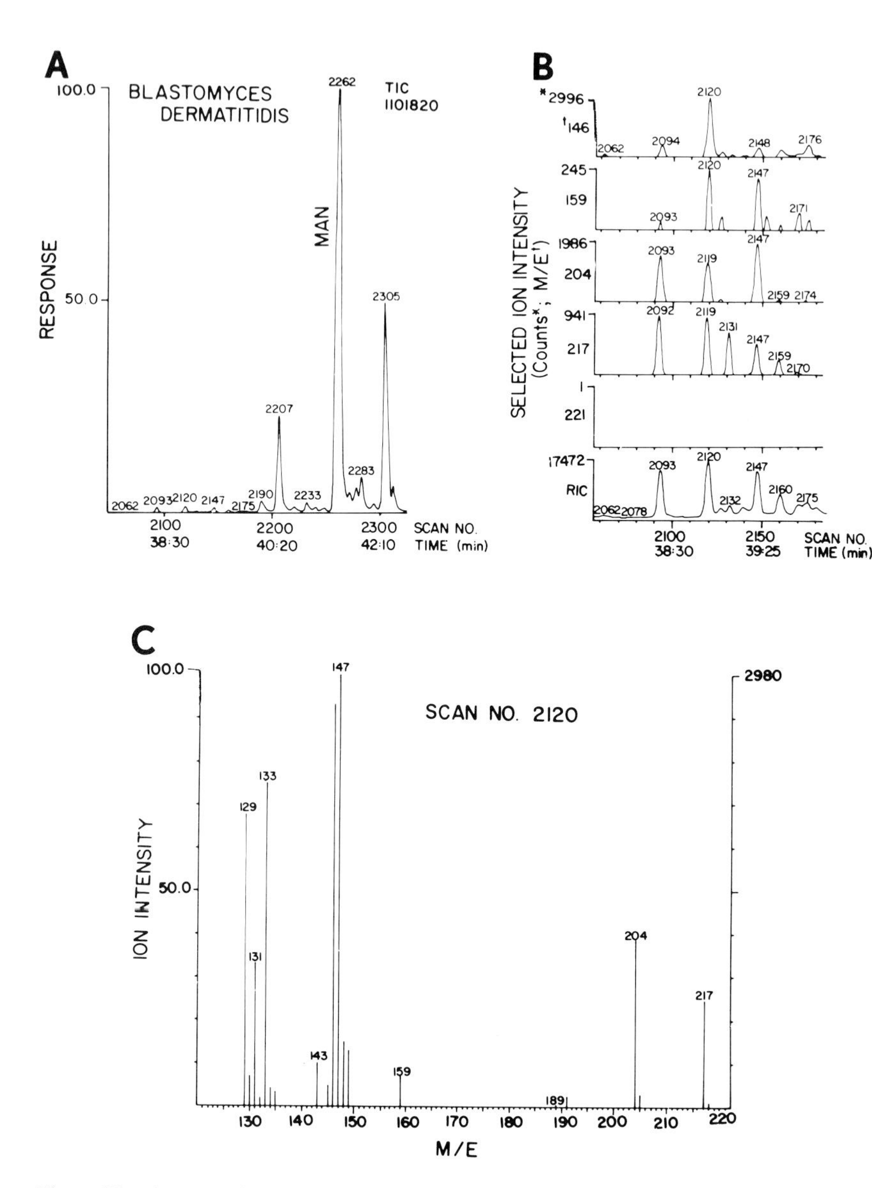

Figure 53. Spectra of TMS derivatives of *Blastomyces dermatitidis* mycelial wall (ASWS extract) (A–C) and *Malbranchea dendritica* conidial wall (D–F) using a 50-m BP5 capillary column and the same temperature program as in Figure 52. Multiple ion scans (B, E) showing the distribution of diagnostic fragment ions (cf. Figure 52B–D) for selected portions of

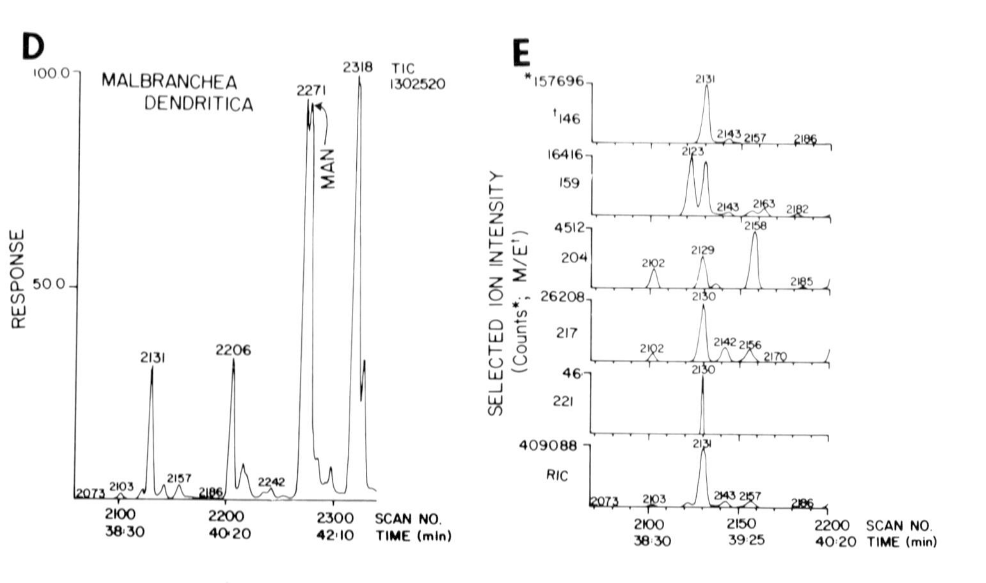

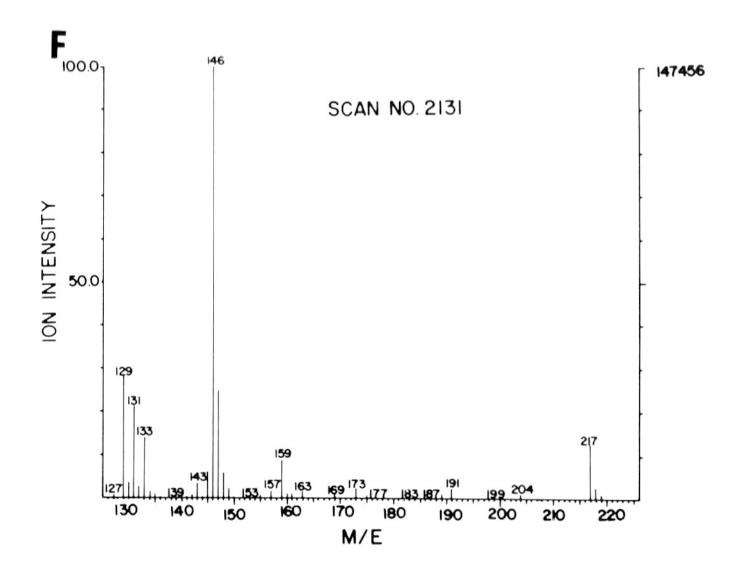

each chromatogram are shown. Positive ion mass spectra of compounds with a comparable difference in retention time between the 3-*O*-methyl-D-mannose standard and mannose (cf. Figure 52A) are presented in (C) and (F) for respective samples. (MAN) Mannose; (RIC) reconstructed ion chromatograph. (From Cole *et al.*, 1985a.)

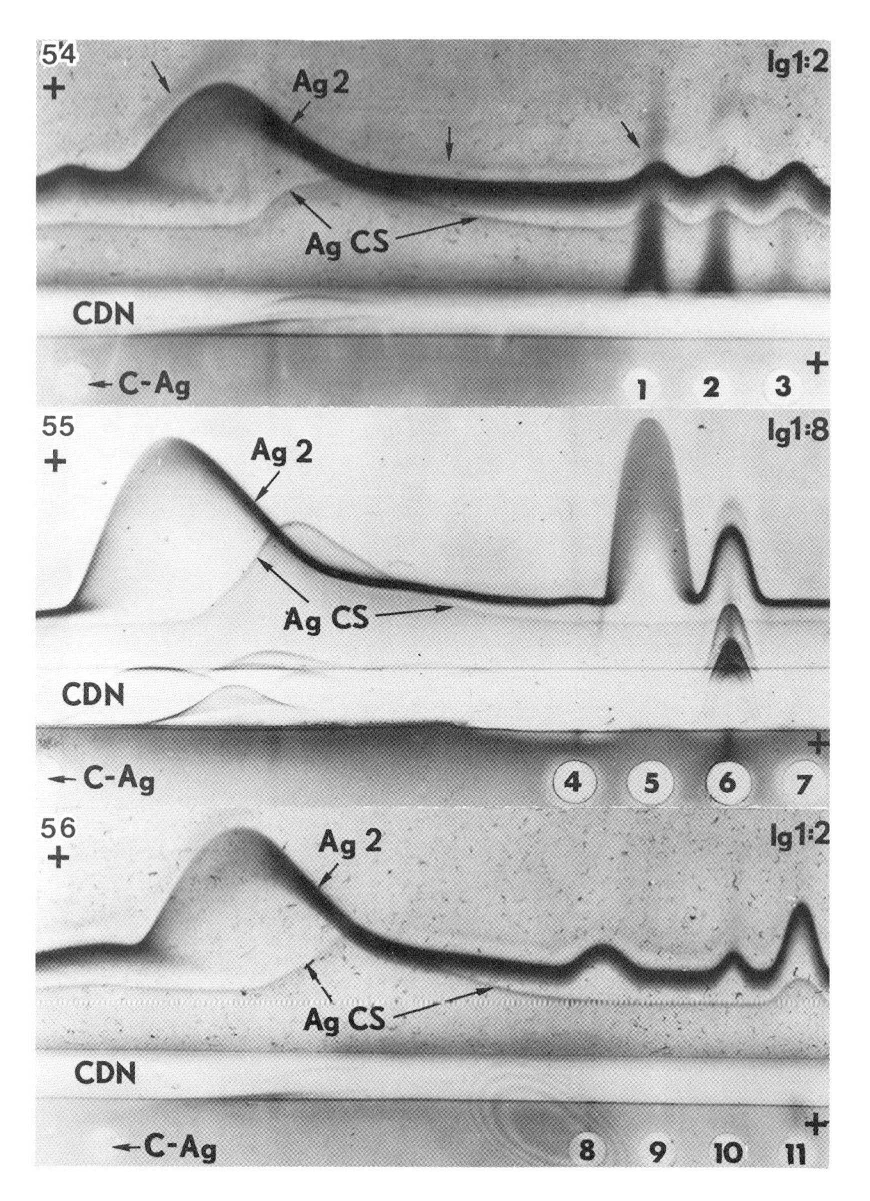

Figures 54–56. Advancing-line IEP gels revealing distribution of two major antigens (Ag 2 and Ag CS) in solubilized wall and cytosol fractions of *C. immitis* (54) and other fungi. (C-Ag) Coccidioidin is the cathodal antigen at a dilution of 1:8 in electrophoresis buffer; (CDN) coccidioidin reference antigen in the intermediate well at a dilution of 1:128; (Ig) immunoglobulin at dilutions of 1:2 and 1:8; (+) indicates anodes and direction of migration in each dimension. The arrows in (54) indicate the suspected polymeric component of Ag 2. Fractions were solubilized in PBS and applied to anodal wells. The anodal wells are numbered 1–11 and contained the following concentrated fractions: (1) ASWS extract of 48-

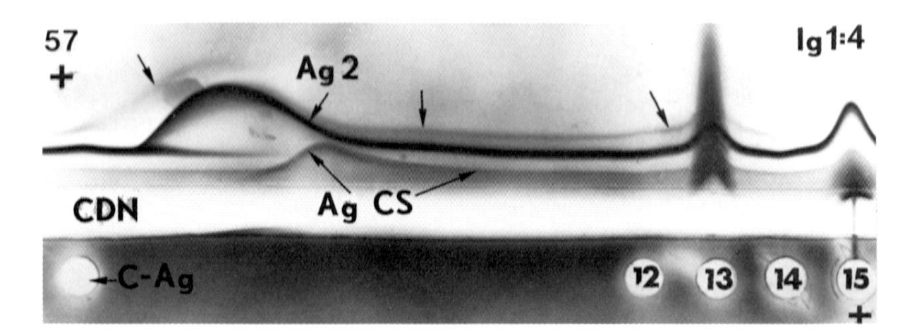

Figure 57. Advancing-line IEP gels using burro immunoglobulin at 1:4 dilution. The arrows indicate the suspected polymeric component of Ag 2. The Anodal wells are numbered 12–15 and contained the following fractions: (12) yeast wall of *B. dermatitidis* (20 mg/ml); (13) ASWS extract of *Aspergillus fumigatus* conidial wall (20 mg/ml); (14) exoantigen of *C. albicans* CA30 (30 mg/ml); (15) 48-hr whole spherule wash (20 mg/ml).

well. A lightly stained precipitin peak and advancing line are visible parallel to and above that of Ag 2 (arrows in Figure 54). This may be a component of Ag 2, which has been suggested to be a polymeric antigen (Cox *et al.*, 1984), or it could be a distinct antigen. A precipitin peak that has migrated beyond that of Ag 2 and forms a distinct advancing line below the Ag 2 line is identified as Ag CS. This antigen is not one of the 26 originally enumerated by Huppert *et al.* (1978, 1979) in their 2D-IEP characterization of CDN. On the basis of electrophoretic differences between Ag CS and Ag 2 in agarose gels using the CDN/anti-CDN reference system, and employing both advancing-line IEP and 2D-IEP techniques, Ag CS is considered a distinct antigen and not simply a component of Ag 2. Results of rocket IEP of samples in the anodal wells (Figure 54) reveal that both Ag 2 and Ag CS are present in solubilized fractions of *C. immitis*. In a recent study (Cole *et al.*, 1985a), we demonstrated that Ag CS was present in all ASWS extracts of different spherule-wall fractions. These results contrast with those of Cox *et al.* (1984), who stated that their ASWS spherule-wall extract contains "antigenic determinants

---

hr spherule exoantigen (0.63 mg/ml); (2) ASWS extract of 72-hr spherule exoantigen (0.63 mg/ml); (3) ASWS extract of 72-hr outer spherule wall fraction II (1.25 mg/ml); (4) ASWS extract of *Histoplasma capsulatum* yeast wall (10 mg/ml); (5) partially purified Ag 2 (supplied by R. A. Cox) (20 mg/ml); (6) endospore cytosol (20 mg/ml); (7) blank; (8) ASWS extract of mixed hyphal and conidial wall of *B. dermatitidis* (20 mg/ml); (9) yeast wall of *H. capsulatum* (10 mg/ml); (10) conidial wall of *Malbranchea dendritica* (10 mg/ ml); (11) filtrate + lysate of CDN (batch Nos. 92–94) diluted 1:64 in electrophoresis buffer.

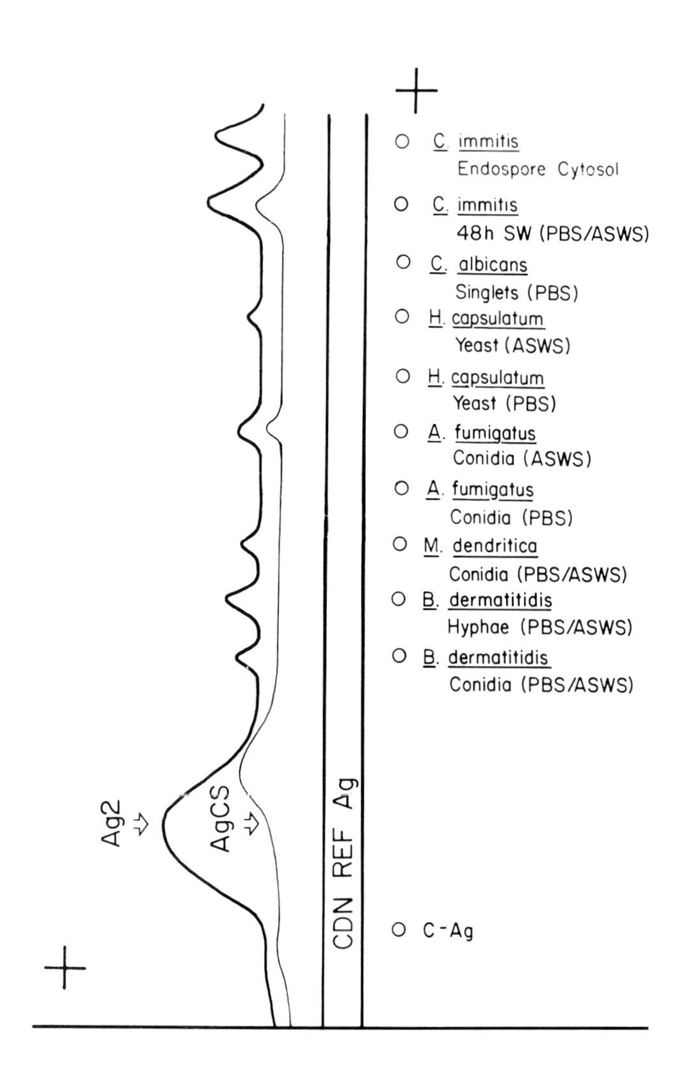

Figure 58. Summary of results of advancing-line IEP analysis of Ag 2 and Ag CS distribution in CDN and solubilized wall and cytosol fractions.

in common with only one antigen present in CDN," which they identified as Ag 2. The partially purified Ag 2 preparation reported by these authors was kindly provided by Dr. R. A. Cox (State Chest Hospital, San Antonio, Texas) and was used in our advancing-line IEP system. The Ag 2 reference precipitin line was clearly distorted above the anodal well (No. 5 in Figure 55), but the Ag CS line was not, which provides additional support that these are distinct antigens. The adjacent anodal well (No. 6) contains the cytosol fraction from isolated and homogenized endospores. In this case, Ag 2 as well as several unidentified antigens are present, but not Ag CS. In fact, Ag CS was not detected in any of the cytosol fractions of *C. immitis* cell types and is therefore considered to be a truly cell-wall-associated antigen. We have used advancing-line IEP to compare the antigenic composition of *C. immitis* fractions to those of *A. fumigatus, B. dermatitidis, H. capsulatum, M. dendritica,* and *C. albicans* (Figures 56 and 57). A summary of the results is presented in Figure 58, which reveals the distribution of both Ag 2 and Ag CS in solubilized wall fractions of these selected pathogenic and nonpathogenic fungi. It is evident that Ag 2 is not unique to *C. immitis* and occurs in wall fractions that have been shown to lack 3-*O*-MM [e.g., *B. dermatitidis* (cf. Figures 53 and 56)]. This suggests that the methylated sugar is not associated with the immunoreactive component of Ag 2. In contrast to the apparent occurrence of Ag 2, in several fungi examined, the newly reported Ag CS was detected only in extracts of *C. immitis* and an ASWS extract of the conidial wall of *A. fumigatus* (Figure 57). This approach to analysis of antigenic composition of fungal cell wall fractions provides the basis for selection and further purification of macromolecules from the cell envelope, which may be of value in the immunodiagnosis of coccidioidomycosis.

REFERENCES

Austwick, P. K. C., 1966, The role of spores in the allergies and mycoses of man and animals, in: *The Fungus Spore* (M. F. Madelin, ed.), Butterworths, London, pp. 321–337.

Axelsen, N. H., 1971, Antigen–antibody crossed electrophoresis (Laurell) applied to the study of the antigenic structure of *Candida albicans, Infect. Immun.* **4**:525–527.

Axelsen, N. H., 1973, Quantitative immunoelectrophoretic methods as tools for a polyvalent approach to standardization in the immunochemistry of *Candida albicans, Infect. Immun.* **7**:949–960.

Axelsen, N. H. (ed.), 1975, *Quantitative Immunoelectrophoresis,* Universitetforlaget, Oslo.

Baker, E. E., and Mrak, E. M., 1941, Spherule formation in culture by *Coccidioides immitis* Rixford and Gilchrist, *Am. J. Trop. Med.* **21**:589–594.

Baker, E. E., Mrak, E. M., and Smith, C. E., 1943, The morphology, taxonomy, and distribution of *Coccidioides immitis* Rixford and Gilchrist 1896, *Farlowia* **1**:199–244.

Baker, O., and Braude, A. I., 1956, A study of stimuli leading to the production of spherules in coccidioidomycosis, *J. Lab. Clin. Med.* **47**:169–181.

Beaman, L., and Holmberg, C. A., 1980, *In vitro* response of alveolar macrophages to infection with *Coccidioides immitis, Infect. Immun.* **28**:594–600.

Beaman, L., Benjamin, E., and Pappagianis, D., 1981, Role of lymphocytes in macrophage killing of *Coccidioides immitis in vitro, Infect. Immun.* **34**:347–353.

Bedell, G. W., and Soll, D. R., 1979, Effects of low concentrations of zinc on the growth and dimorphism of *Candida albicans:* Evidence for zinc-resistant and -sensitive pathways of mycelium formation, *Infect. Immun.* **26**:348–354.

Beever, R. E., and Dempsey, G. P., 1978, Function of rodlets on the surface of fungal spores, *Nature (London)* **272**:608–610.

Beever, R. E., Redgwell, R. J., and Dempsey, G. P., 1979, Purification and chemical characterization of the rodlet layer of *Neurospora crassa* conidia, *J. Bacteriol.* **140**:1063–1070.

Bernstein, D. I., Tipton, J. R., Schoot, S. F., and Cherry, J. D., 1981, Coccidioidomycosis in a neonate; Maternal–infant transmission, *J. Pediatr.* **99**:752–754.

Blank, F., and Burke, R. C., 1954, Chemical composition of cell wall of *Coccidioides immitis, Nature (London)* **173**:829.

Bracker, C. E., 1966, Ultrastructural aspects of sporangiospore formation in *Gilbertella persicaria,* in: *The Fungus Spore* (M. F. Madelin, ed.), Butterworths, London, pp. 39–60.

Bracker, C. E., 1968, The ultrastructure and development of sporangia in *Gilbertella persicaria, Mycologia* **60**:1016–1067.

Brewer, J. H., Parrott, C. L., and Rimland, D., 1982, Disseminated coccidioidomycosis in a heart transplant recipient, *Sabouraudia* **20**:162–265.

Brosbe, E. A., 1967, Use of refined agar for the *in vitro* propagation of the spherule phase of *Coccidioides immitis, J. Bacteriol.* **93**:497–498.

Campbell, D. H., Garvey, J. S., Cremer, N. E., and Sussdorf, D. H., 1970, *Methods in Immunology,* Benjamin, New York.

Carmichael, J. W., Kendrick, W. B., Conners, I. L., and Sigler, L., 1980, *The Genera of Hyphomycetes,* University of Alberta Press, Edmonton.

Catanzaro, A., 1979, Coccidioidin sensitivity in San Diego schools, *Sabouraudia* **17**:85–89.

Chandler, F. W., Kaplan, W., and Ajello, L., 1980, *Histopathology of Mycotic Diseases,* Yearbook Medical Publishers, Chicago.

Ciferri, R., and Redaelli, P., 1936, Morfologia, biologia e posizione sistematica di *Coccidioides immitis* Stiles e delle sue varieta, con notizie sul granuloma coccidioide, *Mem. R. Accad. Ital. Cl Sci Fis Mat. Nat. Chim.* **7**:399–475.

Clutterbuck, A. J., and Roper, J. A., 1966, A direct determination of nuclear distribution in heterokaryons of *Aspergillus nidulans, Genet. Res.* **7**:185–194.

Cole, G. T., 1973, A correlation between rodlet orientation and conidiogenesis in Hyphomycetes, *Can. J. Bot.* **51**:2413–2422.

Cole, G. T., 1975, The thallic mode of conidiogenesis in the Fungi Imperfecti, *Can. J. Bot.* **53**:2983–3001.

Cole, G. T., and Kendrick, W. B., 1968, A thin culture chamber for time-lapse photomicrography of fungi at high magnifications, *Mycologia* **60**:340–344.

Cole, G. T., and Pope, L. M., 1981, Surface wall components of *Aspergillus niger* conidia, in: *The Fungal Spore: Morphogenetic Controls* (G. Turian and H. R. Hohl, eds.), Academic Press, London, p. 195.

Cole, G. T., and Samson, R. A., 1979,. *Patterns of Development in Conidial Fungi,* Pitman, London.

Cole, G. T., and Samson, R. A., 1983, Conidium and sporangiospore formation in pathogenic microfungi, in: *Fungi Pathogenic for Humans and Animals,* Part A, *Biology* (D. H. Howard, ed.), Marcel Dekker, New York, pp. 437–524.

Cole, G. T., Sun, S. H., and Huppert, M., 1982, Isolation and ultrastructural examination of conidial wall components of *Coccidioides* and *Aspergillus, Scanning Electron Microsc.* **1982**(IV):1677–1685.

Cole, G. T., Pope, L. M., Huppert, M., Sun, S. H., and Starr, P., 1983, Ultrastructure and composition of conidial wall fractions of *Coccidioides immitis, Exp. Mycol.* **7**:297–318.

Cole, G. T., Chinn, J. W., Pope, L. M., and Starr, P., 1985a, Characterization and distribution of 3-*O*-methylmannose in *Coccidioides immitis,* in: *Proc. 4th Int. Conf. on Coccidioidomycosis* (H. Einstein and T. Catanzaro, eds.), *Nat. Found. Infect. Dis. Publ.,* Washington, D. C., pp. 130–145.

Cole, G. T., Pope, L. M., Huppert, M., Sun, S. H., and Starr, P., 1985b, Wall composition of different cell types of *Coccidioides immitis,* in: *Proc. 4th Int. Conf. on Coccidioidomycosis* (H. Einstein and T. Catanzaro, eds.), *Nat. Found. Infect. Dis. Publ.,* Washington, D. C., pp. 112–129.

Collins, M. S., and Pappagianis, D., 1973, Effects of lysozyme and chitinase on the spherules of *Coccidioides immitis* and *Histoplasma capsulatum, Contrib. Microbiol Immunol.* **3**:106–125.

Collins, M. S., Pappagianis, D., and Yee, J., 1977, Enzymatic solubilization of precipitin and complement fixing antigen from endospores, spherules and spherule fraction of *Coccidioides immitis,* in: *Coccidioidomycosis: Current Clinical and Diagnostic Status* (L. Ajello, ed.), Symposia Specialists, Miami, pp. 429–444.

Converse, J. L., 1955, Growth of spherules of *Coccidioides immitis* in a chemically defined liquid medium, *Proc. Soc. Exp. Biol. Med.* **90**:709–711.

Converse, J. L., 1956, Effect of physio-chemical environment on spherulation of *Coccidioides immitis* in a chemically defined medium, *J. Bacteriol.* **72**:784–792.

Converse, J. L., 1957, Effect of surface active agents on endosporulation of *Coccidioides immitis* in a chemically defined medium, *J. Bacteriol.* **74**:106–107.

Cox, R. A., and Arnold, D. R., 1979, Immunoglobulin E in coccidioidomycosis, *J. Immunol.* **123**:194–200.

Cox, R. A., and Larsh, H. W., 1974, Isolation of skin test-active preparations from yeast-phase cells of *Blastomyces dermatitidis, Infect. Immun.* **10**:42–47.

Cox, R. A., Huppert, M., Starr, P., and Britt, L. A., 1984, Reactivity of alkali-soluble, water-soluble cell wall antigen of *Coccidioides immitis* with anti-*Coccidioides* immunoglobulin M precipitin antibody, *Infect. Immun.* **43**:502–507.

Deresinski, S. C., 1980, History of coccidioidomycosis: "Dust to dust," in: *Coccidioidomycosis: A Text* (D. A. Stevens, ed.), Plenum Press, New York, pp. 1–20.

Dickson, E. C., 1937, "Valley fever" of the San Joaquin Valley and fungus *Coccidioides, Calif. West. Med.* **47**:151–155.

Dickson, E. C., and Gifford, M. A., 1938, *Coccidioides* infection (coccidioidomycosis), *Arch. Intern. Med.* **62**:853–871.

DiSalvo, A. F., Terreni, A. A., and Wooten, A. K., 1981, Use of the exoantigen test to identify *Blastomyces dermatititidis, Coccidioides immitis,* and *Histoplasma capsulatum* in mixed cultures, *J. Clin. Pathol.* **75**:825–826.

Drutz, D. J. and Catanzaro, A., 1978, Coccidioidomycosis, *Am. Rev. Resp. Dis.* **117**:559–585, 727–771.

Drutz, D. J., and Huppert, M., 1983, Coccidioidomycosis: Factors affecting the host–parasite interaction, *J. Infect. Dis.* **147**:372–390.

Emmons, C. W., 1967, Fungi similar to *Coccidioides immitis,* in: *Coccidioidomycosis,* University of Arizona Press, Tucson, pp. 233–237.

Fiese, M. J., 1958, *Coccidioidomycosis,* Charles C Thomas, Springfield, Illinois.

Flynn, N. M., Hoeprich, P. D., Kawachi, M. M., Lee, K. K., Lawrence, R. M., Goldstein, E., Jordan, G. W., Kundargi, R. S., and Wong, G. A., 1979, An unusual outbreak of windborne coccidioidomycosis, *N. Engl. J. Med.* **301**:358–361.

Galgiani, J. N., Hayden, R., and Rayne, C. M., 1982, Leukocyte effects on the dimorphism of *Coccidioides immitis, J. Infect. Dis.* **146**:56–63.

Gifford, J., and Catanzaro, A., 1981, A comparison of coccidioidin and spherulin skin testing in the diagnosis of coccidioidomycosis, *Am. Rev. Respir. Dis.* **124**:440–444.

Gilardi, G. L., 1965, Nutrition of systemic and subcutaneous pathogenic fungi, *Bacteriol. Rev.* **29**:406–424.

Goldschmidt, E. P., and Taylor, G. W., 1958, Composition of an extracellular polysaccharide fraction produced by *Coccidioides immitis,* in: *Bacteriological Proceedings*, American Society of Microbiology, Baltimore, p. 127.

Hector, R., and Pappagianis, D., 1982, Enzymatic degradation of the walls of spherules of *Coccidioides immitis, Exp. Mycol.* **6**:136–152.

Hess, W. M., 1973, Ultrastructure of fungal spore germination, *Shokubutsu Byogai Kenkyu* **8**:71–84.

Hughes, S. J., 1971a, Percurrent proliferation in fungi, algae and mosses, *Can. J. Bot.* **49**:215–231.

Hughes, S. J., 1971b, On conidia of fungi and gemmae of algae, bryophytes and pteridophytes, *Can. J. Bot.* **49**:1319–1339.

Huppert, M., 1983, Antigens used for measuring immunological reactivity, in: *Fungi Pathogenic for Humans and Animals,* Part B, *Pathogenicity and Detection: I* (D. Howard, ed.), Marcel Dekker, New York, pp. 219–302.

Huppert, M. and Bailey, J. W., 1963, Immunodiffusion as a screening test for coccidioidomycosis serology, *Sabouraudia* **2**:284–291.

Huppert, M., and Sun, S. H., 1980a, Overview of mycology, and mycology of *Coccidioides immitis,* in: *Coccidioidomycosis: A Text* (D. A. Stevens, ed.), Plenum Press, New York, pp. 21–46.

Huppert, M., and Sun, S. H., 1980b, Mycological diagnosis of coccidioidomycosis, in: *Coccidioidomycosis: A Text* (D. A. Stevens, ed.), Plenum Press, New York, pp. 47–61.

Huppert, M., Sun, S. H., and Bailey, J. W., 1967, Natural variability in *Coccidioides immitis,* in: *Coccidioidomycosis: Proceedings of the 2nd Symposium of Coccidioidomycosis* (L. Ajello, ed.), University of Arizona Press, Tucson, pp. 323–328.

Huppert, M., Spratt, N. S., Vukovich, K. R., Sun, S. H., and Rice, E. H., 1978, Antigenic analysis of coccidioidin and spherulin determined by two-dimensional immunoelectrophoresis, *Infect. Immun.* **20**:541–551.

Huppert, M., Adler, J. P., Rice, E. H., and Sun, S. H., 1979, Common antigens among systemic disease fungi analyzed by two-dimensional immunoelectrophoresis, *Infect. Immun.* **23**:479–485.

Huppert, M., Cole, G. T., Sun, S. H., Drutz, D. J., Starr, P., Frey, C. L., and Harrison, J. L., 1983, The propagule as an infectious agent in coccidioidomycosis, in: *Microbiology—1983* (D. Schlessinger, ed.), American Society of Microbiology, Washington, D.C., pp. 262–267.

Kabat, E. A., and Mayer, M. M., 1961, *Experimental Immunochemistry,* Charles C Thomas, Springfield, Illinois.

Keuhn, H. H., Orr, G. F., and Gouri, R. G., 1961, A new and widely distributed species of *Pseudoarachiotus, Mycopathol. Mycol. Appl.* **14**:215–229.

Klotz, S. A., Drutz, D. J., Huppert, M., Sun, S. H., and Demarsh, P. L., 1984, Critical role of CO_2 in the morphogenesis of *Coccidioides immitis* in cell-free subcutaneous chambers, *J. Infect. Dis.* **150**:127–134.

Kwon-Chung, K. J., 1969, *Coccidioides immitis:* Cytological study on the formation of the arthrospores, *Can. J. Genet. Cytol.* **11**:43–53.

Lack, A. R., 1938, Spherule formation and endosporulation of the fungus *Coccidioides in vitro, Proc. Soc. Exp. Biol. Med.* **38**:907–909.

Lecara, G., Cox, R. A., and Simpson, R. B., 1983, *Coccidioides immitis* vaccine: potential of an alkali-soluble, water-soluble cell wall antigen, *Infect. Immun.* **39**:437–475.

Levine, H. B., 1961, Purification of the spherule–endospore phase of *Coccidioides immitis, Sabouraudia* **1**:112–115.

Levine, H. B., Cobb, J. M., and Smith, C. E., 1960, Immunity to coccidioidomycosis induced in mice by purified spherule, arthrospore, and mycelial vaccines, *Trans. N.Y. Acad. Sci.* **22**:436–449.

Li, C. Y., 1983, Melanin-like pigment in zone lines of *Phellinus weirii*-colonized wood, *Mycologia* **75**:562–566.

Lones, G. W., and Peacock, C. L., 1960, Role of carbon dioxide in the dimorphism of *Coccidioides immitis, J. Bacteriol.* **79**:308–309.

Lones, G. W., Peacock, C. L., and McNey, F. A., 1971, Factors affecting the reversion of *Coccidioides immitis* spherules to mycelium, *Sabouraudia* **9**:287–296.

MacNeal, W. J., and Taylor, R. M., 1914, *Coccidioides immitis* and coccidioidal granuloma, *J. Med. Res.* **30**:261–274.

Maddy, K. T., 1958, The geographic distribution of *Coccidioides immitis* and possible ecologic implications, *Ariz. Med.* **15**:178–188.

Maitra, S. K., and Ballou, C. E., 1974, Multiple forms of the methylmannose polysaccharide (MMP) from mycobacteria, *Fed. Proc. Fed. Am. Soc. Exp. Biol.* **33**:1452.

McGinnis, M. R., 1980, Recent taxonomic developments and changes in medical mycology, *Annv. Rev. Microbiol.* **34**:109–135.

McNall, E. G., 1962, Cell wall constituents of pathogenic fungi, in: *Fungi and Fungous Diseases* (G. Dalldorf, ed.), Charles C Thomas, Springfield, Illinois, pp. 139–147.

Nimmich, W., 1970, Occurence of 3-*O*-methylmannose in lipopolysaccharides of *Klebsiella* and *Escherichia coli, Biochim. Biophys. Acta* **215**:189–191.

Olsberg, C. A., and Cox, R. A., 1983, Chemical composition of a mycelial and spherule cell wall antigen from *Coccidioides immitis, Abstr. Annu. Meet. Am. Soc. Microbiol.* **F6**:383.

Ophüls, W., 1905a, Further observations on a pathogenic mould formerly described as a protozoan (*Coccidioides immitis, Coccidioides pyogenes*), *J. Exp. Med.* **6**:443–486.

Ophüls, W., 1905b, Coccidioidal granuloma, *J. Am. Med. Assoc.* **45**:1201–1296.

Ophüls, W., and Moffitt, H. C., 1900, A new pathogenic mould (formerly described as a protozoan: *Coccidioides immitis pyogenes*): Preliminary report, *Philadel. Med. J.* **5**:1471–1472.

Orr, G. F., 1972, Recovery of several arthroaleuriosporous fungi from mice following intraperitoneal inoculation, *Tech. Rep., Desert Test Center, Dugway,* DTC Proj. No. TN-72-542.

Pappagianis, D., 1973, Coccidioidomycosis, in: *Clinical Dermatology,* Vol. 3 (D. J. Demis, R. L. Dobson, and J. McGuire, eds.), Harper and Row, Hagerstown, Maryland, pp. 1–11.

Pappagianis, D., 1980, Epidemiology of coccidioidomycosis, in: *Coccidioidomycosis: A Text* (D. A. Stevens, ed.), Plenum Press, New York, pp. 63–85.

Pappagianis, D., and Kobayashi, G. S., 1958, Production of extracellular polysaccharide in cultures of *Coccidioides immitis, Mycologia* **50**:229–238.

Pappagianis, D., and Kobayashi, G. S., 1960, Approaches to the physiology of *Coccidioides immitis, Ann. N.Y. Acad. Sci.* **89**:109–121.

Pesanti, E. L., 1979, Role of surface wettability in phagocytosis of *Neurospora crassa* spores, *J. Reticuloendothelial Soc.* **26**:549–552.

Porter, J. F., Scheer, E. S., and Wheat, R. W., 1971, Characterization of 3-*O*-methylmannose from *Coccidioides immitis, Infect. Immun.* **4**:660–661.

Posadas, A., 1892, Un nuevo caso de micosis fungoidea con psorospermias, *An. Circ. Med. Argent.* **15**:585–597.

Rao, S., Biddle, M., Balchum, O. J., and Robinson, J. L., 1971, Focal endemic coccidioidomycosis in Los Angeles County, *Am. Rev. Respir. Dis.* **105**:410–416.

Raudaskoski, M., 1970, Occurrence of microtubules and microfilaments and origin of septa in dikaryotic hyphae of *Schizophyllum commune, Protoplasma* **70**:415–422.

Raudaskoski, M., 1972, Occurrence of microtubules in the hyphae of *Schizophyllum commune* during intercellular nuclear migration, *Arch. Microbiol.* **86**:91–100.

Reiss, E., Huppert, M., and Cherniak, R., 1985, Characterization of protein and mannan polysaccharide antigens of yeasts, moulds and Actinomycetes, *Curr. Top. Med. Mycol.* **1** (in press).

Reissig, J. L., Strominger, J. L., and Leloir, L., 1955, A modified colorimetric method for the estimation of *N*-acetylamino sugars, *J. Biol. Chem.* **217**:959–966.

Rixford, E., 1894, A case of protozoic dermatitis, *Occident. Med. Times* **8**:704–707.

Rixford, E., and Gilchrist, T. C., 1896, Two cases of protozoan (coccidioidal) infection of the skin and other organs, *Johns Hopkins Hosp. Rep.* **1**:209–268.

Roberts, R. L., and Szaniszlo, P. J., 1980, Yeast-phase cell cycle of the polymorphic fungus *Wangiella dermatitidis, J. Bacteriol.* **144**:721–731.

Robinow, C. F., 1981, Nuclear behavior in conidial fungi, in: *Biology of Conidial Fungi,* Vol. 2 (G. T. Cole and B. Kendrick, eds.), Academic Press, New York, pp. 357–393.

Roessler, W. G., Herbst, E. J., McCullogh, W. G., Mills, R. C., and Brewer, C. R., 1946, Studies with *Coccidioides immitis.* 1. Submerged growth in liquid culture, *J. Infect. Dis.* **79**:12–22.

Salkin, D., 1961, Pathogenetic classification of coccidioidomycosis, in: *Transactions of the VIth Annual Meeting VA-Armed Forces Coccidioidomycosis Cooperative Study,* pp. 30–34.

San-Blas, G., 1982, The cell wall of fungal human pathogens: Its possible role in host–parasite relationships, *Mycopathologia* **79**:159–184.

Selitrennikoff, C. P., 1976, Easily-wettable, a new mutant, *Neurospora Newslett.* **23**:23.

Sigler, L., and Carmichael, J. W., 1976, Taxonomy of *Malbranchea* and some other hyphomycetes with arthroconidia, *Mycotaxon* **4**:369–488.

Slater, M. L., 1978, Staining fungal nuclei with mithramycin, in: *Methods in Cell Biology* (D. Prescott, ed.), Academic Press, New York, pp. 135–140.

Smith, C. E., 1942, Parallelism of coccidioidal and tuberculous infections, *Radiology* **38**:643–668.

Smith, C. E., 1943, Coccidioidomycosis, *Med. Clin. North Am.* **27**:790–807.

Smith, C. E., Beard, R. R., Rosenberger, H. G., and Whiting, E. G., 1946, Varieties of coccidioidal infection in relation to the epidemiology and control of the disease, *Am. J. Public Health* **36**:1394–1402.

Smith, H., 1977, Microbial surfaces in relation to pathogenicity, *Bacteriol. Rev.* **41**:475–500.

Standard, P. G., and Kaufman, L., 1977, Immunological procedure for the rapid and specific identification of *Coccidioides immitis* cultures, *J. Clin. Microbiol.* **5**:149–153.

Stewart, R. A., and Meyer, K. F., 1932, Isolation of *Coccidioides immitis* from soil, *Proc. Soc. Exp. Biol. Med.* **29**:937–938.

Sun, S. H., and Huppert, M., 1976, A cytological study of morphogenesis of *Coccidioides immitis, Sabouraudia* **14**:185–198.

Sun, S. H., Huppert, M., and Vukovich, K. R., 1976, Rapid *in vitro* conversion and identification of *Coccidioides immitis, J. Clin. Microbiol.* **3**:186–190.

Sun, S. H., Sekhon, S. S., and Huppert, M., 1979, Electron microscopic studies of saprobic and parasitic forms of *Coccidioides immitis, Sabouraudia* **17**:265–273.

Tarbet, J. E., and Breslau, A. M., 1953, Histochemical investigation of the spherule of *Coccidioides immitis* in relation to the host reaction, *J. Infect. Dis.* **92**:183–190.

Thorne, W. S., 1894, A case of protozoic skin disease, *Occident. Med. Times* **8**:703–704.

Van Oss, C. J., 1978, Phagocytosis as a surface phenomenon, *Annu. Rev. Microbiol.* **32**:19–39.

Walch, H. A., 1982, *Coccidioides immitis,* in: *Microbiology* (A. I. Braude, C. E. Davis, and J. Fierer, eds.), W. B. Saunders, Philadelphia, pp. 658–664.

Ward, E. R., Cox, R. A., Schmitt, J. A., Huppert, M., and Sun, S. H., 1975, Delayed-type hypersensitivity responses to a cell wall fraction of the mycelial phase of *Coccidioides immitis, Infect. Immun.* **12**:1093–1097.

Weiner, M. H., 1983, Antigenemia detected in human coccidioidomycosis, *J. Clin. Microbiol.* **18**:136–142.

Wernicke, R., 1892, Ueber einen Protozoenbefund bei *Mycosis fungoides, Zentrabl. Bakteriol.* **12**:859–861.

Wheat, R. W., and Su Chung, K. S., 1977, Antigenic fractions of *Coccidioides immitis,* in: *Coccidioidomycosis: Current Clinical and Diagnostic Status* (L. Ajello, ed.), Symposia Specialists, Miami, pp. 453–460.

Wheat, R. W., and Scheer, E., 1977, Cell walls of *Coccidioides immitis:* Neutral sugars of aqueous alkaline extract polymers, *Infect. Immun.* **15**:340–341.

Wheat, R. W., Tritschler, C., Conant, N. F., and Lowe, E. P., 1977, Comparison of *Coccidioides immitis* arthrospore, mycelium and spherule cell walls, and influence of growth medium on mycelial cell wall composition, *Infect. Immun.* **17**:91–97.

Wheat, R. W., Su Chung, K. S., Ornellas, E. P., and Scheer, E. R., 1978, Extraction of skin test activity from *Coccidioides immitis* mycelia by water, perchloric acid and aqueous phenol extraction, *Infect. Immun.* **19**:152–159.

Wheat, R. W., Woodruff, W. W., and Haltiwanger, R. S., 1983, Occurrence of antigenic (species-specific?) partially 3-*O*-methylated heteromannans in cell wall and soluble cellular (nonwall) components of *Coccidioides immitis* mycelia, *Infect. Immun.* **41**:728–734.

Part V

Dimorphic Mucors

Chapter 13

Mucor racemosus

Clark B. Inderlied, Julius Peters, and Ronald L. Cihlar

1. INTRODUCTION

Mucor racemosus is a member of the order Mucorales of the Zygomyceta. Although *Mucor* exhibits multiple morphologies, interest has focused on vegetative yeast–hyphal dimorphism. Part of the interest in *Mucor* dimorphism concerns their potential as etiological agents of disease. In healthy humans, *Mucor* rarely causes disease, but in the host compromised by immune deficiency, immune suppression, or a serious underlying disease, the incidence of *Mucor* infections is much higher. Although the yeast form of *Mucor* has been observed in human and animal tissue, invariably it is the hyphal form that is associated with disease and pathology (Rippon, 1982). Thus, there may be a very practical reason for understanding the process of dimorphism among *Mucor,* since from such knowledge may emerge improved chemotherapeutic procedures, not only for infections involving *Mucor,* but also for infections involving the other pathogenic dimorphic fungi. In addition to the clinical implication of *Mucor* dimorphism, in the past several years there has been growing interest in *Mucor* as a model system to investigate fundamental

Clark B. Inderlied • Clinical Microbiology, Children's Hospital of Los Angeles, University of Southern California, School of Medicine, Los Angeles, California 90027. **Julius Peters** • Department of Pediatrics, UCLA School of Medicine, Harbor-UCLA Medical Center, Torrance, California 92717. **Ronald L. Cihlar** • Microbiology Department, Schools of Medicine and Dentistry, Georgetown University, Washington, D.C. 20007.

questions of the molecular biology of cellular morphogenesis. In particular, these studies have focused on differential gene expression during *Mucor* development and on the mechanisms that may serve to regulate such expression.

2. BIOLOGY OF *Mucor racemosus*

2.1. Preface

Mucor racemosus is a dimorphic zygomycete commonly found in the soil and on decaying plant material. The organism grows rapidly under either aerobic or anaerobic conditions. In air, the fungus forms a thick gray mycelium that gradually turns brown or black with the accumulation of sporangia that contain numerous dark sporangiospores. Under strictly anaerobic conditions and in the presence of a plentiful source of hexose, *M. racemosus* grows in the yeast form. A high partial pressure of carbon dioxide also favors yeast development (Bartnicki-García and Nickerson, 1962). Under aerobic or microaerobic conditions, the fungus grows in the hyphal form.

2.2. Vegetative Life Cycle

In a complex growth medium containing peptone, glucose, and yeast extract, sporangiospores germinate as hyphae under aerobic conditions and continue to grow by apical extension and eventually form a mycelium from which develop sporangiophores, sporangia, and sporangiospores. The mycelium consists of both aerial and substrate hyphae, and growth is characteristically luxuriant and rapid. In the same medium but under anaerobic conditions, sporangiospores germinate as multipolar budding yeast cells. The morphogenetic process that has been most studied as a model developmental system is the yeast-to-hyphal differentiation. If actively growing yeasts are shifted from an anaerobic, carbon-dioxide-rich environment to an aerobic environment, hyphal tubes emerge from the previously budding yeast cells 3–5 hr after the shift. In terms of understanding the physiological, biochemical, and molecular basis of this developmental system, most of the studies have focused on the period from the time of the shift to 3 or 4 hr after the shift, but before there is an observable morphological change. Presumably, it is during this period that a cascade of biochemical and molecular events occur that lead to the physiological events manifested in the change in both the form and the rate of growth.

3. BIOCHEMISTRY AND PHYSIOLOGY OF *Mucor racemosus*

3.1. Respiration and Fermentation

Interest in the mode of energy production in *M. racemosus* stems from the original observation of Pasteur that the morphological forms of *Mucor* reflect environmental conditions, notably the degree of aerobiosis. A plausible hypothesis is that the mode of energy production is linked to morphogenesis. A number of studies have been directed at defining the possible relationship between energy production and morphology, but the results have been inconclusive and sometimes contradictory. It is clear, however, that under anaerobic conditions, *M. racemosus* produces energy by alcoholic fermentation of glucose, and under aerobic conditions, energy is produced by both fermentation and respiration (Paznokas and Sypherd, 1975; Inderlied and Sypherd, 1978).

Mooney and Sypherd (1976) showed that the morphology of *M. racemosus* growing in a culture sparged with oxygen-free nitrogen gas was dependent on the flow rate of nitrogen through the culture. In a strictly defined system, the hyphal form was observed at low flow rates and the yeast form at high flow rates. Their interpretation of this observation was that hyphal development requires a volatile factor that accumulates in cultures sparged at low flow rates, but is removed from the culture at high flow rates, resulting in yeast development. The implication of these experiments is that oxygen is not required for hyphal development. Since the report of Mooney and Sypherd (1976), several attempts have been made to isolate and identify this putative morphogen, but it has proven to be as elusive as it is volatile. Borgia has reexamined the observations of Mooney and Sypherd (1976). By monitoring the oxidation–reduction potential of the culture with a higher concentration of resazurin than that used by Mooney and Sypherd (1976), he found that the culture was microaerobic under a low flow rate of nitrogen gas (Borgia, personal communication). In addition, Borgia isolated morphological mutants that failed to form hyphae. The mutant selection was carried out under a low flow rate of nitrogen gas rather than in air in an attempt to dissociate morphogenesis and mitochondrial function. However, these mutants have proven to be respiratory-deficient strains with an intact electron-transport chain but with reduced mitochondrial ATPase activity (Borgia, personal communication), suggesting that the low-flow-rate conditions may not be strictly anaerobic.

Other evidence indicates that the differentiation of yeasts to hyphae is primarily a response to the change from anaerobiosis to aerobiosis. Storck and Morrill (1971) isolated respiratory mutants of *M. bacilliformis* that lacked cytochrome oxidase activity and did not form hyphae in air, suggesting that respiratory capacity is associated with hyphal development. Zorzopulos *et al.* (1973) showed that chloramphenicol, an inhibitor of mitochondrial protein synthesis, promotes yeast development of *M. rouxii* and inhibits cytochrome oxidase expression. Clarke-Walker (1973) reported that a high concentration of chloramphenicol promotes yeast development of *M. genevensis* and inhibits cyanide-resistant respiration. Rogers *et al.* (1974), with *M. genevensis,* and Paznokas and Sypherd (1975), with *M. racemosus,* showed that mitochondriogenesis is not repressed by glucose under aerobic conditions.

We conclude from these studies that hyphal morphogenesis is associated with mitochondrial development. However, there is a need to distinguish between respiration and other mitochrondrial functions. Clarke-Walker (1973) showed that chloramphenicol inhibits the growth of *M. genevensis* under microaerobic conditions when the cells apparently lack any respiratory capacity, suggesting that some function other than respiration may be affected. Paznokas and Sypherd (1975) showed with *M. racemosus* that dibutyryl-cyclic AMP blocks hyphal development without affecting respiratory capacity. In addition, experiments with cerulenin, which inhibits phospholipid synthesis (Ito *et al.,* 1982) and consequently mitochondrial membrane development, together with the proposed role of mitochondrial compartmentation in the synthesis of urea (see Section 3.4.1.) suggest that mitochondrial development, though not necessarily respiratory function, may be essential for yeast-to-hyphal differentiation.

3.2. Cyclic 3′,5′-Adenosine Monophosphate

One of the first established and most important biochemical correlates of morphogenesis in *Mucor* is the intracellular cyclic AMP (cAMP) level (Larsen and Sypherd, 1974; Paveto *et al.,* 1975). These studies showed that high intracellular levels of cAMP are associated with yeast cells and low levels are characteristic of hyphal cells. In addition, the differentiation of yeasts to hyphae is blocked by exogenous cAMP or dibutyryl-cAMP. Paznokas and Sypherd (1975) showed that cAMP levels increase during sporangiospore germination in air, but decline to the characteristic low levels of hyphae as germ tubes emerge. More recently, Orlowski (1980) reported that exogenous cAMP prevents the germination of sporangiospores, but not the swelling of spores. The developmental fluctuations in cAMP levels in *M. racemosus* may be accounted for by the fluctuating levels of adenylate cyclase, but probably not phosphodiesterase (Orlowski, 1980). This latter observation contrasts with the earlier report of Paveto *et al.* (1975) that in *Mucor rouxii*, fluctuating phosphodiesterase activities were responsible for the differences in the cAMP levels of yeasts and hyphae. Either this discrepancy may reflect species differences or, alternatively, cAMP levels may be regulated by adenylate cyclase activity during spore germination and by phosphodiesterase activity during the differentiation of yeasts to hyphae. Using the photoaffinity label 8-azido-[^{32}P]-cAMP, Orlowski (1980) also showed that there were changes in cAMP binding, and these changes were reflected in differences in morphology-specific proteins that bind cAMP. The possible regulatory significance of these binding proteins is not known.

In addition, Orlowski (1981) confirmed and extended earlier observations that cAMP levels generally correlate with morphology rather than with carbon dioxide tension, oxygen tension, and growth rate. The single exception to this generalization is that in the presence of phenethyl alcohol, cAMP levels decrease and differentiation is blocked. The cAMP correlation with morphology was important to confirm, since the cAMP effect has been used in turn to validate numerous other biochemical correlates of morphology.

3.3. Lipid Synthesis

In contrast to cell-wall synthesis during the morphogenesis of *Mucor* species (see Chapter 14), little attention has been given to the synthesis of lipids, especially the phospholipids that comprise an integral part of the cell-membrane structure. Recently, Ito *et al.* (1982) showed that in *M. racemosus* there is an increase in lipid synthesis during morphogenesis that parallels the increase in macromolecular synthesis. They examined the changes in phospholipid synthesis and found that the synthesis of all types of phospholipids increases substantially during the differentiation of yeast to hyphae. Perhaps more significant was the finding that a substantial increase in the turnover of phospholipids occurred during morphogenesis. Furthermore, Ito *et al.* (1982) found that a low concentration of cerulenin, an inhibitor of fatty acid synthetases, which inhibited 70% of lipid synthesis, completely blocked morphogenesis. In the presence of cerulenin, yeasts continue to grow by multipolar budding at the same rate as yeast cells growing under anaerobic conditions in the absence of the inhibitor. Cerulenin also inhibited 10–20% of protein and RNA synthesis and specifically inhibited the synthesis of ornithine decarboxylase, another biochemical correlate of morphogenesis. The increase in phospholipid turnover and the dramatic effect of cerulenin on morphogenesis, which can be overcome by the addition of Tween 80 as an exogenous source of fatty acids, suggest that changes in phospholipid synthesis in particular, or lipid synthesis in general, are important in the early stages of the differentiation of yeasts to hyphae. Since dimorphism in *M. racemosus* appears to correlate most strongly with anaerobic vs. aerobic growth conditions, it is of interest that a difference in the lipid composition of aerobically and anaerobically grown *M. genevensis* (Gordon *et al.*, 1971) and *M. rouxii* (Safe and Caldwell, 1975) has been reported.

3.4. Enzyme Synthesis

3.4.1. *Glutamate Dehydrogenase*

Yeast cells of *M. racemosus* are more fastidious than hyphal cells in their nitrogen-source requirements. Hyphae efficiently utilize inorganic nitrogen, whereas yeast cells require organic nitrogen for optimal growth (Bartnicki-García and Nickerson, 1962; Elmer and Nickerson, 1970). In a defined medium, the nitrogen requirement of both morphological types is met by a mixture of alanine, aspartate, glutamate, and ammonium chloride (Peters and Sypherd, 1978). The omission of glutamate drastically reduces the growth rate of yeasts, but not of hyphae, suggesting a morphology-related difference in glutamate metabolism.

Although both NAD- and NADP-glutamate dehydrogenase (GDH) activities are found in *M. racemosus,* only the expression of the NAD form of the enzyme was correlated with morphology (Peters and Sypherd, 1979). NAD-GDH activity is generally an order of magnitude lower in yeasts than in hyphae grown in the same medium. During cellular morphogenesis, the emergence of germ tubes is preceded by an increase in the specific activity of NAD-GDH, while NADP-GDH activity remains constant. When germ-tube formation is blocked by the addition of dibutyryl-cAMP, the increase in NAD-GDH is suppressed. On the basis of these associations with morphology, it was proposed that NAD-GDH is a biochemical correlate of hyphal morphology (Peters and Sypherd, 1979).

Two additional observations bear on the *in vivo* function of NAD-GDH and its role in hyphal differentiation. First, nutritional regulation of NAD-GDH (i.e., carbon catabolite repression by glucose and nitrogen catabolite repression by ammonia) is consistent with a catabolic role for the enzyme (Peters and Sypherd, 1979). Second, a specific exception to the association of high NAD-GDH activity with hyphal cells has been observed when urea or arginine is the nitrogen source. With these nitrogen sources, the NAD-GDH activity is repressed to levels characteristic of yeast cultures (J. Peters, unpublished observation).

It is proposed here that urea is a metabolic signal required for hyphal development. This postulate leads to a model in which the function of NAD-GDH is to provide ammonia for the synthesis of urea. On initiation of the differentiation of yeasts to hyphae, the intracellular cAMP level decreases (Larsen and Sypherd, 1974) and NAD-GDH synthesis is derepressed (Peters and Sypherd, 1979). The mitochondrial pool of ammonia must be generated indirectly, since the mitochondria are impermeable to cytosolic ammonia. Cytosolic glutamate enters the mitochondria and is deaminated by NAD-GDH, an enzyme sequestered within the mitochondria. In turn, this pool of ammonia is a substrate for mitochondrial carbamoyl phosphate synthetase, which is the first enzyme in the arginine biosynthetic pathway (Davis, 1967). The final step in this sequence is the catabolism of arginine via arginase to provide urea during hyphal morphogenesis.

Although this model should be considered as speculative at this point, it has been useful in correlating observations on the regulation of NAD-GDH and is also supported by additional recent findings. First, the low NAD-GDH activity in hyphal cultures grown with urea or arginine as the nitrogen source can be viewed as a form of end-product repression. Second, experiments with respiratory-deficient mutants support the idea that the bulk of NAD-GDH is sequestered within the mitochondria. Two independently isolated morphological mutants of *M. racemosus* (P. Borgia, personal communication), PB103 and PB104, that were selected for impaired hyphal development share a common unselected characteristic: an inability to utilize nonfermentable carbon sources aerobically. These findings are in accord with the earlier results in *M. bacilliformis* that showed that respiratory-deficient mutants are unable to undergo hyphal differentiation (Storck and Morrill, 1971). The initial characterization of the *M. racemosus* mutants PB103 and PB104 showed them to have an intact electron-transport chain but reduced levels of mitochondrial ATPase (P. Borgia, personal communication). On the assumption that NAD-GDH was a mitochondrial enzyme, it was of interest to determine whether the regulation of this enzyme is altered in the respiratory-deficient mutants. It was found that even under aerobic conditions, the NAD-GDH activity remained low in the mutants.

An important question was whether urea could overcome the morphological block in the mutants, since the presumed function of NAD-GDH in morphogenesis is to make ammonia available for urea synthesis. If 10 mM urea is included in the defined growth medium or in a complex growth medium with diminished amounts of yeast extract, then hyphal morpohogenesis takes place. However, urea does not overcome the morphological block when the mutant cells are grown in a yeast-extract-rich medium, most likely because urea transport is repressed under these conditions (D. Logan, personal communication). The metabolic relationship between NAD-GDH activity and urea synthesis has also been tested in the wild-type strain. When growth is maintained in the yeast phase aerobically by the addition of dibutyryl-cAMP to the culture, the NAD-GDH activity remains repressed (Peters and Sypherd, 1979). The question is whether morphogenesis occurs when both urea and dibutyryl-cAMP are added together to a culture when it is shifted from carbon dioxide to air. It was found that the addition of 10 mM urea to the defined medium allowed hyphal morphogenesis in the presence of 1.5 mM dibutyryl-cAMP, but at a slower rate than in defined medium without additional supplementation (J. Peters, unpublished observation). Urea-induced morphogenesis in the respiratory-deficient mutants PB103 and PB104 also occurs at a much reduced rate, suggesting that there may be additional requirements for hyphal morphogenesis not satisfied by adding urea to the medium.

Paznokas *et al.* (1982) have isolated mutants of *M. racemosus* that undergo hyphal morphogenesis even in the presence of dibutyryl-cAMP. It would be expected that the control of NAD-GDH would also be uncoupled from dibutyryl-cAMP. However, the NAD-GDH activity in the mutants was found to be repressed in the presence of dibutyryl-cAMP as it is in the wild-type (Paznokas *et al.*, 1982). This finding appears to be at odds with the model, but further characterization of the mutants may resolve the discrepancy.

Initial experiments have confirmed the role of arginase in this model. Arginase specific activity increases up to 50-fold during hyphal differentiation in both defined and complex media. The arginase appears to be primarily under developmental regulation, rather than nutritional, since the increase in enzyme activity occurs whether arginine is present or absent from the defined medium. This finding is consistent with an increase in arginine catabolism during morphogenesis as would be expected if arginine is the source of urea for hyphal differentiation.

3.4.2. Ornithine Decarboxylase

Ornithine decarboxylase (ODCase) is the first and probably rate-limiting enzyme of the polyamine biosynthetic pathway. Increases in the specific activity of ODCase have been associated with a variety of cellular responses, including increased growth and different types of developmental changes (Tabor and Tabor, 1976). Inderlied *et al.* (1980) showed there is a 40- to 60-fold increase in ODCase activity during the first 3 hr of the yeast-to-hyphal differentiation in *M. racemosus*. Changes in the activity of the enzyme are exquisitely sensitive to environmental changes that lead to morphogenesis. In *M. racemosus,* ODCase appears to be regulated at the level of transcription and translation, since inhibition of RNA synthesis with actinomycin D only partially blocks the increase in ODCase activity. Efforts made to establish the nature of the regulation of ODCase in *M. racemosus,* by measuring the rate of messenger RNA synthesis and degradation of ODCase polypeptide synthesis and degradation, have been thwarted by the failure of several workers to purify the enzyme.

Recently, Fernandez and Inderlied (in prep.) providied evidence for the presence of more than one form of ODCase in *M. racemosus,* and these forms may be morphology-specific. They showed that the yeast enzyme is thermally more unstable than the hyphal enzyme and that there is a clear difference in the Arrhenius plots for yeast and hyphal ODCase. The evidence suggests that there is a yeast enzyme present at low levels that synthesizes putrescine at a rate sufficient for growth. During the yeast-to-hyphal differentiation, a second ODCase enzyme is produced at high levels that may be necessary for the increased growth rate and morphogenesis. Fernandez and Inderlied (in prep.) also showed that the change in ODCase activity is repressed by exogenous putrescine, but there are two levels of repression; i.e., 10–20% of ODCase activity is repressed by low exogenous concentrations of putrescine, and the remaining activity is repressed only by a 100-fold higher concentration of putrescine.

Ito *et al.* (1982) showed that the change in ODCase activity may be linked in some fashion to the synthesis or turnover of phospholipids, since cerulenin, a fatty acid synthetase inhibitor, prevents the increase in ODCase activity that occurs during morphogenesis. The inhibition of the increase in ODCase activity by cerulenin is overcome by the addition of Tween 80, which indicates a close link between changes in the cell membrane and the regulation of ODCase. This observation is consistent with the sensitivity of the enzyme to environmental signals that lead to morphogenesis.

At present, it is unclear how much of the increase in ODCase activity reflects the increase in growth rate and how much reflects a requirement for ODCase in cellular morphogenesis.

3.4.3. Glucosidases

Interest in α- and β-glucosidases of *Mucor* stems from the observation that yeast cells have an absolute requirement for hexose (Bartnicki-García and Nickerson, 1962) and cannot utilize such potentially fermentable carbon sources as maltose or cellobiose that could be cleaved to glucose by the corresponding glucosidase. Aerobic hyphal cultures can grow on a variety of carbon sources including disaccharides (Bartnicki-García and Nickerson, 1962).

The general pattern of control of fungal glucosidase synthesis is by substrate induction and by catabolite repression in the presence of a preferred carbon source such as glucose (Eberhardt and Beck, 1973; Khan and Eaton, 1971). In contrast, β-glucosidase synthesis in *M. racemosus* does not require the presence of exogenous inducers (Borgia and Sypherd, 1977); catabolite repression in the presence of hexoses appears to be the only control mechanism for the synthesis of β-glucosidase. In the absence of hexose, β-glucosidase appears to be maximally derepressed whether β-glucosides (e.g., cellobiose), α-glucosides (e.g., maltose), pentoses (e.g., ribose or xylose), or glycolytic intermediates are provided as the carbon source. Although no published data are available, it has been suggested that β-glucosidase is regulated in a similar fashion in *M. racemosus* (Borgia and Sypherd, 1977). Experiments with RNA-synthesis inhibitors suggest that regulation of α-glucosidase by catabolite repression occurs at the level of transcription.

The addition of cAMP resulted in the inactivation of β-glucosidase *in vivo* (Borgia and Sypherd, 1977); however, cAMP had no effect on glucosidase activity *in vitro* using either permeabilized cells or cell extracts. On removal of cAMP, reactivation of the enzyme occurs in the absence of protein synthesis. This apparently reversible inactivation of the glucosidase is consistent with a mechanism involving phosphorylation by a cAMP-dependent protein kinase and reactivation by dephosphorylation. Although a phosphorylated form of β-glucosidase in *M. racemosus* has not been demonstrated, the presence of a cAMP-stimulated protein kinase has been reported in *M. rouxii* (Moreno *et al.*, 1977).

Several physiological observations are in accord with the expected inverse relationship between β glucosidase activity and the level of cAMP. Carbon-dioxide-grown yeasts that have high internal cAMP levels (Larsen and Sypherd, 1974) and aerobic cultures grown in the presence of exogenous cAMP cannot utilize cellobiose (Borgia and Sypherd, 1977). A rapid increase in β-glucosidase activity occurs at the time of germ-tube formation in aerobically germinating sporangiospores (Borgia and Sypherd, 1977) concomitant with a drop in the cAMP level (Paznokas and Sypherd, 1975). However, the inverse relationship does not hold for nitrogen-grown yeasts that have low levels of cAMP yet fail to grow on cellobiose (Paznokas and Sypherd, 1975). In the latter instance, the predicted derepression of β-glucosidase synthesis and the presence of the enzyme in the active form are apparently insufficient to allow cellobiose utilization.

An additional factor that must be considered is the location of the glucosidases within the cell. Disaccharides apparently are impermeable substrates to *Mucor* (Reyes and Ruiz-Herrera, 1972; Sorrentino *et al.*, 1977), and the corresponding glucosidases must be external to the cell membrane for the substrates to be utilized. Differential localization of α-glucosidase activity in yeasts and hyphae has been reported in *M. rouxii* (Sorrentino *et al.*, 1977). Cytoplasmic α-glucosidase activity accumulated under anaerobic conditions in both yeast and hyphal cultures. However, only in hyphal cultures was there significant α-glucosidase activity measurable in intact cells and hence outside the permeability barrier. This cell-wall fraction constituted 80–90% of the total α-glucosidase activity in hyphal cultures.

A cell-wall-bound and a soluble form of β-glucosidase have been purified from *M. racemosus* (Borgia and Mehnert, 1982). In this study, aerobic hyphal cultures were used, and the possible morphology-specific localization of the enzyme was not examined. Approximately one half the β-glucosidase activity was associated with the cell-wall-bound activity, 40% could be released by incubation of the extract with 2 M NaCl; the unreleased fraction was not characterized further. The soluble form of the enzyme and the high-salt-extractable form were purified to homogeniety. Both forms of the enzyme are glycoproteins of 91,000 daltons and contain approximately 10% carbohydrate. A detailed comparison of the two forms showed them to be indistinguishable in chromatographic and electrophoretic mobilities, antigenicity, enzyme kinetic parameters and substrate specificities, amino acid composition, and the N-terminal amino acid residue (lysine). It is likely that the extraction procedure did not preserve the *in vivo* distribution of the enzyme, since treatment of osmotically stabilized whole cells with chitosanase, a cell-wall-lytic enzyme, released over 80% of the total β-glucosidase activity. This observation indicates that the primary site of localization of the enzyme is in the cell wall (Borgia and Mehnert, 1982).

Sorrentino *et al.* (1977) suggested that the inability of yeasts to utilize maltose is a consequence of the structural differences between yeast and hyphal walls. According to this view, the yeast wall lacks the binding sites necessary for the incorporation of α-glucosidase, whereas these sites are present in the hyphal wall. Borgia and Mehnert (1982) propose an alternative explanation: that the secretory process required for hyphal-wall synthesis and the process of β-glucosidase localization share common steps that are lacking in the process of yeast-wall synthesis. The latter proposal is based in part on analogy with a temperature-sensitive mutant of *Saccharomyces cerevisiae,* which is conditionally deficient in invertase secretion and also is blocked in cell-wall synthesis under the nonpermissive conditions (Novick and Schekman, 1979). Whichever proposal is correct, characterization of glucosidase secretion and insertion into the cell wall may shed light on the processes that control dimorphism.

3.4.4. Pyruvate Kinase

Pyruvate kinase (PK) appeared to be a good candidate for a differentially expressed and possibly morphology-regulating gene product in *Mucor.* This enzyme functions at an important control point in glycolysis, and since yeasts have an absolute requirement for hexose, one could presume that there were morphology-specific differences in the enzymes of glucose metabolism. Tissue-specific isozymes have been found in mammalan cells (Bailey *et al.,* 1968; Cardenas *et al.,* 1973; Costa *et al.,* 1972), and by analogy the possibility that there were yeast- and hyphal-specific enzymes was worth investigating. Indeed, two PK isozymes were found in *M. racemosus:* an A form induced in the presence of glucose and a B form synthesized only in the absence of glucose (Paznokas and Sypherd, 1977). No morphology-specific expression of the two forms of PK could be demonstrated. Yeasts that require hexose had the A form, as did hyphae grown with glucose. Hyphae grown in the absence of glucose possessed the B form of the enzyme. The addition of cAMP to the growth medium had no effect on the level of either enzyme.

Both enzymes have been purified and shown to be homotetramers with monomeric molecular weights of 60,000 for the A form and 62,000 for the B form. The form of the enzyme is regulated allosterically with fructose disphosphate as a positive modifier and ATP as a negative modifier. The B form of the enzyme does not appear to be regulated by either of these modifiers (J. L. Paznokas, personal communication).

Hybrid forms of the enzyme containing both the A and B monomers have been observed in cells grown on nonhexose substrates. Five such forms have been resolved by polyacrylamide gel electrophoresis and DEAE–cellulose chromatography. The homopolymers of the A and B forms do not have significant serological cross-reactivity. Of the five forms of the enzyme, three forms have extensive serological cross-reactivity, indicating that they are hybrids of the A and B monomers.

In summary, these data are consistent with separate genes encoding the two enzymes that are reciprocally regulated by glucose or a glucose-derived metabolite. Inhibitor studies indicate that the control of synthesis of both enzymes is at the level of transcription.

3.5. *S*-Adenosylmethionine Metabolism

A class of developmental mutants, termed *coy,* for *co*nditional *y*east, provided the initial indication that *S*-adenosylmethionine (SAM) metabolism may be involved in yeast–hyphal differentiation. The *coy* mutants do not undergo hyphal development in a minimal medium, but develop normally in a complex medium (Sypherd *et al.*, 1979). The *coy* mutant is capable of producing hyphae in the minimal medium supplemented with methionine. However, the mutant is not a methionine auxotroph or bradytroph (leaky mutant), since yeast cells grow at the wild-type rate without added methionine. From this, it was concluded that methionine is required only for hyphal differentiation. The isolation of the *coy* mutants as well as adenine auxotrophic mutants that undergo hyphal development only in the presence of high concentrations of adenine implicates SAM in the morphogenetic process in *M. racemosus*.

In wild-type cells, the SAM levels increase 3-fold during the first 2 hr of hyphal development (Garcia *et al.*, 1980); in contrast, the SAM levels decrease precipitously by a factor of 10 in the *coy* mutant growing in minimal medium. In the presence of methionine, the SAM levels in the *coy* mutant increase and hyphal development proceeds normally (García and Sypherd, 1984). Furthermore, if cycloleucine, an inhibitor of SAM synthetase, is added to a culture of wild-type cells, the *coy* phenotype is reproduced. In the presence of cycloleucine, the SAM levels decrease when the cells are exposed to air, and they fail to develop hyphae. Thus, the increase in intracellular SAM levels appears to be a correlate to hyphal development, since if the increase in SAM is blocked either by the addition of a SAM synthetase inhibitor or by mutation, the SAM pools are rapidly depleted and hyphal development is blocked.

In wild-type cells, the specific activity of SAM synthetase increases during hyphal development. The amplitude and kinetics of the increase are medium-dependent (García and Sypherd, 1984); for example, SAM synthetase activity increases 2.6-fold in a semidefined medium that contains methionine and 27-fold in a methionine-free medium. In the *coy* mutant, there are similar increases in SAM synthetase. Thus, the biochemical nature of the *coy* mutation is unknown, although an altered SAM synthetase (e.g., an enzyme with a decreased affinity for methionine) seems a reasonable possibility. Further analysis of SAM synthetase including K_m measurements for methionine and measurement of the *in vitro* stability of the enzyme in the *coy* mutant may reveal the nature of this interesting mutation.

In addition to its primary role as a methyl donor, SAM serves a more specialized function as a propylamine donor for the synthesis of the polyamines spermine and spermidine from the diamine putrescine. In this view, the increased level of SAM that occurs during hyphal development could be required for the synthesis of increased amounts of spermidine [filamentous fungi generally lack the higher-molecular-weight polyamine spermine (Nickerson *et al.*, 1977)]. During the yeast-to-hyphal differentiation, the level of putrescine increases while the level of spermidine generally remains constant (Sypherd *et al.*, 1979). Since SAM is required for the synthesis of spermidine but not of putrescine, investigations designed to determine the role of SAM in morphogenesis in *M. racemosus* are now centered on the involvement of SAM in functions other than polyamine biosynthesis.

4. MOLECULAR BIOLOGY OF *Mucor racemosus*

4.1. Preface

While the dimorphism of *Mucor racemosus* may be viewed most fundamentally as a cell-shape change in response to changes in the mechanisms of cell-wall synthesis, considerable evidence, much of which is discussed in this review, suggests that a variety of physiological and biochemical changes not directly involved in cell-wall synthesis are important to the regulation of this simple cell differentiation. It is reasonable to assume that changes in cell-wall synthetic activity are determined by changes in the expression of genes as well as changes in the activities of gene products. On the basis of this assumption, several studies have been directed at understanding the molecular biology and genetic organization of *M. racemosus* in relation to morphogenesis. Because of the fundamental nature of these studies, the results are relevant not only to our understanding of dimorphism, but also to our understanding of the regulation of gene expression.

4.2. Protein Synthesis

As a prelude to more detailed studies of the regulation and function of specifically identified structural and catalytic proteins that are differentially expressed during morphogenesis, initial experiments defined general features of protein synthesis in *M. racemosus.* Orlowski and Sypherd (1977) examined protein synthesis by both pulse-labeling and steady-state labeling techniques during the yeast-to-hyphal differentiation. Their results showed that the instantaneous rate of protein synthesis increases immediately after the shift from carbon dioxide to air, peaks at 4 hr after the shift, and declines to preshift levels by 6 hr. This change was not reflected in the steady-state labeling of proteins, and an attempt to resolve this paradox was unsuccessful (Orlowski and Sypherd, 1978a).

While this paradox remains unresolved, the nature of the increase in the instantaneous rate of protein synthesis was examined further

(Orlowski and Sypherd, 1978b). The conclusion was that there are two changes in the mechanism of protein synthesis that occur during yeast-to-hyphal differentiation: (1) a decrease in the number of active ribosomes and (2) an increase in the velocity of polypeptide chain elongation. More recent evidence (Orlowski, 1981) confirms the conclusion that the rate of polypeptide synthesis in *M. racemosus* is regulated by the availability of ribosomes and the rate of elongation. However, these changes are no longer considered a correlate to morphogenesis (Orlowski and Ross, 1981; Ross and Orlowski, 1982a,b). Nevertheless, an understanding of the mechanisms that regulate the rate of polypeptide synthesis in *M. racemosus* is important to our understanding of this fundamental process as it occurs in eukaryotic cells.

Other efforts have been expended to determine whether posttranslational modifications in structural or catalytic proteins involved in the translation mechanism correlate with morphogenesis. In this regard, the assumption has been that modifications in the translation apparatus provide a mechanism for changes in gene expression at the level of translation. Larsen and Sypherd (1979) analyzed ribosomal proteins of *M. racemosus* for evidence of modification that correlated with morphogenesis. The composition of ribosomal proteins from yeast and hyphae was identical, except for the S6 protein of the 40 S subunit. The S6 protein is modified by phosphorylation, and Larsen and Sypherd (1979) showed that the degree of phosphorylation was different in yeast compared to hyphae and the protein was not phosphorylated in sporangiospores. Two other ribosomal proteins, S10 and L34, were shown to be phosphorylated, but the significance of the phosphorylation of these proteins is unknown. A subsequent study (Larsen and Sypherd, 1980) showed that the degree of phosphorylation of S6 increases with the growth rate of the organism and is not a morphological correlate. Indeed, a correlation was established between the intracellular ATP pool size and the degree of S6 phosphorylation. The intriguing idea that the change in the modification of the S6 ribosomal protein regulates the rate of polypeptide elongation has not been investigated further.

Two types of evidence suggest that methylation reactions might be important to the morphogenetic process. First, Sypherd *et al.* (1979) isolated a morphological mutant that converted from the yeast to the hyphal form in a defined medium only if methionine was included in the medium. As already described, this mutant is referred to as *coy* to indicate *co*nditional *y*east. Second, García *et al.* (1980) showed that SAM levels increase 3-fold during morphogenesis and that [methyl-3H]methionine is incorporated into protein by a posttranslational mechanism. There was a quantitative change in the number of proteins methylated as well as a change in the degree of methylation of certain proteins during morphogenesis. No assessment was made of the role of methylation reactions in the conversion of cell types.

One of the methylated proteins was characterized further by Hiatt *et al.* (1982). This protein is one of the most abundant polypeptides in both yeast and hyphae, comprising 0.5 and 1.6% of the total cell protein, respectively. The molecular weight of the protein is 53,000 and the isoelectric point is 9.5. From these data, as well as a partial amino acid sequence and use of this protein in an *in vitro* assay, the protein was identified as the α-subunit of protein synthesis elongation factor 1 (EF-1α). Most remarkable is the extent to which the protein is methylated; as many as 16 methylated polypeptide fragments were observed in tryptic digests of the protein. This is in contrast to the more common situation in which no more than two sites within a specific protein are methylated (Weisback and Ochoa, 1976). The methylated amino acids were mono-, di-, and trimethylated lysine. A comparison of EF-1α methylation in sporangiospores and hyphae showed that whereas 16.6% of EF-1α lysine residues were methylated in hyphae, only 1.2% of the lysine residues were methylated in spores. The possibility that the methylation of EF-1 serves to regulate the polypeptide elongation activity is a subject of current interest (Fonzi *et al.*, 1985).

On the basis of the assumption that differential gene expression might be reflected in the differential synthesis of polypeptides, Hiatt *et al.* (1980) examined the pattern of polypeptides synthesized by yeast and hyphae. In each case, samples were pulse-labeled with [^{35}S]methionine and the polypeptides were extracted and then separated by two-dimensional polyacrylamide gel electrophoresis. From the rather limited number of polypeptides resolved ($<$500), it appeared that the major change in polypeptide synthesis that occurs during morphogenesis is an increase or decrease in the synthesis of various polypeptides. There was some evidence that 10–15 polypeptides were specific to one cell type or the other. It was not clear, however, whether the observed quantitative and qualitative differences in polypeptide synthesis reflected solely the difference in morphology, the difference in growth rate, or both.

In summary, an understanding of the mechanisms of regulation of protein synthesis in *M. racemosus* is beginning to emerge. A change in the elongation rate, a change in the availability of ribosomes, and modifications of the protein components of the translation apparatus may be important in the regulation of the rate of protein synthesis. These mechanisms appear to respond primarily to physiological and environmental conditions and are not directly related to the morphogenetic process.

4.3. Gene Organization

To understand the mechanisms involved in the regulation of gene expression in *M. racemosus,* a knowledge of the genetic organization is essential. In this regard, several studies in which recombinant DNA methodologies were used have been done in an effort to understand the genetic organization of this fungus.

From an *M. racemosus* gene library constructed with the plasmid vector pBR322, DNA sequences encompassing the entire ribosomal DNA (rDNA) region were isolated and characterized by Cihlar and Sypherd (1980). The rDNA is contained on a 10.2-kilobase (kb) tandem repeat unit spanned by two *Bam*HI restriction fragments. As with other eukaryotes examined to date, the arrangement of the rDNA in *M. racemosus* was found to be: 18 S–5.8 S–25 S. In contrast to most other organisms, the 5 S encoding sequence was found to reside within the basic repeat unit. The overall organization of the rDNA of *M. racemosus* more closely resembles the arrangement seen in *Saccharomyces cerevisiae* (Russell and Wilkerson, 1980). In addition, a number of other clones have been isolated that harbor recombinant plasmids encoding transfer RNAs (tRNAs) (Cihlar and Sypherd, unpublished observations).

Attempts have also been made to complement auxotrophic mutant strains of *E. coli* directly with cloned *M. racemosus* DNA. In this regard, a single recombinant plasmid has been isolated that complements the *leu*B6 mutation in *E. coli* (Cihlar and Sypherd, 1982). The recombinant plasmid is comprised of two *Hind*III-generated restriction fragments of 3.0 and 1.7 kb, both of which are seen in a blot of total *Hind*III digest of genomic DNA. The nature of the *leu*B6 complementation is unknown. The *Hind*III fragment probably does not encode for the isopropyl malate dehydrogenase gene of *M. racemosus,* analogous to the *leu*B6 of *E. coli,* since the fragments do not complement other *leu*B alleles. Suppression of a missense or a nonsense mutation by a cloned *Mucor* tRNA is possible, but a tRNA was not detected on the insert. The plasmid does direct the synthesis of several small peptides of unknown identity in minicells.

Recently, a repeated DNA sequence has been isolated from the *M. racemosus* geonomic library (Dewar *et al.,* 1985). In light of the potential importance of repeated DNA in the regulation of gene expression (Davidson and Britten, 1979; Zuker and Lodish, 1981), preliminary experiments have been performed to characterize the sequence. The sequence comprises a portion of an 8-kb *Hind*III, *Bam*HI-generated restriction fragment from a plasmid designated PMu140. When a 0.9-kb portion of the fragment was labeled by nick translation (Maniatis *et al.,* 1975) and used to probe *Hind*III-digested genomic DNA of *Mucor mucedo, M. hiemalis, and M. genevensis,* fragments homologous to the repeated sequence were detected in the genome of each species. While the apparent number and chromosomal position of the repeated sequence vary from strain to strain, it is clear that at least portions of the element have been conserved within the genus. Analysis of this interesting DNA sequence is continuing.

4.4. DNA Synthesis and Nuclear Division

Although there have been several studies of protein and RNA synthesis during the growth and morphogenesis of *M. racemosus,* very little is known about the synthesis of DNA. Recently, Lin and Inderlied (in prep.) used a quantitative fluorimetric assay employing diaminobenzoic acid to measure the rates of DNA synthesis during yeast and hyphal growth and during the differentiation of yeast to hyphae. During vegetative growth of either form of the fungus, there is good coordination between DNA and protein synthesis; however, during hyphal morphogenesis, the rate of DNA synthesis actually exceeds the rate of protein synthesis as measured by a Folin phenol assay.

Using the fluorescent dye 5,6-diamidinophenylindole, Lin and Inderlied (in prep.) also examined the division and distribution of nuclei during morphogenesis. During the first 3 hr after a shift from carbon dioxide to air, there is an increase in nuclear division as evidenced by an increase in the density of nuclei (the number of nuclei per unit cell area as observed in photomicrographs) within the cells and an increase in the number of nuclei actually seen in the process of division (i.e., the number of dumbbell-shaped nuclei). The density of nuclei appears to peak as hyphal tubes are formed and then decreases as nuclei appear within the hyphal tubes. These observations are consistent with the measurements of the rate of DNA synthesis and indicate that DNA synthesis and the division and distribution of nuclei are important early parts of the differentiation process.

Lin and Inderlied (in prep.) also showed that in a preparation of sporangiospores, a majority (90%) of the spores contain a single nucleus, and that an early event in spore germination is nuclear division, since spores that have swollen only twice their original size have at least two nuclei. By carefully counting and sizing the spores with a Coulter particle-size analyzer and extracting and quantitating the DNA, they calculated the *M. racemosus* genome size as 12.8×10^{-14} g per haploid genome. This value agrees with the value of 8.5×10^{-14} g per haploid genome obtained by Storck and Morrill (1977) using a diphenylamine assay.

Comparing these values to the value for the genome size based on hybridization kinetics (Storck and Morrill, 1977) there is approximately 10–15% repetitive DNA in the *M. racemosus* genome.

5. MULTIPLE DRUG RESISTANCE OF *Mucor racemosus*

Mucor racemosus is able to resume growth in the presence of various drugs that are intitally fungistatic (T. Leathers, personal communication), and this response has been referred to as adaptive drug resistance. When an actively growing culture is treated with a growth-inhibiting concentration of cycloheximide, trichodermin, or amphotericin B, growth ceases for a period that varies directly with the concentration of the drug. During this period, however, the entire population of cells adapts to the drug and eventually growth resumes, but at a slower rate than an untreated culture. This phenomenon has been previously described in the ciliated protozoan *Tetrahymena pyriformis* (Frankel, 1970; Roberts and Orias, 1974) and in the myxomycete *Physarum polycephalum* (Gorman, 1977).

On the basis of current studies of the mechanism of drug adaptation in *M. racemosus* (T. Leathers and P. Sypherd, personal communication), it appears that adaptation is inducible and does not involve the selection of resistant mutants. The phenomenon is reversible, since an adapted cell population becomes susceptible after several generations in drug-free medium. Drug inactivation does not appear to be involved in this process.

There is strong evidence that adaptation involves a common mechanism for drugs that are structurally dissimilar and that affect different cellular target sites. First, exposure to a low dose of one drug confers adaptive resistance to a second drug; i.e., the growth delay that would normally occur with the challenge dose is reduced or abolished. Second, two types of mutants have been isolated with altered sensitivity to cycloheximide: a hypersensitive mutant that is also hypersensitive to amphotericin B and trichodermin and a cycloheximide-resistant mutant that is also resistant to amphotericin B and trichodermin and appears to be constitutively adapted to all three drugs. These mutants should prove useful in establishing the biochemical basis of adaptive drug resistance.

6. CONCLUSION

From the studies reviewed in this chapter, several salient points emerge concerning our understanding of dimorphism in *M. racemosus*. Certain observations and hypotheses have not stood the test of time and must be set aside. An explanation of morphology in terms of a simple association with the mode of energy production, i.e., hyphal morphology and respiration vs. yeast morphology and fermentation, is inadequate.

The contention that hyphal development can occur in the absence of oxygen is untenable in the light of recent observations. Hyphal development can occur under microaerobic but not strictly anaerobic conditions. We believe that it is important to distinguish between the role of oxygen as a terminal electron acceptor and as an inducer of mitochondriogenesis. Mitochondrial functions other than respiration appear to be important in hyphal development. The morphologically relevant role of mitochondria may be in the compartmentation of metabolic reactions.

Finally, the phenomenon of multiple drug resistance that has been demonstrated in *M. racemosus* may have broad clinical significance. It is common for fungal infections to respond initially to chemotherapy but eventually to recrudesce. Although there may be a variety of reasons for a chemotherapeutic failure, the recrudescence of fungal infections may reflect an adaptive type of drug resistance such as described here, especially since chronic fungal infections often fail to respond to a variety of drugs.

ACKNOWLEDGMENTS. We would like to thank our mentor, Paul S. Sypherd, who introduced us to dimorphism in *Mucor racemosus* and has encouraged and supported our interest and investigations in this field. We would also like to express our appreciation to Peter Borgia, John Paznokas, Roberto Garcia, David Logan, and Timothy Leathers, who communicated to us the results of unpublished experiments.

REFERENCES

Bailey, E., Stripe, F., and Taylor, C. B., 1968, Regulation of rat liver pyruvate kinase, *J. Biochem.* **108:**427–436.

Bartnicki-García, S., and Nickerson, W. J., 1962, Induction of yeast-like development in *Mucor* by carbon dioxide, *J. Bacteriol.* **84:**829–840.

Borgia, P. I., and Mehnert, D. W., 1982, Purification of a soluble and wall-bound form of β-glucosidase from *Mucor racemosus, J. Bacteriol.* **149:**515–522.

Borgia, P., and Sypherd, P. S., 1977, Control of β-glucosidase synthesis in *Mucor racemosus, J. Bacteriol.* **130:**812–817.

Cardenas, J. M., Dyson, R. D., and Strandholm, J. J., 1973, Bovine pyruvate kinase: Purification and characterization of the skeletal muscle enzyme, *J. Biol. Chem.* **248:**6931–6937.

Cihlar, R. L., and Sypherd, P. S., 1980, The organization of the ribosomal RNA genes in the fungus *Mucor racemosus, Nucleic Acids Res.* **8:**793–804.

Cihlar, R. L., and Sypherd, P. S., 1982, Complementation of the *leu*B6 mutation of *Escherichia coli* by cloned DNA from *Mucor racemosus, J. Bacteriol.* **151:**521–523.

Clarke-Walker, G. D., 1973, Relationship between dimorphology and respiration in *Mucor genevensis* studies with chloramphenicol, *J. Bacteriol.* **116:**972–980.

Costa, L., Jimenez de Asna, L., Rozengurt, E., Bade, E. G., and Carminatti, H., 1972, Allosteric properties of the isozymes of pyruvate kinase from rat kidney cortex, *Biochim. Biophys. Acta* **289:**128–136.

Davidson, E. H., and Britten, R. J., 1979, Regulation of gene expression: Possible role of repetitive sequences, *Science* **204:**1052–1059.

Davis, R. H., 1967, Channeling in *Neurospora* metabolism, in: *Organizational Biosynthesis* (J. O. Lampen and V. Bryson, eds.), Academic Press, New York, pp. 305–310.

Dewar, R., Katayama, C., Sypherd, P. S., and Cihlar, R. L., 1985, Dispersed repetitive DNA sequence of *Mucor, J. Bacteriol.* **162** (in press).

Eberhardt, B. M., and Beck, R. S., 1973, Induction of β-glucosidases in *Neurospora crassa, J. Bacteriol.* **116:**295–303.

Elmer, G. W., and Nickerson, W. J., 1970, Nutritional requirements for growth and yeast-like development of *Mucor rouxii* under carbon dioxide, *J. Bacteriol.* **101:**595–602.

Fonzi, W. A., Katayama, C., Leathers, T., and Sypherd, P. S., 1985, Regulation of protein synthesis factor EF-1α in *Mucor racemosus, Mol. Cell. Biol.* **5:**1100–1103.

Frankel, J., 1970, An analysis of the recovery of *Tetrahymena* from the effects of cycloheximide, *J. Cell. Physiol.* **76:**55–63.

García, J. R., Hiatt, W. R., Peters, J. and Sypherd, P. S., 1980, *S*-Adenosylmethionine levels and protein methylation during morphogenesis of *Mucor racemosus, J. Bacteriol.* **142:**196–201.

García, J. R., and Sypherd, P. S., 1984, S-Adenosyl methionine and morphogenesis in *Mucor racemosus, Curr. Top. Microbiol. Immunol.* **10:**111–116.

Gordon, P. A., Stewart, P. R., and Clarke-Walker, G. D., 1971, Fatty acid and sterol composition of *Mucor genevensis* in relation to dimorphism and anaerobic growth, *J. Bacteriol.* **107:**114–129.

Gorman, J. A., 1977, Adaptation to trichodermin and anisomycin in *Physarum polycephalum, J. Cell. Physiol.* **92:**447–456.

Hiatt, W. R., Inderlied, C. B., and Sypherd, P. S., 1980, Differential synthesis polypeptides during morphogenesis of *Mucor, J. Bacteriol.* **141:**1350–1359.

Hiatt, W. R., García, R., Merrick, W. C., and Sypherd, P. S., 1982, Methylation of elongation factor 1α from the fungus *Mucor, Proc. Natl. Acad. Sci. U.S.A.* **79:**3433–3437.

Inderlied, C. B., and Sypherd, P. S., 1978, Glucose metabolism and dimorphism in *Mucor, J. Bacteriol.* **133:**1282–1286.

Inderlied, C. B., Cihlar, R. L., and Sypherd, P. S., 1980, Regulation of ornithine decarboxylase during morphogenesis of *Mucor racemosus, J. Bacteriol.* **141:**699–706.

Ito, E. T., Cihlar, R. L., and Inderlied, C. B., 1982, Lipid synthesis during morphogenesis of *Mucor racemosus, J. Bacteriol.* **152:**880–887.

Khan, N. A., and Eaton, N. R., 1971, Genetic control of maltase formation in yeast I. Strains producing high and low basal levels of enzyme, *Mol. Gen. Genet.* **112:**317–322.

Larsen, A. D., and Sypherd, P. S., 1974, Cyclic adenosine 3′,5′ monophosphate and morphogenesis in *Mucor racemosus, J. Bacteriol.* **117:**432–438.

Larsen, A. D., and Sypherd, P. S., 1979, Ribosomal proteins of the dimorphic fungus, *Mucor racemosus, Mol. Gen. Genet.* **175:**99–109.

Larsen, A. D., and Sypherd, P. S., 1980, Physiological control of phosphorylation of ribosomal protein S6 in *Mucor racemosus, J. Bacteriol.* **141:**20–25.

Maniatis, T., Jeffrey, A., and Kleid, D. G., 1975, Nucleotide sequence of the rightward operator of phage λ, *Proc. Natl. Acad. Sci. U.S.A.* **72:**1184–1188.

Mooney, D. T., and Sypherd, P. S., 1976, Volatile factor involved in the dimorphism of *Mucor racemosus, J. Bacteriol.* **126:**1266–1270.

Moreno, S., Paveto, C., and Passeron, S., 1977, Multiple protein kinase activities in the dimorphic fungus *Mucor rouxii:* Comparison with a cyclic adenosine 3′,5′-monophosphate binding protein, *Arch. Biochem. Biophys.* **180**:225–231.

Nickerson, J. W., Dunkle, L. D., and Van Etten, J. L., 1977, Absence of spermine in filamentous fungi, *J. Bacteriol.* **129**:173–176.

Novick, P., and Schekman, R., 1979, Secretion and cell-surface growth are blocked in a temperature sensitive mutant of *Saccharomyces cerevisiae, Proc. Natl. Acad. Sci. U.S.A.* **76**:1858–1862.

Orlowski, M., 1980, Cyclic adenosine 3', 5'-monophosphate and germination of sporangiospores from the fungus *Mucor, Arch. Microbiol.* **126**:133–140.

Orlowski, M., 1981, Growth-rate-dependent adjustment of ribosome function in the fungus *Mucor racemosus, J. Biochem.* **196**:403–410.

Orlowski, M., and Ross, J. F., 1981, Relationship of internal cyclic AMP levels, rates of protein and synthesis and *Mucor* dimorphism, *Arch. Microbiol.* **129**:353–356.

Orlowski, M., and Sypherd, P. S., 1977, Protein synthesis during morphogenesis of *Mucor racemosus, J. Bacteriol.* **132**:209–218.

Orlowski, M., and Sypherd, P. S., 1978a, A location of protein synthesis during morphogenesis of *Mucor racemosus, J. Bacteriol.* **133**:399–400.

Orlowski, M., and Sypherd, P. S., 1978b, Regulation of translation rate during morphogenesis in the fungus *Mucor, Biochemistry* **17**:569–575.

Paveto, C., Epstein, A., and Passeron, S., 1975, Studies on cyclic adenosine 3′,5′-monophosphate levels, adenylate cyclase and phosphodiesterase activities in the dimorphic fungus, *Mucor rouxii, Arch. Biochem. Biophys.* **169**:449–457.

Paznokas, J. L., and Sypherd, P. S., 1975, Respiratory capacity, cyclic adenosine 3′,5′-monophosphate, and morphogenesis of *Mucor racemousus, J. Bacteriol.* **124**:134–139.

Paznokas, J. L., and Sypherd, P. S., 1977, Pyruvate kinase isozymes of *Mucor racemosus:* Control of synthesis by glucose, *J. Bacteriol.* **130**:661–666.

Paznokas, J. L., Tripp, M. L., and Wertman, K. F., 1982, Mutants of *Mucor racemosus* insensitive to dibutyryl cAMP-mediated changes in cellular morphology, *Exp. Mycol.* **6**:185–189.

Peters, J., and Sypherd, P. S., 1978, Enrichment of mutants of *Mucor racemosus* by differential freeze-killing, *J. Gen. Microbiol.* **105**:77–81.

Peters, J., and Sypherd, P. S., 1979, Morphology associated expression of nicotinamide adenine dinucleotide-dependent glutamate dehydrogenase in *Mucor racemosus, J. Bacteriol.* **137**:1134–1139.

Reyes, E., and Ruiz-Herrera, J., 1972, Mechanism of maltose utilization of *Mucor rouxii, Biochim. Biophys. Acta* **273**:328–335.

Rippon, J. W., 1982, *Medical Mycology,* W. B. Saunders, Philadelphia.

Roberts, C. T., and Orias, E., 1974, On the mechanism of adaptation to protein synthesis inhibitors by *Tetrahymena, J. Cell Biol.* **62**:707–716.

Rogers, P. J., Clarke-Walker, G. D., and Stewart, P. R., 1974, Effects of oxygen and glucose on energy metabolism and dimorphism of *Mucor genevensis* growth in continuous culture: Reversibility of yeast–mycelium conversion, *J. Bacteriol.* **119**:282–293.

Ross, J. F., and Orlowski, M., 1982a, Growth-rate dependent adjustment of ribosome function in chemostat grown cells of the fungus *Mucor racemosus, J. Bacteriol.* **149**:650–653.

Ross, J. F., and Orlowski, M., 1982b, Regulation of ribosome function in the fungus *Mucor:* Growth rate vis-à-vis dimorphism, *FEMS Microbiol. Lett.* **13**:325–328.

Russell, P. J., and Wilkerson, W. M., 1980, The structure and biosynthesis of fungal cytoplasmic ribosomes, *Exp. Mycol.* **4**:281–337.

Safe, S., and Caldwell, J., 1975, The effect of growth environment on the chloroform–methanol and alkali extractable cell wall and cytoplasm lipid levels of *Mucor rouxii, Can. J. Microbiol.* **21:**79–84.

Sorrentino, A. P., Zorzopulos, J., and Terenzi, H. F., 1977, Inducible α-glucosidase of *Mucor rouxii:* Effects of dimorphism on the development of the wall bound activity, *Arch. Biochem. Biophys.* **180:**232–238.

Storck, R., and Morrill, R. C., 1971, Respiratory deficient, yeast-like mutant of *Mucor, Biochem. Gen.* **5:**467–479.

Storck, R., and Morrill, R. C., 1977, Nuclei, nucleic acids and protein in sporangiospores of *Mucor bacilliformis* and other *Mucor* species, *Mycologia* **69:**1031–1041.

Sypherd, P. S., Orlowski, M., and Peters, J., 1979, Models of fungal dimorphism: Control of dimorphism in *Mucor racemosus,* in: *Microbiology—1979* (D. Schlessunger, ed.), American Society for Microbiology, Washington, D.C., pp. 224–227.

Tabor, C. W., and Tabor, H., 1976, 1,4-Diaminobutane (putrescine), spermidine and spermine, *Annu. Rev. Biochem.* **45:**285–306.

Weisback, H., and Ochoa, S., 1976, Soluble factors required for eukaryotic protein synthesis, *Annu. Rev. Biochem.* **45:**191–216.

Zorzopulos, J. Jobbagy, A. J., and Terenzi, H. F., 1973, The effects of ethylenediaminetetraacetate and chloramphenicol on mitochondrial activity and morphogenesis in *Mucor rouxii, J. Bacteriol.* **115:**1198–1204.

Zuker, C., and Lodish, H. F., 1981, Repetitive DNA sequences cotranscribed with developmentally regulated *Dictyostelium discoideum* mRNAs, *Proc. Natl. Acad. Sci. U.S.A.* **78:**5386–5390.

Chapter 14

Dimorphism in *Mucor* Species with Emphasis on *M. rouxii* and *M. bacilliformis*

José Ruiz-Herrera

1. INTRODUCTION

Different species of Mucorales are characterized by their alternative growth as either hyphae or yeasts depending on the culture conditions; i.e., they are dimorphic. However, not all Mucorales are dimorphic; in fact, some species grow only as hyphal organisms (they are monomorphic), and among these, some grow only aerobically. Yeast growth among some dimorphic species may be induced by anaerobiosis, whereas others require high CO_2 tension plus anaerobiosis to grow in the yeast morphology. These different patterns of growth and some representative mucoraceous species are listed in Table I. However, it must be anticipated that this grouping of species is an oversimplification and represents only a broad guideline for discussion. Factors such as the carbon and nitrogen sources, inhibitors, and others may severely affect the growth patterns of the different species listed.

The transition of hyphal (cylindrical) to yeast (spherical) growth may be considered a simple model to explore the biochemical bases of mor-

José Ruiz-Herrera • Department of Genetics and Molecular Biology, Center for Investigation and Advanced Studies, I.P.N., and Institute for Investigation in Experimental Biology, Faculty of Chemistry, University of Guanajuato, Guanajuato, Gto. 36000, Mexico.

Table I
Growth Patterns of Mucorales

Group	Characteristics	Representative species
I	Grow only aerobically as hyphae.	*Phycomyces blakesleeanus, Zygorhynchus* spp., *Circinella* spp., *Mortierella* spp., *Sporodinia* spp., *Cunninghamella verticillata, Gilbertella* spp.
II	Grow aerobically and anaerobically as hyphae.	*Rhizopus oryzae, R. arrhizus, R. fusiformis, R. nigricans*
III	Grow aerobically and anaerobically as hyphae, but CO_2 in anaerobiosis induces yeast growth.	*Mucor rouxii, M. racemosus*
IV	Grow aerobically as hyphae and anaerobically as yeasts.	*Mucor bacilliformis, M. subtillissimus* (some strains)

phogenesis. Thus, several species of *Mucor* have been studied for many years.

2. GROWTH CHARACTERISTICS OF *MUCOR* SPECIES

2.1. Spore Germination

Independent of environmental conditions, cultured sporangiospores enter into a phase that has been described as "spherical growth" (Bartnicki-García *et al.,* 1968). In this phase I of growth, the sporangiospore increases its diameter from 5–6 μm to about 18–20 μm by an active process involving macromolecule and organelle biosynthesis. Simultaneously, the cell wall of the spore is stretched and eventually fractured. Whether the fracturing process occurs by mechanical means or by the action of lytic enzymes is not known. Completion of phase I of growth involves the synthesis of a new wall with a different chemical composition (see below) beneath the original spore wall.

After this phase of isotropic sporangiospore growth, which takes about 4–5 hr under aerobic conditions or 8–10 hr under anaerobiosis, phase II of germination starts by the emergence of either a germ tube or a bud, depending on the environmental conditions. The cell wall of the emerging hypha or bud is continuous with the new wall synthesized below the original spore coat, which is finally ruptured. Although incipient buds are not morphologically different from emerging germ tubes (Lara and Bartnicki-García, 1974), they quickly terminate extension and rapidly become spherical. Septation of the bud occurs when the cell has grown to about half the diameter of the germinating spore. This process occurs at the junction of mother and daughter cells by the invagination of the plasmalemma, followed by deposition of two layers of electron-dense material in the space delimited by the double layer of plasmalemma. Finally, a double septum is created. Abscission of the daughter cell occurs as a result of the breakage of the original neck wall of the budding cell.

2.2 Hyphal and Yeast Growth

Once established, the pattern of growth (i.e., hyphal or yeast) is maintained until a transition is induced by either autogenous or exogenous factors. For example, in submerged cultures, sporogenesis does not occur, even under aerobic conditions, since this process requires formation of aerial mycelium outside the aqueous environment. However, if yeast cells are placed under appropriate conditions, they are able to give rise to aerial hyphae and spores (Bartnicki-García and Nickerson, 1962a).

Aged cultures of *Mucor* develop arthrospores. Arthrosporogenesis was studied by Barrera (1983), who found that arthrospores are formed in a random manner in terminal and internal regions of the hyphae. Septal walls are usually formed by centripetal growth of the internal layer of the hyphal-cell wall. Arthrospores eventually increase in volume and adopt a spherical shape and then detach from the hypha. Although arthrospores have a morphology similar to that of yeasts, they can be differentiated by the fact that arthrospores do not bud. Hyphal development is characterized by apical growth, whereas yeast growth is isotropic. This aspect will be discussed more thoroughly below.

2.3. Hyphal–Yeast Transitions

Alterations in environmental conditions may give rise to transition from yeasts to hyphae or vice versa. Transition of yeasts to hyphae is a rapid process, occurring in 1–3 hr (see, for example, Mooney and Sypherd, 1976; Gutierrez and Ruiz-Herrera, 1979). Hyphae normally develop from young buds, but they may also originate directly from mother cells. The transition of yeasts to hyphae is inhibited by cycloheximide (Haidle and Storck, 1966) and thus appears to be dependent on *de novo* protein biosynthesis. The hyphal wall is formed as an extension of the yeast wall, despite their difference in thickness, and apparently develops from the most internal layer of the yeast wall (Bartnicki-García *et al.,* 1968). In contrast to the rapid yeast–hyphal transition, the opposite morphogenesis is a slow process (Mooney and Sypherd, 1976; Gutierrez and Ruiz-Herrera, 1979), taking more than 6–8 hr, and may not be quantitative; a few hyphae still remain after prolonged incubation in conditions that favor yeast development. It is apparent that growth polarization is more easily gained than lost.

3. FACTORS THAT AFFECT MORPHOLOGY IN MUCORALES

3.1. Atmospheric Environment

From the initial studies of *Mucor* during the last century (for a review, see Bartnicki-García, 1963), it became evident that the atmosphere of growth is of primary importance to the morphology of some species. Pasteur, Reese, and Fitz independently concluded that *Mucor* grows as hyphae under aerobiosis and as yeasts under anaerobic conditions. In addition, Brefeld concluded that CO_2 tension is more important than anaerobiosis.

More recently, Bartnicki-García and Nickerson (1962a) rediscovered the role of CO_2 in *Mucor* morphogenesis. These authors observed that *M. rouxii* is able to grow as a mycelium under both aerobic and anaerobic conditions. Increasing concentrations of CO_2 give rise to gradual yeast development, and when 30% CO_2 is reached, homogeneous yeast growth results. This effect of CO_2 is strictly dependent on the lack of oxygen; exposure to oxygen completely eliminates yeast growth. Mooney and Sypherd (1976) discovered that changes in the flow rate of nitrogen, or other inert gases such as argon, influence the morphology of *M. racemosus* and *M. rouxii.* At 22°C, flow rates higher than 4 ml gas/min per ml medium give rise to 100% yeast growth, whereas flow rates below 1.0 ml gas/min per ml medium induce homogeneous hyphal growth. These authors attributed this behavior to the production of a volatile compound necessary to maintain the hyphal morphology. However, more recently, Borgia and Sypherd (personal communication) discovered that the volatile factor is in fact oxygen that leaked into the anerobic culture system through the Tygon tubing.

3.2. Nutritional Factors

A key factor in *Mucor* dimorphism is the carbon source. Bartnicki-García and Nickerson (1962b) observed that *M. rouxii* utilizes anaerobically only hexoses as carbon sources. Subsequently, it was repeatedly observed that yeast growth requires a fermentable carbon source. Bartnicki-García (1968a) reported that depending on the glucose concentration in an anaerobic environment, *M. rouxii* could develop hyphal or yeast growth. When glucose concentration is decreased below 0.05%, the fungus displays hyphal growth even at high CO_2 tensions. On the other hand, at high concentrations of glucose (8%), *M. rouxii* grows in the yeast morphology under a nitrogen atmosphere. An interesting observation was that the higher the glucose concentration, the greater the diameter of the hyphae that develop, suggesting a gradual loss of the mechanisms of growth polarization. Similarly, high concentrations of glucose induce an aberrant yeast growth of *M. genevensis* in continuous culture (Rogers *et al.*, 1974).

Nitrogen source also seems to be an extremely important factor in the dimorphic transition of *Mucor.* Bartnicki-García and Nickerson (1962b) noticed that the use of individual nitrogen sources, such as threonine, ammonium, or nitrate salts, in contrast to complex sources, such as peptone, gives rise to significant hyphal formation in CO_2-induced yeast cells of *M. rouxii.* Elmer and Nickerson (1970) observed that whereas good growth of the hyphal phase of the fungus occurs with ammonium salts, growth of the yeast form requires complex nitrogen sources. Sypherd *et al.* (1978) found that with a combination of ammonium salts, alanine, aspartate, and glutamate, there is good growth of the yeast form of *M. racemosus.* These results suggest that the nitrogen source, in interplay with other factors, also has an important role in the dimorphic transition. A possible explanation for this phenomenon is discussed below.

3.3 Effect of Inhibitors

The morphology of *Mucor* may be altered by different chemical compounds. It was found that in *M. rouxii,* several chelating agents of the *N*-acetic acid type, such as ethylenediamine tetraacetate (EDTA), iminodiacetate, iminotriacetate, 1,2-diaminocyclohexane-*N,N*-tetraacetate, and diethylaminotriaminopentaacetate, which inhibit the growth of the fungus, also abolish the effect of CO_2, giving rise to hyphal growth under a pure atmosphere of carbon dioxide (Bartnicki-García and Nickerson, 1962b). The effect is apparantly due to the chelating properties of the compounds, since different transition group metal ions, but not alkaline earth metals, reverse their effect, both inhibitory and morphogenetic. However, the phenomenon appears somewhat specific, since other chelating agents, such as 8-hydroxyquinoline and *O*-phenanthroline, inhibit growth without affecting morphology. On the other hand, Zn^{2+} is able to release the inhibitory effect of EDTA, but not its morphogenetic effect.

Zorzopulos *et al.* (1973) also observed that EDTA induces hyphal growth of *M. rouxii,* but concluded that the effect is not related to chelation, since it is not reproduced by elimination of metallic ions from the medium. However, because complex nitrogen sources are often contaminated with metals, an unequivocal interpretation of these experiments is not possible.

Terenzi and Storck (1969) observed that phenethyl alcohol at a concentration of 0.2–0.3% enhances yeast growth in aerobic conditions in the presence of hexoses (2.5%). When xylose, maltose, or a mixture of amino acids is employed as the carbon source, growth is hyphal. Higher concentrations of the alcohol severely inhibit growth. Data from Fisher (1977) indicate that diverse fungicides and inhibitors as different as ethidium bromide, tyrocidine, azauracil, actinomycin D, and glutathione all induce yeast growth in *M. pusillus* and *Actinomucor elegans.* The diverse nature of the inhibitors suggests that multiple sites are involved in the induction of the dimorphic phenomenon. In our laboratory, L. E. Sosa (unpublished results) has observed that the addition of low concentrations of different toxic agents, such as mercuric salts, ethionine, and fungicides, gives rise to severe morphological alterations in *M. rouxii.* These results suggest that drastic alterations in the metabolic balance induce morphological changes. However, in these cases, the treated cells are "sick" and are in no way relevant to the elucidation of the morphogenetic phenomenon.

4. METABOLIC AND BIOCHEMICAL ALTERATIONS RELATED TO DIMORPHISM

4.1. General Considerations

During the transition of hyphae to yeasts and vice versa of dimorphic Mucorales, there occurs a series of alterations in metabolism. Some of these alterations seem to be related only to a change in habitat: aerobic to anaerobic or the reverse. A clear example of these changes is the requirement for thiamine and niacin by *M. rouxii* when cultivated anaerobically, whereas both vitamins are synthesized by the fungus in aerobic conditions (Bartnicki-García and Nickerson, 1961).

Aspects of metabolic alterations not related to the obligate changes induced by the aerobic-anaerobic shift, but strictly associated with, or responsible for, the morphological change, have been exhaustively explored by the different groups interested in *Mucor* dimorphism. These explorations have not been simple, since the relationships between cause and effect are not always clear and their interplay may be so subtle, or so intricate, that they are almost impossible to distinguish. For these rea-

Table II
Changes That Accompany the Morphological Transition of *Mucor*[a]

Metabolic parameter	Observed alteration
Flow and regulation of carbon metabolism	Fermentation/respiration ratio
	EMP/HMP shunt flow ratio
	cAMP levels
	cAMP phosphodiesterase levels
	Levels of cAMP-binding proteins
	Differential synthesis of pyruvate kinase isozymes
	Capacity for disaccharide utilization
	Levels of CO_2 fixation
Respiratory enzymes	Cytochrome biosynthesis
Nitrogen metabolism	Inorganic-nitrogen-source utilization
	Levels of glutamate dehydrogenase
	Levels of ornithine decarboxylase
Protein and nucleic acid biosynthesis	Rate of protein biosynthesis
	Levels of RNA polymerases
Cell-wall structure and biosynthesis	Content of mannans
	Mannosyl transferase levels
	Polarization of cell-wall biosynthesis
	Stability of chitin synthetase *in vitro*

[a]For details and references, see the text.

sons, I consider it more fruitful to proceed to a general description of the known alterations, independent of the importance they may eventually be found to have on the morphogenetic process. A summary of these alterations appears in Table II.

4.2. Carbon Metabolism

As mentioned above, it is known that yeast growth in *Mucor* requires a fermentable carbon source. Rogers *et al.* (1974) found that as glucose concentrations are increased in aerobic continuous cultures of *M. genevensis,* the transition of yeasts to hyphae is inhibited. At the same time, the cells develop a fermentative metabolism. Transition of yeasts to hyphae is also inhibited in *M. rouxii* by high glucose concentrations (García and Villa, 1980). Under these conditions, fermentative metabolism increases with production of higher amounts of ethanol. Interestingly, it was also found that as the size of the inoculum is increased, the transition of yeasts to hyphae is inhibited. This observation led to the suggestion that a product that blocks the morphological transition accumulates in the medium.

Inderlied and Sypherd (1978) reported that yeast growth in *M. racemosus* is associated with fermentative metabolism. In their studies, most of the glucose in the medium was catabolyzed to ethanol, CO_2, and glycerol through the Embden–Meyerhoff–Parnas (EMP) pathway, with only 14–20% of the glucose being channeled through the hexose monophosphate (HMP) shunt. In contrast, aerobic cells had a higher aerobic metabolism and a more significant flow of glucose through the hexose monophosphate shunt.

These data clearly indicate the importance of fermentative metabolism for yeast development. However, it must be warned that fermentative metabolism is not unique to the yeast morphology. As mentioned above, depending on the gaseous atmosphere, flow rate, and glucose concentration, some *Mucor* species may develop hyphae under anaerobic conditions. As would be expected, these anaerobically grown hyphae utilize a fermentative pathway; thus, it was shown that *M. rouxii* grown anaerobically produces the same amount of ethanol and CO_2 independent of morphology (Bartnicki-García, 1963) and also that anaerobically grown hyphal and yeast forms of *M. racemosus* utilize almost exclusively the EMP pathway (Inderlied and Sypherd, 1978).

Considering the relationship found in bacteria between carbon source and levels of cyclic AMP (cAMP), it is not surprising that considerable investigation of the effects of cAMP on *Mucor* morphology has been carried out. Larsen and Sypherd (1974) found that CO_2-grown yeasts of *M. racemosus* contain 4 times more cAMP than aerobically grown hyphae and that exogenously added dibutyryl-cAMP inhibits the transition of yeasts to hyphae when such cultures are transferred to aerobic conditions. Dibutyryl-cAMP also induces the yeast morphology from aerobically grown mycelium. These results are obtained only when the fermentable carbon source, glucose, is employed, and not when succinate or maltose is used. Similar results have been obtained with *M. rouxii*. Paveto *et al.* (1975) found that the alterations in cAMP levels are correlated with changes in cAMP phosphodiesterase activity, whereas adenylate cyclase activity is not appreciably affected. Interestingly, when the morphology of *M. racemosus* is controlled by the N_2 flow rate, Paznokas and Sypherd (1975) found similar levels of cAMP in both yeasts and mycelium and were unable to induce morphological alterations by addition of dibutyryl-cAMP to the growth medium.

While trying to investigate the mode of action of cAMP, Moreno *et al.* (1977) described the presence of two cAMP-binding proteins in hyphal cells of *M. rouxii,* one of which is associated with a fraction with protein kinase activity. No difference exists between aerobically and anaerobically grown cells. On the other hand, Forte and Orlowski (1980) observed a decrease in the amount of two cAMP-binding proteins from *M. racemosus* and *M. genevensis* during the transition of CO_2-grown yeasts to hyphae induced by aerobiosis. Orlowski (1980) observed that the levels of cAMP-binding proteins in germinating spores of *M. genevensis* and *M. mucedo* decrease to a minimal level just before germination. These results suggest that cAMP plays an important role in the morphogenetic process, although its effect apparently depends on different factors, such as the carbon source and the metabolic state of the cell. In this regard, it is pertinent to cite data from Jones and Bu'Lock (1977), who found that dibutyryl-cAMP inhibits growth of *M. hiemalis* and *M. mucedo* and that after recovery, the hyphae grow with an altered morphology by exhibiting swellings, septations, and multiple branching. Accordingly, it may be tentatively suggested that high cAMP concentrations induce the loss of apical growth. It is possible that cAMP does not act directly on the phenomenon *in vivo,* but is only one among the multiple effectors involved.

The study of some key enzymes of carbohydrate metabolism led to the discovery of three pyruvate kinase isozymes in *M. rouxii,* which were resolved by ion-exchange chromatography (Passeron and Terenzi, 1970; Passeron and Roselino, 1971; Terenzi *et al.,* 1971). Isozymes I and II are synthesized by glucose-grown cells, have the same molecular weight, display positive cooperative effects for phosphoenol-pyruvate, fructose diphosphate, and Mn^{2+} ions, and are allosterically activated by ADP. However, isozyme I is present in ungerminated spores and yeast cells, whereas enzyme II appears in aerobically grown hyphae. Levels of pyruvate kinase I in yeast cells are higher than those of isozyme II in mycelium, in agreement with the role expected for the enzyme in a key step for energy conservation in glycolysis. Isozyme III is synthesized in the absence of glucose, is sensitive to dilution, and is not activated by fructose diphosphate or pyruvate. In *M. racemosus,* two isozymes, A and B, are detected (Paznokas and Sypherd, 1977). Form A is synthesized in the presence of glucose, being similar in this respect to isozymes I and II from *M. rouxii,* whereas form B is repressed by glucose in a similar fashion to enzyme III from *M. rouxii.* No correlation was found by the authors between the synthesis of either enzyme and fungal morphology.

An interesting characteristic of *Mucor* species is their inability to ferment disaccharides (Bartnicki-García and Nickerson, 1962b). While studying this phenomenon in *M. rouxii,* Flores-Carreon *et al.* (1970) found that most of the α-glucosidase is bound to the cell wall, suggesting that maltose is hydrolyzed outside the permeability barrier of the fungus. It was later determined that *M. rouxii* protoplasts are unable to utilize maltose regardless of whether they are prepared from glucose or maltose-grown cells (Reyes and Ruiz-Herrera, 1972). Addition of cell walls prepared from maltose-grown cells, but not from glucose-grown cells, allows for the utilization of the disaccharide. It was proposed that the cell-wall-bound α-glucosidase is obligatorily required for maltose utilization. It was also suggested that the enzyme is not induced or secreted during anaerobiosis. This requirement seems to be merely energetic, since the addition of small amounts of glucose permits the synthesis of α-glucosidase under anaerobic conditions (E. Reyes and J. Ruiz-Herrera, unpublished observations). Sorrentino *et al.* (1977) suggested as an alternative hypothesis that α-glucosidase is synthesized under anaerobic conditions, but not incorporated into the yeast wall, due to the different architecture of the hyphal wall. In this regard, it seems pertinent that in our laboratory, mutants of *M. rouxii,* which metabolize maltose under anaerobiosis and keep their yeastlike morphology, have been isolated (G. A. Gonzalez and L. E. Sosa, unpublished results). These results are in contradiction to the hypothesis of Sorrentino *et al.* (1977).

Borgia and Sypherd (1977) found that β-glucosidase biosynthesis is repressed by hexoses in *M. racemosus,* but not by nonfermentable substrates. Repression by hexoses is correlated with high levels of cAMP. Addition of exogenous cAMP repressed the biosynthesis of the enzyme and produced its reversible inactivation. More recently, Borgia and Mehner (1981) demonstrated that similar to the α-glucosidase from *M. rouxii,* the β-glucosidase from *M. racemosus* is mostly a wall-bound enzyme. These results suggested that the synthesis or secretion or both of disaccharidases is a phenomenon controlled by catabolyte repression, which is related to, but may be dissociated from, the morphogenetic phenomenon.

Because of the importance of CO_2 as a morphogenetic agent, Bartnicki-García and Nickerson (1962c) studied the fate of fixed CO_2 by anaerobically grown *M. rouxii* yeasts. They suggested that CO_2 is fixed by malic enzyme. The main product of CO_2 incorporation is aspartic acid, although minor incorporation into threonine and glutamic acid also occurs. The relationship between the fixation of CO_2 into these amino acids (which were incorporated into protein) and the morphogenetic effect of CO_2 remains obscure.

4.3. Respiratory Enzymes

As would be expected, anaerobic conditions induce alterations in the pattern of respiratory enzymes. Aerobically grown *M. rouxii* shows differential spectra suggestive of the presence of cytochromes *a, b,* and *c* (Terenzi and Storck, 1969). When cells are grown anaerobically, almost no cytochrome peaks are found. Terenzi and Storck (1969) observed that addition of phenethyl alcohol induces yeastlike growth, together with a decrease in the level of cytochrome *a*. *Mucor genevensis* also contains cytochromes *a*, *b*, and *c* when grown aerobically. When oxygen tension is severely reduced (0.1 μM), the cytochrome *b* band disappears, but cells still contain significant amounts of the *a*-type cytochrome (Rogers *et al.*, 1974). In *M. bacilliformis*, anaerobiosis causes a 10-fold decrease in cytochromes a–a^3 but cytochrome *b* is less severely affected (Ruiz-Herrera *et al.*, 1983). These data suggest that a functional respiratory chain is required for hyphal growth. However, other results are contradictory. Anaerobic hyphae, for example, can be obtained from several species of *Mucor*, and addition of chloramphenicol to aerobically grown *M. genevensis* induced fermentative capacities, development of cyanide-resistant respiration, and impairment of mitochondrial biogenesis, but hyphal growth was unaffected (Rogers *et al.*, 1974).

4.4. Nitrogen Metabolism

Bartnicki-García and Nickerson (1962b) noticed that individual nitrogen sources such as ammonium or nitrate salts, threonine, or serine give rise to significant hyphal formation in CO_2-induced yeasts of *M. rouxii*. Elmer and Nickerson (1970) observed that whereas good growth of hyphae occurs with ammonium salts, growth of yeasts requires complex nitrogen sources. These results suggested that nitrogen assimilation in both forms is different and prompted Peters and Sypherd (1979) to analyze the alterations of glutamate dehydrogenase during the yeast–hyphal transition of *M. racemousus*. These authors demonstrated the presence of two glutamate dehydrogenases, one NAD-dependent and the other NADP-dependent. Both enzymes are repressed by glucose. Whereas levels of the NADP-dependent glutamate dehydrogenase were slightly higher in yeast cells, the NAD-dependent enzyme was an order of magnitude higher in hyphae. Transition of yeasts into hyphae, induced by CO_2-to air or CO_2-to-N_2 shifts, is preceded by a rise in NAD-dependent glutamate dehydrogenase. When hyphal induction by air is prevented by dibutyryl-cAMP addition, a rise in the level of the enzyme is also inhibited. According to these results, it appears that NAD-glutamate dehydrogenase is directly correlated with the morphology of the fungus. Similar results were obtained with *M. bacilliformis* (Ruiz-Herrera *et al.*, 1983). Hyphae of this species contain two orders of magnitude more of the NAD-dependent than of the NADP-dependent glutamate dehydrogenase. In yeast cells induced by anaerobic growth, levels of NAD-dependent enzyme drop to 10% of the aerobic value, whereas the NADP-dependent enzyme is unaffected. It has been observed that NAD-dependent glutamate dehydrogenase from *M. rouxii in vitro* catalyzes only the reductive amination of ketoglutarate, and not the oxidation of glutamate, and that the growth in glutamate does not induce higher levels of the enzyme (Ruiz-Herrera, *et al.,* 1983). These data and those demonstrating the presence of much higher levels of the NAD-dependent vs. the NADP-dependent enzyme in the cells suggest that the NAD-dependent, rather than the NADP-dependent, glutamate dehydrogenase may be responsible for ammonia utilization in these species. This would explain the necessity for an organic nitrogen source for best growth during anaerobiosis, conditions in which the NAD-dependent glutamate dehydrogenase activity drops in very low levels.

It has been observed that ornithine decarboxylase from *M. racemosus* increases during yeast-to-hyphal transition induced by both CO_2-to-air and CO_2-to-N_2 shifts. Cycloheximide, but not actinomycin D or metropsin, blocks induction, which suggests that control of the enzyme operates at the translational level (Inderlied *et al.,* 1980). Despite these results, Marshall *et al.* (1979) found no significant difference in the levels of polyamines between the yeast and hyphal phases of several fungi, including *Mycotypha* spp., *Microspora* spp., and *Mucor bacilliformis.* We observed that ornithine decarboxylase from *M. bacilliformis* is about 3.5 times higher in the hyphal phase than in the yeast phase. Much lower values of the enzyme are found in yeast monomorphic mutants (Ruiz-Herrera *et al.,* 1983) (see below).

4.5. Biosynthesis of Proteins and Nucleic Acids

During the transition from yeast to hyphal growth of *Mucor* spp., there are significant changes in the rate of protein and nucleic acid biosynthesis (Orlowski and Sypherd, 1978). However, since most biosynthetic studies of protein and nucleic acids have been carried out in *M. racemosus,* a much more thorough presentation of the corresponding data can be found in Chapter 13. Nevertheless, for *M. rouxii,* it is important to mention results of Young and Whiteley (1975), who found that during yeast-to-hyphal transition induced by aerobiosis, there is an increase in the levels of DNA-dependent RNA polymerases, mainly enzyme I (the nucleolar enzyme responsible for ribosomal RNA biosynthesis) and enzyme II (nucleoplasmid enzyme involved in messenger RNA biosynthesis), whereas enzyme III (nucleoplasmic enzyme involved in the synthesis of 5S and transfer RNA) is almost unaffected. Haidle and Storck (1966) observed that during the transition of yeasts to hyphae in *M. rouxii,* there is an accelerated biosynthesis of RNA.

5. CELL-WALL STRUCTURE AND BIOSYNTHESIS DURING THE DIMORPHIC TRANSITION

5.1. Chemical Composition

Considering that the shape of a fungal cell is dictated by the cell wall, studies of its chemical composition and its mechanism of biosynthesis have been pursued among Mucorales by several groups. Cell walls of *M. rouxii,* as well as those from other Zygomycetes (for a review, see Bartnicki-García, 1968b), contain chitin as structural polysaccharide and are characterized by the presence of the deacetylated polymer chitosan. Chitin is present in the cell wall in the form of microfibrils (see, for example, Bracker and Halderson, 1971). The cell walls of *Mucor* also contain mannan, polyuronides, protein, and polyphoshate. However, unlike many other fungi, the vegetative walls of *Mucor* lack significant amounts of glucans, although more than 40% of the spore wall is glucan. Few qualitative differences have been found between the compositions of yeast and hyphal walls (Table III). The only major quantitative difference is in the amount of mannose, which is about 8 times higher in the cell wall of the yeast (Bartnicki-García and Nickerson, 1962d). This difference is considered important because many ascomycetous, basidiomycetous, and imperfect yeasts generally have high cell-wall mannose contents (for a review, see Bartnicki-García, 1968b). Accordingly, it was suggested that incorporation of an aspartic-acid-rich mannoprotein into the cell wall was responsible for an alteration in the pattern of wall formation and that

Table III
Chemical Composition of the Cell Wall from Different Stages of *M. rouxii*[a]

Wall component	Yeasts	Hyphae	Sporangiophores	Spores
Chitin	8.4	9.4	18.0	2.1
Chitosan	27.9	32.7	20.6	9.5
Mannose	8.9	1.6	0.9	4.8
Fucose	3.2	3.8	2.1	0.0
Galactose	1.1	1.6	0.8	0.0
Glucuronic acid	12.2	11.8	25.0	1.9
Glucose	0.0	0.0	0.1	42.6
Protein	10.3	6.3	9.2	16.1
Lipid	5.7	7.8	4.8	9.8
Phosphate	22.1	23.3	0.8	2.6
Melanin	0.0	0.0	0.0	10.3

[a]From Bartnicki-García (1968b).

this resulted in the morphological change from hyphae to yeasts (Bartnicki-García, 1963). How this could be achieved remains unknown. In contrast to the large body of information existing on mannan structure in the Saccharomycetaceae (for a review, see Ballou, 1976), the knowledge of mannan structure in *Mucor* is very scant. However, it has been demonstrated that mucoran, an acid heteropolymer extracted from the yeast-cell walls of *M. rouxii,* contained mannose and glucuronate in alternating sequence, and also fucose (Bartnicki-García and Reyes, 1968; Bartnicki-García and Lindberg, 1972).

Dow and Rubery (1977) confirmed the higher content of mannose in the walls of the yeast form of *M. rouxii* and also studied the several polysaccharides extracted from the cell walls of both forms of the fungus. They demonstrated the presence of at least three types of compounds: high-molecular-weight and acidic polysaccharides, high-molecular-weight glycoproteins, and low-molecular-weight glycopeptides. Mannose is more abundant in the latter two polymers extracted from yeast-cell walls. The difference in mannose content in the cell walls of *M. rouxii* is not correlated with activity of mannosyl transferase (Gutierrez and Ruiz-Herrera, 1979), since hyphal cells contain higher activity than yeast cells.

5.2. Cell-Wall Biosynthesis and Polarization

The lack of significant differences in chemical composition of the cell walls of yeast and hyphal forms of *Mucor,* which could explain their difference in morphology, prompted investigations into the mechanisms of cell-wall biosynthesis. Bartnicki-García and Lippman (1969) gave short pulses of [^{3}H]-*N*-acetylglucosamine ([^{3}H]-GlcNAc) to growing hyphae or yeasts of *M. rouxii* and then followed by autoradiography the distribution of incorporated radioactivity (chitin) into the cell wall. They found that whereas wall biosynthesis in yeasts occurs homogeneously over the whole surface, cell-wall growth in hyphae is confined to the apical zone. Moreover, the rate of cell-wall synthesis decreases sharply over a distance that corresponds to the apical dome of the hyphal tip. It was suggested that this difference in wall growth is responsible for the ultimate shape of the fungus. Isotropic wall growth as it occurs in yeasts generates a spherical cell, whereas polarized wall growth gives rise to an extending cylinder. The hyphal type of growth thus seems to require a gradient of wall growth at the apex, which is maximal at the tip and decreases sharply as a function of the angle (α) formed between the longitudinal axis of the hypha and a line drawn to a particular point in the apical wall. Considering the apical dome of a hypha as a hemisphere, the specific rate of area expansion was considered proportional to the cosine of the angle (Green, 1969).

However, since hyphal tips approximate half-ellipsoids rather than hemispheres, the specific rate of wall-area increase seems to be proportional to the cotangent of the angle (Trinci and Saunders, 1977). It was further demonstrated that prior to bud or germ-tube emergence, spores of *M. rouxii* show a period of nonpolarized wall growth during which spores grow into larger spheres, and that prior to germ-tube emergence, there is a gradual polarization, which concentrates the wall growth at the site of germination and then displaces it to the tip of the emerging hyphal tube (Bartnicki-García and Lippman, 1977). Although such autoradiographic studies were very conclusive (Bartnicki-García and Lippman, 1969; Gooday, 1971), a large body of evidence demonstrating apical growth in fungi had already accumulated (for a review, see Bartnicki-García, 1973). It is not surprising, then, that cytologists made an exhaustive search for the apical structures involved in polarized growth. It is now generally agreed that vesicles, which accumulate at the apical portion of hyphae (Girbardt, 1969; Brove and Bracker, 1970) and which may be equivalent to the so-called "Spitzenkorper" (Brunswick, 1924), are responsible for the transfer of enzymes and precursors necessary for the synthesis of the new cell wall. According to this concept, cell shape would be the result of the vectorial components that determine the directionality of vesicle migration to the cell surface.

To explain the gradient of wall synthesis at the hyphal tip, and taking into consideration the importance of chitin in maintaining cell-wall rigidity, a temporal control was suggested (Ruiz-Herrera and Bartnicki-García, 1976), by which proteolytic activation of chitin synthetase occurs after discharge of the enzyme at the apical pole. This would be followed by proteolytic inactivation of the enzyme as it moves down to the lateral surface of the cell. A similar mechanism, which guarantees apical growth in *Saprolegnia monoica* by proteolytic inactivation of $\beta(1\rightarrow4)$-glucan synthetase, has been proposed by Fevre (1981). In yeast cells, this mechanism of inactivation would not be operative, and the long-lived chitin synthetase, which is discharged to the whole surface of the cell, would account for the synthesis of a thicker cell wall (Ruiz-Herrera and Bartnicki-García, 1976).

Evidence to sustain this hypothesis *in vivo* is extremely difficult to obtain because of the small size of the growing region of hyphae. Autoradiography of cell-wall fragments from *M. rouxii* (McMurrough *et al.*, 1971) and *Phycomyces* (Jan, 1974) gave evidence that chitin synthetase accumulates in the apical region of these fungi. A more decisive result was obtained with the giant sporangiophore of *Phycomyces,* which has a growing zone about 2 mm long. By cutting young sporangiophores into 1-mm sections, we found that most chitin synthetase is confined to the first millimeter of the apical zone (Herrera-Estrella and Ruiz-Herrera, 1983). Considering the dynamic nature of the sporangiophore, it can be anticipated that the second and successive 1-mm sections were each once the tip and that at that time each contained most of the chitin synthetase of the cell. Since these sections contained only traces of the enzyme at the time the sporangiophores were cut, one may conclude that the chitin synthetase is inactivated after a brief period of activity.

This idea leads, then, to a hypothesis that may explain how chitin synthetase is delivered to specific sites of the cell surface. We have isolated from the cytoplasm of the yeast form of *M. rouxii* (Bracker *et al.*, 1976; Ruiz-Herrera *et al.*, 1977), as well as from other fungi representative of the different taxonomic groups (Bartnicki-García *et al.*, 1978), specialized microvesicles measuring about 40–70 mm in diameter that, on proteolytic activation and incubation with UDP-GlcNAc and GlcNAc, synthesize chitin microfibrils. Considering the importance of vesicles in cell growth, it was proposed that chitosomes are responsible for the delivery of chitin synthetase at the cell surface (for a review, see Bartnicki-García *et al.*, 1979).

It is generally accepted that vesicles are transported intracellularly by means of microtubules. Experiments on fungi with antimicrotubule agents both support (Howard and Aist, 1980) and deny (Herr and Heath, 1982) the involvement of microtubules in the migration of apical vesicles. An alternative possibility is the involvement of microfilaments as suggested in other systems (Mollenahauer and Morre, 1976). Involvement of electrical fields in the mechanism of polarization has also been suggested in several systems (Jaffe and Nuccitelli, 1977), and DeVries and Wessels (1982) found that outgrowth of protoplasts of *Schizophyllum commune* can be polarized in an external electrical field.

In regard to the biosynthesis of other cell-wall components, it was mentioned above that the wall from the yeast form of *M. rouxii* contains higher amounts of mannose than the hyphal form of the fungus. An analysis of the levels of mannosyl transferase present in both forms and their alterations during the transition from yeasts to hyphae or vice versa has been made (Guitierrez and Ruiz-Herrera, 1979). The results showed that activity is higher in hyphae, mainly at the onset of germination. Mannosyl transferase activity in the yeasts increases late in the growth cycle, and this increase appears related to cell-wall thickening. Transition from yeasts to hyphae is accompanied by a rise in activity coincident with germ-tube emergence, whereas the reverse transition causes a sudden drop in activity. It thus appears that variations in mannosyl transferase are not directly related to morphology, but the rate of cell-wall biosynthesis.

6. GENETIC APPROACHES TO THE STUDY OF DIMORPHISM

It can be anticipated that a full understanding of the phenomena that underlie dimorphism will require isolation of morphological mutants and their biochemical and genetic characterization. These goals are hampered by the extreme genetic stability of several species of *Mucor* and the problems involved in recombinational analysis due to the long period of dormancy of zygospores, the lack of strains with a clean genetic background, and the absence of a stock of auxotrophic or resistant mutant strains. In the specific case of *M. rouxii,* the situation is made worse by the fact that the fungus does not exhibit heterothallism.

We feel the need to establish with *Mucor* a joint effort similar to the one that has made *Phycomyces* such a beautiful model of genetic analysis. For the time being, however, the minor attempts to isolate morphological mutants have been only partially successful. Storck and Morril (1971) studied a spontaneous yeast mutant of *M. bacilliformis.* This mutant is similar to "petite" strains of *Saccharomyces* or "poky" strains of *Neurospora crassa* in the sense that it lacks both *b* and *a* cytochromes and has no respiratory activity. The authors made the interesting observation that the rate of spontaneous appearance of yeastlike colonies of the fungus is extremely high (about 1 in every 3000). These data contrast with our painful attempts to isolate morphological mutants of *M. rouxii.* Most of the morphological mutants we have obtained are extremely unstable and are lost after two or three subcultures (J. Ruiz-Herrera, unpublished results). Perhaps this can be explained by extrapolation of the results of DNA analysis of spores from several species of *Mucor.* These analyses led Storck and Morrill (1977) to suggest that *M. bacilliformis* is the only haploid species of the genus. More recently, we have observed that nuclear division in *M. rouxii* precedes initiation of DNA biosynthesis (C. Cano and J. Ruiz-Herrera, unpublished results). These results suggest an alternative hypothesis concerning the difficulty in obtaining stable mutants: that *Mucor* spores are in the G_2 phase of the cell cycle.

We have isolated a significant number of stable yeastlike mutants from *M. bacilliformis* after nitrosoguanidine treatment of mycelium that was then left to sporulate. Biochemical analyses were included in studies of the mutants and the various factors that have been suggested to be involved in *Mucor* dimorphism (Ruiz-Herrera *et al.,* 1983). Our results can be summarized as in Table IV. The data show that (1) the mutants are unable to grow on nonfermentable carbon sources; (2) they respire with glucose as substrate; and (3) in all but one, respiration is resistant to cyanide. Apparently, the mutants utilize a flavoprotein bypass for respiration, since all of them exhibit respiration sensitive to salicylic acid

Table IV
General Characteristics of Monomorphic Mutants of *M. bacilliformis*

Parameter	Number of mutants tested	Number with abnormal behavior
Growth in nonfermentable substrates	14	14
Respiration with glucose	14	0
Cyanide-resistant respiration[a]	14	13
Respiration sensitive to SHAM	14	14
Cytochrome pattern	14	13
NAD-glutamate dehydrogenase	10	2
Levels of cAMP	14	3
Ornithine decarboxylase	7	7

[a]Variable degree.

hydroxamate (SHAM). Interestingly, the only mutant with respiration sensitive to cyanide shows a normal cytochrome pattern. The rest of the mutants have different alterations in their cytochrome pattern, and four of them lack both cytochromes *a* and *b* (Table V). These particular mutants are similar to the one described by Storck and Morrill (1971). Only two and three of the total number of monomorphic mutants have low levels of NAD-dependent glutamate dehydrogenase and high levels of cAMP, respectively. These results suggest that the two alterations may go together with a morphological change of the fungus, but either the alterations are not a prerequisite to morphogenesis or they represent early steps in the morphogenetic pathway. Finally, it has been observed that all the mutants have low levels of ornithine decarboxylase. This points out an interesting association between polyamine metabolism and morphogenesis. However, it must be mentioned that addition of polyamines

Table V
Characteristics of Cytochromes from *M. bacilliformis* Mutants as Deduced from Their Spectra

Characteristics	Number of mutants
Normal	1
Normal, but cytochrome *a* displaced	2
Cytochrome *a* decreased or absent	2
Cytochrome *a* decreased and displaced	1
Cytochrome *b* decreased or absent	4
Cytochromes *a* and *b* absent	4
TOTAL	14

either singly or in mixtures does not induce mycelial growth of the mutants. It is likely that if a correlation exists with morphology, then it is more complex than we originally expected.

7. GENERAL CONCLUSIONS AND PERSPECTIVES

From the material discussed above, one may conclude that the study of dimorhism of *M. rouxii* and *M. bacilliformis* in particular and of *Mucor* in general has involved the following three main approaches:

1. Study of the metabolic alterations that occur during the morphological transition. The main fruits of this approach have been (a) to demonstrate that yeast growth requires hexoses as the carbon source and a fermentative metabolism (a word of caution must be raised in this regard, however, since there are several *Mucor* species that grow in the hyphal morphology if CO_2 is removed and hexose level is kept low); (b) to demonstrate an interplay between CO_2 and glucose to induce yeast growth; (c) to demonstrate that yeast growth requires a mixture of complex nitrogen sources, possibly because of an alteration in the levels of NAD-dependent glutamate dehydrogenase that appears involved in ammonia utilization; and (d) to suggest a possible role of polyamine metabolism in the dimorphic transition.
2. Molecular biology approach, directed mainly toward detecting alterations in the rate and specificity of transcription and translation process. This approach has revealed several interesting apsects, including (a) the occurrence of alterations in the levels of cAMP during the dimorphic transition; (b) the suggestion that the regulation of synthesis of specific proteins present in either morpholgy occurs at the level of translation; and (c) the demonstration that changes in the rate of translation during the dimorphic transitions are due to changes in the methylation of one of the elongation factors (Hiatt *et al.*, 1982).
3. Study of the cell wall, mainly the mechanism of biosynthesis of its polymers and its polarization. These studies have revealed that (a) cell shape is dictated by polarization in cell-wall biosynthesis; (b) polarization involves a discharge of specific vesicles carrying both enzymes and precursors (among which chitosomes occupy a central role, since they are involved in the biosynthesis of chitin, the structural component of the cell wall); and (c) chitin synthetase exists mainly in an inactive (zymogenic) form and is acti-

vated by proteolysis, which gives a temporal control of chitin biosynthesis.

These different approaches are not mutually exclusive, and one may anticipate that an understanding of dimorphism will require investigations that will bring all together. For instance, one may ask what is the relationship between CO_2 or glucose concentration and the polarization process, or what is the role of an accelerated rate of protein biosynthesis in vesicle migration? It is also feasible that the use of alternative species of Mucorales will help us to understand the phenomenon of dimorphic transition. Accordingly, there are only a few species of Mucorales able to grow anaerobically. What allows these facultative species to grow anaerobically? There are also species that grow anaerobically as yeasts independent of CO_2 tension. Do these species lack some restrictive mechanism that is present in the other species that require CO_2 to grow as yeasts? Analysis of such species may help us to understand the relationship between cause and effect in themorphogenetic process. Last, it seems clear to me that more efforts will be made in the near future to develop genetic systems for the analysis of *Mucor* species. These will be invaluable for the separation of those factors that only accompany the dimorphic transition from those that are directly involved in the process.

REFERENCES

Ballou, C. 1976, Structure and biosynthesis of the mannan component of the yeast cell envelope, *Adv. Microb. Physiol.* **14**:93–158.

Barrera, C. R., 1983, Formation and ultrastructure of *Mucor rouxii* arthrospores, *J. Bacteriol.* **155**:886–895.

Bartnicki-García, S., 1963, Mold–yeast dimorphism of *Mucor, Bacteriol. Rev.* **27**:293–304.

Bartnicki-García, S., 1968a, Control of dimorphism in *Mucor* by hexoses: Inhibition of hyphal morphogenesis, *J. Bacteriol.* **96**:1586–1594.

Bartnicki-García, S., 1968b, Cell wall chemistry, morphogenesis, and taxonomy of fungi, *Annu. Rev. Microbiol.* **22**:87–108.

Bartnicki-García, S., 1973, Fundamental aspects of hyphal morphogenesis, in: *Microbial Differentiation* (J. M. Ashworth and J. E. Smith, eds.), Cambridge University Press, Cambridge, pp. 245–267.

Bartnicki-García, S., and Lindberg, B., 1972, Partial characterization of mucoran, the glucuronomannan component, *Carbohydr. Res.* **23**:75–85.

Bartnicki-García, S., and Lippman, E., 1969, Fungal morphogenesis: Cell construction in *Mucor rouxii, Science* **165**:302–304.

Bartnicki-García, S., and Lippman, E., 1977, Polarization of cell wall synthesis during spore germination of *Mucor rouxii, Exp. Mycol.* **1**:230–240.

Bartnicki-García, S., and Nickerson, W. J., 1961, Thiamine and nicotinic acid: Anaerobic growth factors of *Mucor rouxii, J. Bacteriol.* **82**:142–148.

Bartnicki-García, S., and Nickerson, W. J., 1962a, Induction of yeastlike development in *Mucor* by carbon dioxide, *J. Bacteriol.* **84**:829–840.

Bartnicki-García, S., and Nickerson, W. J., 1962b, Nutrition, growth and morphogenesis of *Mucor rouxii, J. Bacteriol.* **84**:841–858.

Bartnicki-García, S., and Nickerson, W. J., 1962c, Assimilation of carbon dioxide and morphogenesis of *Mucor rouxii, Biochim. Biophys. Acta* **64**:548–551.

Bartnicki-García, S., and Nickerson, W. J., 1962d, Isolation, composition and structure of cell walls of filamentous and yeast-like forms of *Mucor rouxii, Biochim. Biophys. Acta* **58**:102–119.

Bartnicki-García, S., and Reyes, E., 1968, Polyuronides in the cell walls of *Mucor rouxii, Biochim. Biophys. Acta* **170**:54–62.

Bartnicki-García, S., Nelson, N., and Cota-Robles, E., 1968, Electron microscopy of spore germination and cell wall formation in *Mucor rouxii, Arch. Mikrobiol.* **63**:242–255.

Bartnicki-García, S., Bracker, C. E., Reyes, E., and Ruiz-Herrera, J., 1978, Isolation of chitosomes from taxonomically diverse fungi and synthesis of chitin microfibrils *in vitro, Exp. Mycol.* **2**:173–192.

Bartnicki-García, S., Ruiz-Herrera, J., and Bracker, C. E., 1979, Chitosomes and chitin synthesis, in: *Fungal Walls and Hyphal Growth* (J. H. Burnett and A. P. J. Trinci, eds.), Cambridge University Press, Cambridge, pp. 149–168.

Borgia, P., and Mehnert, D. W., 1981, Purification of a soluble and a wall-bound form of β-glucosidase from *Mucor racemosus, J. Bacteriol.* **149**:515–522.

Borgia, P., and Sypherd, P. S., 1977, Control of β-glucosidase synthesis in *Mucor racemosus, J. Bacteriol.* **130**:812–817.

Bracker, C. E., and Halderson, N. K., 1971, Wall fibrils in germinating sporangiospores of *Gilbertella persicaria* (Mucorales), *Arch. Microbiol.* **77**:366–376.

Bracker, C. E., Ruiz-Herrera, J., and Bartnicki-García, S., 1976, Structure and transformation of chitin synthetase particles (chitosomes) during microfibril synthesis *in vitro, Proc. Natl. Acad. Sci. U.S.A.* **73**:4570–4574.

Brunswick, H., 1924, Untersuchungen über Geschlechts und Kernverhältnisse bei der Hymenomyzetengattung *Coprinus,* in: *Botanische Abhandlungen,* Vol. 5 (K. Goebel, ed.), Gustav Fisher, Jena, pp. 1–152.

De Vries, S. C., and Wessels, J. G. H., 1982, Polarized outgrowth of hyphae by constant electrical fields during reversion of *Schizophyllum commune* protoplasts, *Exp. Mycol.* **6**:95–98.

Dow, J. M., and Rubery, P. H., 1977, Chemical fractionation of the cell walls of mycelial and yeast-like forms of *Mucor rouxii:* A comparative study of the polysaccharide and glycoprotein components, *J. Gen. Microbiol.* **99**:29–41.

Elmer, G. W., and Nickerson, W. J., 1970, Nutritional requirements for growth and yeast-like development of *Mucor rouxii* under carbon dioxide, *J. Bacteriol.* **101**:595–602.

Fevre, M. 1981, Regulation of glucan synthetase activities and its implication in fungal cell wall growth, in: *Cell Walls '81* (D. G. Robinson and H. Quader, eds), Wissenschaftliche Verlagsgellschaft mbH, Stuttgart, pp. 143–152.

Fisher, D. J., 1977, Induction of yeast-like growth in Mucorales by systemic fungicides and other compounds, *Trans. Br. Mycol. Soc.* **68**:397–402.

Flores-Carreon, A., Reyes, E., and Ruiz-Herrera, J., 1970, Inducible cell wall-bound α-glucosidase in *Mucor rouxii, Biochim. Biophys. Acta* **222**:354–360.

Forte, J. W., and Orlowski, M., 1980. Profile of cyclic adenosine 3′,5′ monophosphate-binding proteins during the conversion of yeasts to hyphae in the fungus *Mucor, Exp. Mycol.* **4**:78–86.

García, R., and Villa, V., 1980, A correlation between glucose concentration, accumulation of ethanol, and germ tube biogenesis in the dimorphic mold *Mucor rouxii, Exp. Mycol.* **4**:65–77.
Girbardt, M., 1969, Die Ultrastrucktur der Apikalregion von Pilzhyphen, *Protoplasma* **67**:413–441.
Gooday, G. W., 1971, An autoradiographic study of hyphal growth of some fungi, *J. Gen. Microbiol.* **99**:1–11.
Green, P. B., 1969, Cell morphogenesis, *Annu. Rev. Plant Physiol.* **20**:365–394.
Grove, S. N., and Bracker, C., 1970, Protoplasmic organization of hyphal tips among fungi: Vesicles and spitzenkorper, *J. Bacteriol.* **104**:989–1009.
Gutierrez, F., and Ruiz-Herrera, J., 1979, Mannosyl transferase from yeast and hyphal forms of *Mucor rouxii, Exp. Mycol.* **3**:351–362.
Haidle, C. W., and Storck, R., 1966, Control of dimorphism in *Mucor rouxii, J. Bacteriol.* **92**:1236–1244.
Herr, F. B., and Heath, M. C., 1982, The effect of antimicrotubule agents on organelle positioning in the cowpea rust fungus, *Uromyces phaseoli* var. *vignae, Exp. Mycol.* **6**:15–24.
Herrera-Estrella, L., and Ruiz-Herrera, J., 1983, Light response in *Phycomyces blakesleeanus:* Evidence for roles of chitin biosynthesis and breakdown, *Exp. Mycol.* **7**:362–369.
Hiatt, W. R., García, R., Merrick, W. C., and Sypherd, P. S., 1982, Methylation of EF-1 from the fungus *Mucor, Proc. Natl. Acad. Sci. U.S.A.* **790**:3433–3437.
Howard, R. J., and Aist, J. R., 1980, Cytoplasmic microtubules and fungal morphogenesis: Ultrastructural effects of methyl benzimidazole-2-ylcarbamate determined by freeze-substitution of hyphal tip cells, *J. Cell Biol.* **87**:55–64.
Inderlied, C. B., and Sypherd, P. S., 1978, Glucose metabolism and dimorphism in *Mucor, J. Bacteriol.* **133**:1282–1286.
Inderlied, C. B., Cihlar, R. I., and Sypherd, P. S., 1980, Regulation of ornithine decarboxylase during morphogenesis of *Mucor racemousus, J. Bacteriol.* **141**:699–706.
Jaffe, L. F., and Nuccitelli, R., 1977, Electrical controls of development, *Annu. Rev. Biophys. Bioeng.* **6**:445–476.
Jan, Y. N., 1974, Properties and cellular localization of chitin synthetase in *Phycomyces blakesleeanus, J. Biol. Chem.* **249**:1973–1979.
Jones, B. E., and Bu'Lock, J. D., 1977, The effect of N_6,O_2-dibutyryladenosine-3′,5′-cyclic monophosphate on morphogenesis in Mucorales, *J. Gen. Microbiol.* **103**:29–36.
Lara, S. L., and Bartnicki-García, S., 1974, Cytology of budding in *Mucor rouxii:* Wall ontogeny, *Arch. Microbiol.* **97**:1–16.
Larsen, A. D., and Sypherd, P. S., 1974, Cyclic adenosine 3′,5′-monophosphate and morphogenesis in *Mucor racemosus, J. Bacteriol.* **117**:432–438.
Marshall, M., Russo, G., Van Etten, J., and Nickerson, K., 1979, Polyamines in dimorphic fungi, *Curr. Microbiol.* **2**:187–190.
McMurrough, I. Flores-Carreon, A., and Bartnicki-García, S., 1971, Pathway of chitin synthesis and cellular localization of chitin synthetase in *Mucor rouxii, J. Biol. Chem.* **15**:3990–4007.
Mollenhauer, H. H., and Morre, D. J., 1976, Cytochalasin B, but not colchicine, inhibits migration of secretory vesicles in root tips of maize, *Protoplasma* **87**:39–48.
Mooney, D. T., and Sypherd, P. S., 1976, Volatile factor involved in the dimorphism of *Mucor racemosus, J. Bacteriol.* **126**:1266–1270.

Moreno, S., Paveto, C., and Passeron, S., 1977, Multiple protein kinase activities in the dimorphic fungus *Mucor rouxii:* Comparison with a cyclic adenosine 3′,5′-monophosphate binding protein, *Arch. Biochem. Biophys.* **180**:225–231.

Orlowski, M., 1980, Cyclic adenosine 3′,5′-monophosphate and germination of sporangiospores from the fungus *Mucor, Arch. Microbiol.* **126**:133–140.

Orlowski, M., and Sypherd, P. S., 1978, Regulation of translation rate during morphogenesis of the fungus *Mucor, Biochemistry* **17**:569–575.

Passeron, S., and Roselino, E., 1971, A new form of pyruvate kinase in mycelium of *Mucor rouxii. FEBS Lett.* **18**:9–12.

Passeron, S., and Terenzi, H., 1970, Activation of pyruvate kinase of *Mucor rouxii* by manganese ions, *FEBS Lett.* **6**:213–216.

Paveto, C., Epstein, A., and Passeron, S., 1975, Studies on cyclic adenosine 3′,5′-monophosphate levels, adenylate cyclase and phosphodiesterase activities in the dimorphic fungus *Mucor rouxii, Arch. Biochem. Biophys.* **169**:449–457.

Paznokas, J. L., and Sypherd, P. S., 1975, Respiratory capacity, cyclic adenosine 3′,5′-monophosphate and morphogenesis of *Mucor racemosus, J. Bacteriol.* **124**:134–139.

Paznokas, J. L., and Sypherd, P. S., 1977, Pyruvate kinase isozymes of *Mucor racemosus:* Control of synthesis by glucose, *J. Bacteriol.* **130**:661–666.

Peters, J., and Sypherd, P. S., 1979, Morphology-associated expression of nicotinamide and adenine dinucleotide-dependent glutamate dehydrogenase in *Mucor racemosus, J. Bacteriol.* **137**:1134–1139.

Reyes, E., and Ruiz-Herrera, J., 1972, Mechanism of maltose utilization by *Mucor rouxii, Biochim. Biophys. Acta* **273**:328–335.

Rogers, P. J., Clark-Walker, G. D., and Stewart, P. R., 1974, Effects of oxygen and glucose on energy metabolism and dimorphism of *Mucor genevensis* grown in continuous culture: Reversibility of yeast-mycelium conversion, *J. Bacteriol.* **119**:282–293.

Ruiz-Herrera, J., and Bartnicki-García, S., 1976, Proteolytic activation and inactivation of chitin bythetase from *Mucor rouxii, J. Gen. Microbiol.* **97**:241–249.

Ruiz-Herrera, J., Lopez-Romero, E., and Bartnicki-García, S., 1977, Properties of chitin synthetase in isolated chitosomes from yeast cells of *Mucor rouxii, J. Biol. Chem.* **252**:3338–3343.

Ruiz-Herrera, J., Ruiz, A. and Lopez-Romero, E., 1983, Isolation and biochemical analysis of *Mucor bacilliformis* monomorphic mutants, *J. Bacteriol.* **156**:264–272.

Sorrentino, A. P., Zorzopulos, J., and Terenzi, H. F., 1977, Inducible α-glucosidase of *Mucor rouxii:* Effect of dimorphism on the development of the wall-bound activity, *Arch. Biochem. Biophys.* **180**:232–238.

Storck, R., and Morrill, R. C., 1971, Respiratory-deficient, yeastlike mutant of *Mucor, Biochem. Genet.* **5**:467–479.

Storck, R., and Morrill, R. C., 1977, Nuclei, nucleic acids and protein in sporangiospores of *Mucor bacilliformis* and other *Mucor* species, *Mycologia* **69**:1031–1041.

Sypherd, P. S., Borgia, P. T., and Paznokas, J. L., 1978, Biochemistry of dimorphism in the fungus *Mucor, Adv. Microb. Physiol.* **18**:67–104.

Terenzi, H. F., and Storck, R., 1969, Stimulation of fermentation and yeast-like morphogenesis in *Mucor rouxii* by phenethyl alcohol, *J. Bacteriol.* **97**:1248–1261.

Terenzi, H. F., Roselino, E., and Passeron, S., 1971, Two types of pyruvate kinase: Changes in the enzymatic pattern related to aerobic development, *Eur. J. Biochem.* **18**:342–350.

Trinci, A. P. J., and Saunders, P. T., 1977, Tip growth of fungal hyphae, *J. Gen. Microbiol.* **103**:243–248.

Young, H. A., and Whiteley, H. R., 1975, Changes in the levels of DNA-dependent RNA polymerases during the transition of the dimorphic fungus *Mucor rouxii* from yeast-like to mycelial growth, *Exp. Cell Res.* **91**:216–227.

Zorzopulos, J., Jobbagy, J., and Terenzi, H. F., 1973, Effects of ethylendiaminotetraacetate and chloramphenicol on mitochondrial activity and morphogenesis in *Mucor rouxii, J. Bacteriol.* **115**:1198–1204.

Index